Praise for *The Autism Sourcebook*

"In the storm that is autism, Karen Siff Exhorn's *The Autism Sourcebook* is a welcome port."   —Joe Mantegna, actor

"For children with autism, parents must become behavior therapists, physical therapists, linguists, pharmacists, nutritionists, mind-readers, and occasional saints. By providing guidance through the maze of options and services, *The Autism Sourcebook* gives every parent a head start on becoming an expert for his or her child."   —Tom Insel, M.D.

"A much-needed guide to the world of autism for parents and professionals alike who are involved in the care and treatment of children on the autism spectrum."   —Margaret L. Bauman, M.D.

"A comprehensive reference for parents and professionals who are dealing with the complexities of autism spectrum disorders."
                —Lee Grossman, president and CEO, Autism Society of America

"Clearly written, with the intimacy and urgency that perhaps only a parent could bring to the topic, *The Autism Sourcebook* is a gem of book that no one who knows a young child with [an] ASD should be without."
                —Peter Gerhardt, chair, scientific council,
                The Organization for Autism Research

"Easy to read and chock-full of practical information, *The Autism Sourcebook* is a vital resource that I wish my parents had when I was diagnosed on the autism spectrum as a toddler."
                —Stephen Shore, author of *Beyond the Wall: Personal Experiences with Autism and Asperger Syndrome*

"A *must have* for parents of children with autism. Siff Exkorn has put her heart and soul and a bit of her own experience into this book. I truly wish it had been around when my son was diagnosed with autism."
                —Karen Simmons, founder and president, Autism Today

"A clear, concise road map for parents navigating those first few dark and confusing years with autism. Easy to pick up and read all the way through, or use as a reference when moments for reading and research are few and far between. A must have for your autism library."

—Shelley Hendrix Reynolds, president, Unlocking Autism

"Every parent who has a child with autism should read this book. Furthermore, I would advise such parents to ask their pediatrician if he or she has read it. If the answer is no, this would make a great holiday gift."

—Marianne E. Felice, M.D., physician-in-chief,
UMass Memorial Children's Medical Center

"Wow! I wish *The Autism Sourcebook* had been available when my daughter was diagnosed. This book is the ultimate resource guide, providing clarity and guidance for parents who don't know where to go or what to do when handed this diagnosis."

—Ann DiChiara, president, Foundation for
Educating Children with Autism, Inc.

THE AUTISM SOURCEBOOK

EVERYTHING YOU NEED TO KNOW
ABOUT DIAGNOSIS, TREATMENT,
COPING, AND HEALING

KAREN SIFF EXKORN

ReganBooks
An Imprint of HarperCollins*Publishers*

Story credits: pages 175–176, "Welcome to Holland," © 1987 by Emily Perl Kinsley, all rights reserved, reprinted by permission of the author; page 274, "The Mountain" by Jim Stovall.

HarperCollins books may be purchased for educational, business, or sales promotional use. For information please write: Special Markets Department, HarperCollins Publishers Inc., 10 East 53rd Street, New York, NY 10022.

FIRST EDITION

618.92
ExK
8/06

Designed by Kris Tobiassen

Printed on acid-free paper

Library of Congress Cataloging-in-Publication Data has been applied for.

ISBN 0-06-079988-9

05 06 07 08 09 QWF 10 9 8 7 6 5 4 3 2

To Franklin and Jake
with love

The children and their families profiled in this book are based on actual people. With the exception of our son, Jake; my husband, Franklin; and parents who gave permission to be identified, all names, identities, and some details have been changed to respect the privacy of the families.

Throughout the book, I've tried to be sensitive with regard to ascribing different gender labels (such as using *he or she* to describe a nonspecific child or individual) whenever possible, but in some cases, I ascribe only one gender to a subject to preserve the flow of the text. I also use the word *parents* in the book. Please know that this is done for purposes of simplicity and is not meant to exclude single parents, caretakers, guardians, significant others, and partners.

CONTENTS

FOREWORD

Although autism was first defined by psychiatrist Leo Kanner more than sixty years ago, it has only been in the last decade that public interest in this developmental disorder has so dramatically increased. There is more research and a greater knowledge about the importance of intervention than ever before. As public awareness has increased, more cases of autism have been identified, and autism is now being diagnosed earlier in life. Whereas a four-year-old child with autism used to be considered a young case, specialized centers are now seeing children between the ages of twelve and eighteen months fairly frequently. Consequently, more parents are beginning to search for intervention programs for their children.

Not surprisingly, as the number of identified cases has increased, the number of treatments proposed for autism (and related conditions) has also skyrocketed. We now have a much stronger basis of understanding autism, yet the research that's necessary to evaluate treatments properly has not kept up with the basic research. This is why, in many instances, treatments are proposed with little or no scientific basis. In other instances, a strong scientific basis does exist, but parents are unaware of it. In making treatment decisions, it is important that parents carefully evaluate their options and look for treatments with scientifically proven effectiveness and safety.

Given the myriad treatments for autism that are now available, how are parents to make informed choices for their children? Fortunately, parents who have been through the process have come forward to help. *The Autism Sourcebook* reflects the dedication of one mother who, having searched extensively for effective treatment for her own child, is willing to share her knowledge and expertise with other parents. Thus this book is born out of Karen's efforts to help her son, Jake, whose story is a testament to the importance of early intervention in autism; it will be an invaluable resource for parents who want basic, comprehensive information about what treatments are available today.

In *The Autism Sourcebook*, Karen provides a compelling and highly moving account of her own experiences as a mother of a child with autism. She introduces and describes the many treatments she came across in a nonjudgmental and even-handed manner. As she notes, some treatments for autism now have a strong scientific basis, whereas others are backed only by a handful of case reports. Some of these unproven treatments will be researched over the coming years—and only some of them will be shown to be effective. For parents who are struggling to decide which treatments are right for their children, this book will be an invaluable aide.

As *The Autism Sourcebook* also emphasizes, the child with autism does not exist in a vacuum. The birth of a child with any disability strikes at the heart of family functioning. Fortunately, the burden that autism places on a family, although still significant, is much less than it was fifty years ago, when few (if any) supports were available. There are now many resources and coping methods for parents who are struggling to keep their families healthy and whole. As Karen explains, parents must take care of themselves and their other children as well. By taking care of themselves and one another, parents can also become better, more effective advocates for their autistic children.

It is important to emphasize the enormous range of autism spectrum disorders and the many differences that exist between children on the spectrum. It is important that we not lose sight of the individual in our search to treat autism. While there is no single right formula for a given child, we should recognize the importance of programming treatments to meet the particular needs of a child and his or her family. The goal is to help children enter adulthood with capacities for social and personal self-sufficiency. This book will be of great interest to parents and professionals alike. It addresses common concerns and is written in language that parents will understand. It also shows that advocacy and interventions have produced a major revolution in the autism field, where what was once a philosophy of despair has given way to one of hope and optimism. It is a great pleasure for me to recommend to you *The Autism Sourcebook*.

FRED R. VOLKMAR, M.D.
Irving B. Harris Professor
Child Psychiatry, Pediatrics, and Psychology
Yale University School of Medicine
New Haven, CT

NOTE TO READER

Dear Reader,

The Autism Sourcebook was born as a result of my own frustration in trying to understand and get help for our son, Jake, when he was diagnosed with autism. At the time, I found that I had to wade through hundreds of books and articles that left me feeling confused and overwhelmed. I wasn't looking for complex theories; I was looking for simple answers to basic questions such as the following:

What is autism?
Why does my son have autism?
Who are the right people to diagnose my son?
What treatments are available, and which are the most effective?
What results can I expect?

The diagnosis of Jake's autism came as a shock to both me and my husband, Franklin. Up until then, our knowledge of the disorder was based on the movie *Rain Man,* but Jake didn't have any of the behavioral anomalies that the Dustin Hoffman character did. Franklin and I assumed that our seventeen-month-old son had developed a hearing problem or some kind of speech delay when Jake had stopped speaking and become totally unresponsive to us. When I finally did receive a diagnosis for what was wrong with our son, I resisted believing what the doctors told me. I fought with doctors to give Jake any diagnosis other than autism. Autism carried a stigma. Autism meant no hope. Autism meant our son had slipped into a world by himself, a world whose parameters are silence and isolation.

Every aspect of our lives metamorphosed with Jake's diagnosis. Days and nights were filled exclusively with trying to help our son; Franklin and I had no time for each other. We felt as if we'd been involuntarily enrolled in graduate school with heavy duty multiple majors—crash courses in medicine, law, and business education. We learned which doctors and specialists to listen to in order to get Jake the right diagnosis and treatment program. We learned how to negotiate for Jake's treatment services and how to exercise our legal rights, as we would eventually have to go through two lawsuits to get services for our son.

I also desperately needed advice on how to cope with my own personal and emotional issues. It seemed nearly impossible to maintain hope for our son who had a condition for which there was said to be no cure. So I found myself on an emotional roller coaster of denial, acceptance, and pure rage— and I couldn't figure out a way to stop it. Where was the advice for how to deal with the blows that our marriage was taking under the stress of our son's diagnosis, not to mention the impending financial stress? Giving up my consulting business meant the loss of a second income, which we would most likely need for Jake's treatment. How was I supposed to function in the outside world when all I wanted to do was sit at home and cry? I couldn't imagine how I would interact with parents of fully functioning typical children toward whom I felt bitter resentment. And how could I handle the reality that it was no longer possible for us to be a typical family?

I kept hearing the words "early intervention" over and over again from all of the experts on autism, which I quickly learned meant that Jake should be treated as soon as possible. But which treatment? There were too many treatment options scattered around in too many books. I would become hopeful about a particular treatment described in one book, only to find that the same treatment was dismissed in another one. The clock was ticking. Each day spent on research meant another day Jake wasn't being treated. We needed to make a quick decision that was not rash. The wrong choice could be costly, both financially and in terms of Jake's overall development and healing potential.

We ended up trying different treatments for Jake. Some worked better than others. Ultimately, through intensive early intervention, Jake blossomed. He learned how to speak. He learned how to make friends. Today, Jake no longer meets any of the criteria for autism. Indistinguishable from his peers, he is currently in third grade at a local private school.

Not all children with autism have the same outcome as Jake because every child on the autism spectrum has his or her own set of unique challenges to overcome. What we do know is that hope exists for all children on the spectrum.

While none of us can predict the outcome for our children, whether they have autism or not, there are ways we can help them along their journeys. In the case of autism, we know a few simple facts. Early diagnosis and early treatment are the keys to helping a child with autism. Parents have the power to make things happen—to get their children proper diagnoses and the right treatment services to meet their children's needs. Even though no one really knows what the future holds, parents have the power to set their children on paths to growth.

The Autism Sourcebook focuses on children under the age of twelve who have been diagnosed with autism. I recognize that autism also affects adolescents and adults, but the needs of each age group are different, and I want to provide information that is comprehensive yet not overwhelming. That's why I decided to set parameters. However, if you are the parent of an adolescent or adult with autism, you may find that reading this book will help you understand your loved one better, no matter how long ago he or she was diagnosed. There is much more information now than there was even seven years ago when Jake was diagnosed. There are more treatments, resources, and studies that point to more hopeful futures for individuals and families who are affected by autism. My mission is to compile a resource for families of children with autism; but along the way, this book has also become a snapshot of where the health industry and science are today in addressing a developmental disorder that is picking up steam for reasons we do not understand.

Like many parents of newly diagnosed children with autism, I felt inordinate pressure to read every book, article, and website on autism. To make matters worse, many of the available books were written in such technical language that I couldn't fully grasp what the authors were trying to say. What I really wanted was *one* book to help guide me on my way.

The Autism Sourcebook can become your one-stop shopping center for autism information—or, at the very least, a comprehensive guidebook to help direct you to other resources. It's written in user-friendly language that explains what your child's diagnosis means, what treatment options exist, and how to help you cope with personal problems that arise as a result of your child's diagnosis.

Because the goal of *The Autism Sourcebook* is to provide comprehensive, accessible information, it's organized according to the following basic chronology:

Part I: Diagnosis
Part II: Treatment
Part III: Coping
Part IV: Healing

Its format has been designed to help you easily access the specific information you need at any point during the course of helping your child. Each section includes questions and answers based on questions most frequently asked by parents of newly diagnosed children. You'll learn everything from cutting-edge, scientific research to practical advice from parents. A recommended reading list, glossary, resource guide, descriptions of current treatments, and a list of national and international autism organizations are included at the end of the book, providing you with comprehensive information that will help you understand autism better and guide you through the process of helping your child.

In the years since Jake's recovery, I've kept up with the latest advances in autism, as well as the most important issues that concern families and loved ones of children with autism. Combining my skills as a business consultant and my background in psychology, I currently consult with families of newly diagnosed children, helping them make treatment decisions, coaching them on their legal rights to services, and offering advice on how to handle marital, family, professional, and community relationships.

Through our odyssey with Jake, my research for the book, and speaking with countless parents and professionals who work with children who have autism, I've acquired a privileged view of what a parent really needs to know—from diagnosis and treatment to coping and healing. As a result, I've come to certain realizations.

- Respect and value your instincts about your child—never ignore them, no matter what anyone tells you.

- Holding a loved one's life in your hands means that you have to accept a position of power even when you don't want it.

- You must become an advocate for your child, even if it means standing alone against the world.

Finally, I've learned that ordinary and motivated parents can overcome seemingly impossible hurdles and make an extraordinary difference in their children's lives.

I wish you luck on your journey.

KAREN SIFF EXKORN

PART I:
DIAGNOSIS

There is nothing either good or bad, but thinking makes it so.

—WILLIAM SHAKESPEARE

Don't ask for a light load, but rather ask for a strong back.

—UNKNOWN

At his second birthday party, we found our son, Jake, lying facedown in the driveway, his cheek pressed into the gravel. He did not look at us or talk to us. It was as if we—his own mother and father—were not there.

Two weeks later, Jake was diagnosed with autism.

In the first seventeen months of his life, Jake hit every developmental milestone: he crawled, he walked, and he talked. He was within the age-appropriate weight and height percentiles. By all accounts, he was a typical child. And then, over a six month period, Franklin and I watched as our once active and talkative toddler gradually developed into a lethargic and silent little boy. It was as if, one by one, all of the circuit breakers in his brain were clicking off.

Something was affecting Jake's overall development. His coordination was off. He couldn't keep his balance while running or going down the slide. His behavior changed. Jake no longer showed any interest in playing with other children—he hardly even played with his toys. Apart from turning light switches on and off and opening and closing all the doors in the house, his favorite activity was lying on the floor and staring. He also began to have full-blown, horrific tantrums that looked and sounded like nothing I'd ever seen—complete with shrieking and sobbing that caused him to hyperventilate. But aside from the tantrums, Jake was quiet. And honestly, I think what disturbed us the most was his silence. Our house used to be filled with the sounds of his laughter and his raspy, little voice. But the house became so much quieter as Jake's vocabulary dwindled to only a few words. Then, shortly after his second birthday, Jake stopped speaking entirely.

Franklin and I were alarmed and confused. We tried talking more, filling in the silence with empty chatter in the hopes of motivating Jake to start talking again. But nothing happened. Then we tried talking less, thinking that maybe Jake needed more space to express himself. Still nothing. Jake stopped responding in general, not even looking at us when we called out his name. The affectionate boy who freely gave us hugs and kisses was gone. Now, Jake's whole body stiffened whenever we tried to hug him. He could no longer tell us what he wanted—not even by pointing. Jake would shake his whole hand in the direction of the kitchen cabinet to let us know that he was hungry. We'd end up pulling out box after box of cookies, crackers, and snack foods to try to figure out what he wanted. Sometimes his grunting indicated that we'd found the right snack. Other times his sobbing indicated that we hadn't, usually after we had emptied out the entire cabinet. We just couldn't figure out how to give our son what he wanted— whether it was food or anything else.

"He's a boy. Boys develop later than girls," our family pediatrician replied when I expressed our concerns. For each of Jake's symptoms, he had an explanation. Jake didn't speak because he was either shy or obstinate. He didn't play or behave like other children because all children are different. "You should stop being so competitive by comparing him to other children on the playground," he told me. When I was concerned that Jake's tantrums bordered on hysterics, the pediatrician said, "Move the furniture so he won't get hurt." He repeatedly told me not to worry, chalking up Jake's behaviors to the "terrible twos."

But I did worry. Something wasn't right with Jake. He was drifting further and further away from us.

For months, I listened with gnawing uncertainty to the pediatrician. Then, one day, I stopped listening. I was Jake's mother, after all, and I knew my own son better than anyone—including the doctor. That's when I started listening to what my instincts had been telling me for months. I took Jake to another doctor and *another one after that. When I finally got to the bottom of it, when I finally found the right doctor to tell me what was the matter with our son, I heard the words that no parent wants to hear: "Your son has autism."*

At that moment, I wished nothing more fervently than that our family pediatrician had been right all along. . . .

1
THE MANY
FACES OF AUTISM

His parents called Nathan their "gentle giant." At age six, he was big for his age but wouldn't hurt a fly. He appeared to be shy and fearful at all social activities—from playing with other kids to looking his mom and dad in the eye. Nathan's favorite activity was jumping on the trampoline all by himself in his backyard. He seemed to live in a world of his own and had never uttered a word in his life.

At age four, Michael could tell you everything about the life cycle and migratory patterns of the monarch butterfly. He'd even taught himself about photosynthesis. Although clearly intellectually gifted, Michael could not hold a two-way conversation. Instead, he preferred to lecture nonstop about a subject with which he was obsessed, such as butterflies or train schedules.

Blonde-haired, blue-eyed Samantha, age three, was a bundle of energy—always racing aimlessly around the house and flapping her hands. She had an uncanny habit of echoing people's language—using the exact same words and intonation—and could recite entire passages from a Disney video after having seen it only once.

At age two, Jake, who used to be messy and throw his toys around like most kids his age, was now lining up his trains in perfectly neat rows. He would often take a train, lie down on his belly, and push the train on an imaginary three-inch track, his eyes carefully following the wheels of the train. He could entertain himself in this manner for hours.

These children seem so different, yet they have one thing in common: They were all diagnosed with autism.

A BRIEF HISTORY OF AUTISM

The word *autism* comes from the Greek word *autos,* which means *self.* Even though autism seems like a fairly new diagnosis, some of the earliest published descriptions of behaviors that resemble autism date back to the eighteenth century. It wasn't until 1911 that Swiss psychiatrist Eugen Bleuler coined the term *autism* in his work with schizophrenic patients. He observed that his patients were isolated from the outside world and extremely self-absorbed.

Dr. Leo Kanner and Dr. Hans Asperger are considered the pioneers in the field of autism as we know it today. In the early 1940s, unbeknownst to each other, both men conducted research in which they described children as autistic—not in reference to schizophrenics, but to what we now know as the more classic definition of the word. Kanner conducted his research on children in the United States, Asperger in Austria. It's a remarkable coincidence that these studies happened to occur at the same time in different parts of the world, and that both researchers used the word *autistic* to describe the children in their studies. Kanner's definition of autism was referred to as *early infantile autism* or *childhood autism.* Now we just use the word *autism.* Kanner's explanation is what we would consider to be the classic definition, where children display symptoms of impaired social interaction, lack of imaginative play, and verbal communication problems. Asperger described children with similar traits, except that his children seemed to have higher IQs and precocious language skills—they spoke like little adults. In the 1980s, Dr. Lorna Wing, psychiatric consultant for the National Autistic Society in the United Kingdom, coined the term *Asperger's Syndrome* to differentiate the condition from classic autism.

What Does Autism Mean Today?

The word autism is the catch-all term that many people use when referring to the spectrum of autistic disorders. The more current term for autism is ASDs, or Autism Spectrum Disorders, and includes the following five diagnoses: Autistic Disorder, Asperger's Disorder, Childhood Disintegrative Disorder

(CDD), Rett's Disorder, and PDD-NOS (Pervasive Developmental Disorder-Not Otherwise Specified).

Many people used to subscribe to the myth that everyone with an ASD behaved like the Dustin Hoffman character in the movie *Rain Man,* who had the uncanny ability to remember complex combinations of numbers but couldn't perform simple tasks like making toast. Or people subscribed to the myth that all children with ASDs were aloof and unresponsive, rejected hugs, and never showed affection. We now know that ASDs are much more complex, with a variety of symptoms and characteristics that can occur in different combinations and in varying degrees of severity. We also know that each individual with an ASD is unique, with a distinctive personality and individual character traits.

An ASD is not a disease, such as pneumonia or high blood pressure. (A *disease* is defined as an illness or sickness where typical physiological function is impaired). An ASD is a developmental disorder—a condition in which there is a disturbance of some stage in a child's typical physical and/or psychological development, often retarding development. An ASD shows up in the first few years of a child's life. It can affect a child's abilities to communicate, use his or her imagination, and connect with other people—even parents and siblings.

As the name implies, ASDs are spectrum disorders, ranging from mild to severe. A child on the severe end of the spectrum may be unable to speak and also have mental retardation. A child on the mild end of the spectrum may be able to function in a regular classroom and even reach the point where he or she no longer meets the criteria for autism. No two children with ASDs are alike, even if they have the same diagnosis. One child with an ASD may be nonverbal and have a low IQ. Another child with the exact same diagnosis may have an above-average IQ. A third child may be verbally and intellectually precocious. The terms *high-functioning* and *low-functioning* are sometimes used to describe where a child is on the autism spectrum.

You can't tell that a child has an ASD simply by looking at a picture of him or her. A two-year-old with an ASD can be the same height and weight and be just as adorable as a "typical" two-year-old. ("Normal" is not used in this book because it is a relative term, and one that is not widely accepted in the ASD world. The Autism Network International introduced a new term, *neurologically typical* or NT, to describe people without ASDs, which has been shortened to *typical* as the acceptable term in many publications). What distinguishes a child with an ASD from a typical peer is what you can't see: the brain. This is why ASDs are known as invisible disabilities.

Because there is no medical test for an ASD, a child is diagnosed based on either the absence or presence of certain behaviors and skills. For example, if a child is still not speaking by the age of three, that is considered the absence of an age-appropriate behavior. If a three-year-old child engages in odd or idiosyncratic behavior, such as excessive hand flapping, grimacing, or aimlessly running back and forth across a room, that may be an indication of a developmental disorder.

What Are Early Signs of ASDs?

Most parents notice that something is not right with their children when the children are two or three years old. In some cases, parents pick up signs even earlier, when their children are in infancy. They may notice that their babies don't look at them or seem to recognize familiar faces. Perhaps their babies don't cry when they leave the room, exhibit anxiety around strangers, make babbling sounds, imitate gestures such as clapping and pointing, or enjoy playing games like peekaboo—all signs of a typically developing infant.

There's no single personality type that represents the model of an ASD baby. Some parents of children with ASDs look back and describe their children as having been angels when they were babies, hardly making a peep and demanding very little attention. Others describe their children as screamers. Still others describe their babies' behavior as typical—nothing out of the ordinary. According to the National Institute of Mental Health (NIMH), some possible early indicators of ASDs include the following:

- does not babble, point, or make meaningful gestures by one year of age

- does not speak one word by sixteen months

- does not combine two words by two years of age

- does not respond to his or her name

- loses language or social skills

- avoids eye contact

- doesn't seem to know how to play with toys

- excessively lines up toys or other objects

- is attached to one particular toy or object

–doesn't smile

–at times seems to be hearing impaired[1]

Parents may also notice that their child doesn't meet the physical, mental, language, and social developmental standards that most typical children reach. Their one-year-olds may not imitate their actions when they clap or wave, or respond to their smiles, as most one-year-olds do. Their two-year-olds may not be able to understand simple two-step instructions ("Go get your cup, and put it on the table.") or do such things as point to basic body parts (nose, ears, or eyes), identify objects, ask simple questions (or even speak at all), engage in common physical activities (jumping, running, or climbing), or draw circles and lines on paper—as most typical two-years-olds do. Typical three- and four-year-olds drive their parents crazy with constant "Why?" and "What?" questions, eagerly answer simple "Where?" and "Who" questions, enjoy picture books and being read to, and like to play with other children, whereas most three- and four-year-olds with ASDs do not. As toddlers, children with ASDs may not show their curiosity by leaning out of their strollers to look at things that interest them or pointing things out to their parents.

Sometimes a child with an ASD will develop unevenly—early in some areas, yet late in others—which can add to parents' confusion. Children may walk early and talk later or talk early but have trouble with basic motor skills such as running and jumping. Or children may develop appropriate imitation skills as an infant, but then, as they reach toddler age, they may take their imitation skills to the extreme—copying and repeating the exact actions of other people without really understanding what they're doing (a condition known as *echopraxia*).

Some parents have an easier time detecting very early signs of an ASD because they have other typical children at home with whom they can compare their child.

"How do we know what's normal?" Franklin asked me when Jake stopped speaking.

He had a point. Jake was our first child. How did we know what was considered typical development? We had read the parenting books and had a sense of typical developmental milestones, but the books said there were always exceptions.

"You're overreacting," our pediatrician tried to reassure me when I expressed concerns about Jake's loss of speech and his sudden lethargy.

While Jake's loss of speech was the biggest red flag for us, it wasn't until after Jake was diagnosed with an ASD that we were able to look back at what were identified as other early infancy red flags. Jake had trouble nursing (an early sign of oral motor issues), had an unusual combat crawl where he dragged himself across the floor (an early sign of gross motor issues, which involve the larger muscle groups), and didn't walk until he was sixteen months old (quite late according to developmental charts). Other parents report not noticing infancy or toddler warning signs until years later when they watched early home videos of their children. It was only then they observed that their children didn't imitate or engage in pretend play or know how to grip a crayon when they were supposed to.

Researchers are now convinced that the earlier children are diagnosed, the greater the chances that they will receive the maximum benefit from treatment intervention. A report from the National Research Council (NRC) of the National Academies of Science urges the National Institutes of Health (NIH) and the U.S. Department of Education to promote early routine screening of children for ASDs, similar to the routine screening that is done for hearing and vision problems.[2]

Which signs should you look for? Here is a list of questions that can help you detect the signs of ASDs. It's crucial to keep in mind that a child who exhibits one or two of the listed behaviors is not necessarily on the autism spectrum. What makes these behaviors significant is that they occur frequently, intensely, and in clusters. This list should be used to alert you to some of the early signs of an ASD; it should not be used for official diagnostic purposes. I compiled this list based on information from the Centers for Disease Control and Prevention (CDC), the Autism Society of America (ASA), and from speaking with doctors and experts in the field of autism spectrum disorders:

DOES YOUR TWO- TO FIVE-YEAR-OLD CHILD . . .

- ☐ not respond when you call his or her name or seem generally unresponsive?
- ☐ not use his or her index finger to point to objects to indicate what he or she wants or to show you something?
- ☐ have intermittent or no eye contact?

☐ still not speak?

☐ not speak anymore?

☐ demonstrate odd or idiosyncratic speech or language—such as endlessly repeating nursery rhymes, echoing or repeating words or phrases, or making unusual sounds?

☐ demonstrate odd or idiosyncratic behavior—such as hand flapping, finger flicking, or constant spinning?

☐ demonstrate a regression in overall behavior—including communication, play, and social skills?

☐ experience emotional volatility and tantrums that are out of control?

☐ have poor motor coordination when it comes to physical activities such as running or climbing?

☐ fixate on objects such as ceiling fans or bright lights or parts of objects such as the wheels of a toy car?

☐ seem highly distracted or "spaced out"?

☐ show an inappropriate attachment to objects (such as always carrying around a statue or piece of string) or frequently put objects into his or her mouth?

☐ engage in obsessive, repetitive behaviors such as opening and closing doors, turning light switches on and off, or lining up cars?

☐ display ritualistic behaviors such as lining up books on the floor in a specific order at specific times?

☐ engage in little or no spontaneous pretend play?

☐ constantly play by him or herself, showing no interest in peers?

☐ never bring or show you toys?

☐ show no separation anxiety when you leave?

☐ resist change and insist on sticking to specific routines or rituals?

☐ engage in self-injurious behavior such as head banging or hand biting?

☐ show no apparent fear of danger or pain?

☐ not like to be hugged, cuddled, or touched?

☐ have unanimated facial expressions and/or a monotone voice?

☐ demonstrate extreme over- or underactivity?

☐ display a lack of sensitivity or oversensitivity to sound, touch, or visual stimuli (such as loud noises, rough fabrics, or bright lights)?

☐ have unusual sleep patterns (such as trouble falling asleep or not sleeping through the night)?

☐ eat only limited, specific foods?

Sometimes parents notice that their children are engaging in behaviors that they suspect are not typical but don't recognize them as symptoms of an ASD until after their children are diagnosed. In an extensive questionnaire I gave to parents of children with ASDs, one of the questions I asked was, "Before your child was diagnosed, did you suspect something was wrong? If so, what symptoms did your child exhibit?" I asked them to describe any behaviors that were out of the ordinary. Here's what a few had to say.

– We had always considered our son "different" from other children we know, but had chalked it up to boy/girl differences. Besides, he was an easy child, preferring to be on his own for significant amounts of time, even as an infant. We were concerned about his hearing because at eighteen months, he didn't turn if you called his name. He also could not be carried or cuddled—he would squirm out of any grasp to get away.

– Our daughter was precocious and spoke at an early age. She counted and knew her alphabet by age one. She recited poetry and remembered every word to every book. We thought she was just clever. I was unable to get her to notice other children, and she had very limited eye contact. She began to have tantrums and became fixated on strange objects for extended periods of time.

– There was no back and forth communication with our son and minimal eye contact. He stared at ceiling fans, brick walls, garage doors. He also hit his head often, he was a toe walker, and he hated sand, grass, and cold water. We would walk for hours up and down the alley behind our house looking at rows of garage doors. He would constantly walk away from us and was always hyper, running back and forth without stopping.

– We suspected something was wrong with our daughter when she was sixteen months old, mostly because we had an older daughter to compare her with. She didn't form any emotional bond to us as she developed. She had no language and no interest in the world around her. We thought she was deaf. But when she walked on her toes and flapped her hands, we thought she was so cute!

– At the toddler music group, my son ran to the middle of the circle, looked up at the ceiling lights, and shook his head back and forth. Later in the music group, he ran around the room. As he ran, he would stop at every door, touch it, and then continue on. While the other kids, even the active ones, would sing and clap their hands to the music, my little boy could not sit, could only shake his head at the lights, and try to get away to hit the doors. He also had these obsessions with things like water-bottle tops, clocks, and the blow sticks that go with bubble cans (he didn't care about the bubbles—he just wanted the plastic stick).

– When I would rock my son at night, he would stare at his hands, as if examining them, flipping them back and forth. I remember my mother-in-law commenting on how sweet it was.

Do any of these characteristics sound familiar? You may recognize some of these same or similar behaviors in your own child. Some behaviors are not immediately alarming, such as toe walking or running back and forth without stopping, and therefore don't serve as red flags to parents. But when there is a combination of these behaviors or behaviors that seem obviously out of the ordinary, such as continually not responding when called by name, fixating on certain topics or objects, or not speaking at all, parents begin to worry.

If your child has not yet been diagnosed, but you suspect an ASD, ask your pediatrician for help. Your pediatrician can recommend a specialist, and can also provide you with the CHAT (Checklist for Autism in Toddlers) or the M-CHAT (Modified-Checklist for Autism in Toddlers), which include questions to help determine if your child exhibits behaviors characteristic of an ASD. The M-CHAT is actually an American, expanded version of the CHAT from the United Kingdom. According to Dr. Deborah Fein, one of the researchers who developed the M-CHAT, it is not designed to detect all possible developmental disorders, and not all children who fail the checklist will meet the criteria for ASDs. If you are at all concerned about your child, regardless of his or her score on the M-CHAT, you should bring your child in for a more in-depth developmental evaluation by a physician or specialist (see Appendix A).

You can also access valuable information on early detection of ASDs by requesting information from the CDC. Call 1-800-CDC-INFO or go to the CDC National Center on Birth Defects and Developmental Disabilities website at www.cdc.gov/ncbddd/autism/actearly/.

OFFICIAL DIAGNOSES

The official names of the ASD diagnoses and their definitions may seem technical and confusing—especially if you're still feeling emotionally overwhelmed about the news of your child's diagnosis. This section will break it down for you so that you can easily identify the five subcategories of diagnoses, and you'll be able to read case studies illustrating the common behaviors and characteristics of children with these particular diagnoses.

The Diagnostic and Statistical Manual, Fourth edition, Text Revision (DSM-IV-TR) is the official manual used by physicians and mental health professionals for diagnosing children on the autism spectrum. (While parents may obtain copies of this manual, it's not necessary. The information that you'll need from the DSM-IV-TR is listed in Appendix B). The DSM-IV-TR presents these five subcategories of diagnoses.

- Autistic Disorder

- Asperger's Disorder

- Childhood Disintegrative Disorder (CDD)

- Rett's Disorder

- Pervasive Developmental Disorder-Not Otherwise Specified (PDD-NOS)

These five disorders are listed under the heading *PDD* or *Pervasive Developmental Disorders,* which is the classic umbrella term for autism spectrum disorders that was first used in the 1980s. The term *pervasive* indicates that a child's overall behavior and development is affected. The term *developmental disorder* indicates that there is a disordered or disorganized way in which a child is developing.

At the time of diagnosis, you may hear both the terms *PDD* and *ASDs*. Don't be confused by these terms, as they are often used interchangeably. The term ASDs is used in this book because it is more current.

Each of the five disorders has its own set of criteria, and yet all of them fall under the heading of PDD. All of them share a common "triad of symptoms." No matter which diagnosis a child receives on the autism spectrum, a child with an ASD displays examples of the following behaviors to some degree before the age of three:

1. Qualitative Impairment in Social Interaction

What this means: While typical children show an intense interest in other children, children with ASDs often show an intense interest in objects. Compared with typical children who play together at the playground, children with ASDs will be noticeably solitary and detached, often engaged in repetitive, odd behaviors. Toddlers with ASDs don't use body language to indicate what they want; they don't point or reach their arms up to indicate they want to be picked up. Nor do they share what they're doing—you won't hear "Watch me!" from a child with an ASD. Other signs of social impairment include little to no eye contact, flat or unemotional facial expressions, and no real sense of empathy toward others.

"Most children come into the world set up to be experts on people," states Dr. Fred Volkmar, Director of the PDD at the Yale Child Study Center, *"but children with autism don't have this. They're set up to be experts on things, their inanimate environment."*[3]

2. Qualitative Impairments in Communication

What this means: Children with ASDs may have no speech, delayed speech, or idiosyncratic or repetitive speech. It has been estimated that 40 percent or more of children with ASDs do not speak at all. Those who can speak may be unable to initiate or hold a two-way conversation. Another sign of communication impairment is being unable to engage in make-believe play, which involves nonverbal communication (e.g., extending the arms out to the sides while pretending to be an airplane) and verbal communication (e.g., making airplane sounds).

"All children and adults with autistic disorders have problems with communication," states Dr. Lorna Wing. *"Their language (that is grammar, vocabulary, even the ability to define the meanings of single words) may or may not be impaired. The problem lies with the way they use whatever language they do have."*[4]

3. Restricted, Repetitive, and Stereotyped Patterns of Behavior, Interests, and Activities

What this means: Children with ASDs may obsess about a certain topic (e.g., trains or bus schedules) or object (e.g., piece of string or bottle cap) to the point where nothing or no one else seems to exist. They may have a tendency to fixate on a specific routine or ritual (e.g., touching each wall of the bedroom before bedtime), have stereotyped or repetitive actions or movements (e.g., hand flapping or rocking) known as *stereotypies,* or fixate on parts of objects (e.g., wheels of a toy car). Children also may have heightened sensitivities to certain sounds, sights, smells, tastes, or textures (e.g., insisting on wearing only certain clothes or eating only certain foods).

"Stereotypies are not just present in movements, but also in thoughts, and hence can be invisible," states Uta Frith, Professor of Cognitive Development at the Institute of Cognitive Neuroscience at University College, London.[5]

UNDERSTANDING THE FIVE SUBCATEGORIES OF PDD

Here are the five subcategories of PDD with parent-friendly definitions and accompanying case studies. (For official DSM-IV-TR definitions, see Appendix B.) Keep in mind that each of these children exhibits some, but not all, of the characteristics of his or her particular disorder. So, for example, if your child has been diagnosed with Autistic Disorder, he or she may not have a sensitivity to certain sounds like Nathan or talk a blue streak like Sam. If you revisit the triad of symptoms, you'll see that there are different characteristics under each category.

There is, however, one area where all children with ASDs share similarities. "If you were in a room with one hundred autistic patients, first you'd be struck by how different they are from one another, but then you would quickly realize how similar they are," says Dr. Volkmar. What's similar is an overpowering disability in social interactions.[6]

According to the executive summary report by the NRC entitled, "Educating Children with Autism" (2001), "the manifestations of autism spectrum disorders can differ considerably across children and within an individual child over time. Even though there are strong and consistent commonalities, especially in social deficits, there is no single behavior that is always typical of autism or any of the autistic spectrum disorders and no behavior that would automatically exclude an individual child from diagnosis of autistic spectrum disorder."[7]

1. Autistic Disorder

Autistic Disorder was once known as *Kanner's Syndrome* or *Infantile Autism* and is often referred to simply as *autism*. Children with Autistic Disorder can display a wide range of deficiencies in moderate to severe communication skills, social skills, and behavioral problems. Some children with Autistic Disorder also have mental retardation.

The three most common early symptoms of Autistic Disorder are a lack of eye contact, a lack of pointing, and a lack of responding.

Many children with Autistic Disorder have little or no interest in making friends or establishing relationships and often seem more interested in objects than in people. They don't engage in typical play activities like pretend play, and they use toys differently from typical children—preferring to put them in their mouths, line them up, or else focus on parts of a toy (e.g., twirling the string on a pull-toy or spinning the wheels of a toy car). Some children always have to have a toy or object in each hand—when they walk around the house, go out, or even go to sleep at night. If someone removes a toy from one hand, they will quickly reach for the nearest object to replace it. Other children don't actually play with toys, but repeatedly flip them over.

While most typical children will say, "Look at me!" when enjoying an activity, most children with Autistic Disorder do not share their interests. Many of these children have trouble communicating, either because they have limited or no speech or repetitive, idiosyncratic language. They also tend to engage in rigid routines or rituals and repetitive, stereotyped motor mannerisms such as hand flapping or rocking.

Even though the criteria for Autistic Disorder are quite detailed and specific, remember that two children with the exact same diagnosis can appear quite different. You'll see what I mean when you read the profiles of Nathan and Samantha, both of whom were diagnosed with Autistic Disorder.

Nathan's Story

As a baby, Nathan was completely the opposite of his older sister. Nathan's older sister had been extremely active and verbal, while Nathan was quiet and reserved. But their parents had heard that siblings could be quite different from one another, and that boys often developed later than girls, so they weren't initially concerned with Nathan's behavior. They considered Nathan to be an easy-going infant and toddler and were somewhat relieved Nathan was not the high-maintenance baby his sister had been.

Nathan's parents didn't have to constantly play games or entertain him. He was quite independent and preferred just to be on his own. He never cried if either or both parents left the room. His parents worked from home, and Nathan would lie quietly on his back on the floor just staring at the ceiling while they worked. He would entertain himself with finger games for hours—constantly touching his fingers together and flicking them. Nathan also liked to pull off the fringe on the area rug and rub the material between his fingers. He'd pull loose threads from his mother's blouse or father's pants and play with those as well. Even when his parents took turns taking breaks during the workday to play with Nathan, they found that Nathan preferred staring at a ceiling fan or out the window to engaging with them in a play activity. When his father did try to coax him out of the room for some fun, Nathan would usually only get as far as the door. He liked to slowly open and close the door while focusing on the shiny hinges. In the summertime, the one thing that could get Nathan out of the house was the little inflatable swimming pool in the backyard. He could sit and splash for an entire afternoon.

Nathan's parents did notice that he had sensitive hearing. Certain noises upset him, such as the roar of a motorcycle or the ringing of the doorbell. When he heard these sounds, he'd cover his ears and rock back and forth. Sometimes, he'd hit his head with both fists. His parents tried to make the house into a "quiet zone" by turning off the ringers on the phones and lowering the volume on the television.

They were somewhat concerned that by the time he was fifteen months old, Nathan was not yet speaking. The family pediatrician said that Nathan's frequent ear infections may have contributed to his lack of speech, but suggested that the parents take Nathan to a developmental pediatrician, just to have him checked out. Nathan's parents decided to wait.

One afternoon at an outing at the local playground, when he was nineteen months old, Nathan was engaged in his usual bird imitation; he forcefully flapped his hands and spun around, eyes wide, face tilted toward the sky. It was amazing to his mother that he did not get dizzy. He'd spin round and round and stop and flick his fingers as if trying to remove dirt. Then he'd begin his bird imitation again. In the past, other children would try to join in, but Nathan did not acknowledge them. His mother assumed that it was because he was so focused on his own activity that he did not realize they were there. On this particular day as they were leaving the playground, another mother approached Nathan's mother and handed her a note and smiled. Nathan tugged at his mother's hand and pulled her toward the exit. Nathan's mother thanked the woman and opened the note in the car.

The note said, "Look up PDD."

Thinking that this was some special code word, Nathan's mother went home and looked up PDD on the Internet. What she found caught her off guard.

In reading the definition of PDD and Autistic Disorder, she recognized her own son. Nathan, whom she had thought was simply shy, perhaps aloof, independent, focused, and idiosyncratic in an artistic way, was not typical.

When Nathan was nineteen months old, his parents brought him to both a pediatric neurologist and a developmental pediatrician. When tested, Nathan had an IQ of 68—a score that, coupled with the fact that he showed significant deficits in communication skills, social skills, and everyday adaptive behavior, qualified him as mentally retarded. Nathan was ultimately given a diagnosis of Autistic Disorder.

Samantha's Story

Samantha was given the nickname "Sam" by her older sister on the day she was born because her older sister wanted a baby brother. From that day on, Samantha was known as Sam.

Sam was diagnosed at age three with Autistic Disorder, much to her mother's surprise, who had brought Sam in for testing because she thought she was gifted. As a toddler, while her peers were first learning their ABCs, Sam appeared to be reading at a first-grade level. Her mother simply had to read a story to her once, and Sam was able to recite it back to her word for word. When Sam recited sections of dialogue from her Disney videos, she used the same intonation that the characters used.

Sam's pediatrician became concerned when he saw Sam running frantically around the examination room and banging into the walls. Her mother said that this behavior was typical for Sam. She'd learned it from her older sister, a tomboy who roughhoused with her. Her mother reported that Sam barely noticed when she was hurt. While she wasn't fond of her mother's gentle hugs, she liked when her sister wrestled with her and held her tightly in a bear hug.

When the doctor asked, "Sam, how are you today?" Sam responded with "How are you today?" as if mimicking the doctor. Her mother said that Sam always acted silly.

At first, the pediatrician suspected that Sam had ADHD (Attention Deficit/Hyperactivity Disorder), but by the end of the visit, he was concerned about Sam's other behaviors. He suggested that Sam see a pediatric neurologist.

The pediatric neurologist agreed that Sam was hyperactive but took into account her other symptoms as well. His first clue was Sam's speech patterns. Sam exhibited classic echolalia—that is, she echoed what others said without necessarily comprehending what she was saying. Sam also engaged in *perseverative behaviors* (obsessive, repetitive behaviors); she would repeat phrases or nursery rhymes over and over to herself. While Sam's mother and the doctor spoke, Sam sat in the corner and chanted the phrase "Twinkle, twinkle little star" again and again. Sam didn't play with toys appropriately; she began licking the toys and moved on to sucking on the electrical cord of a lamp in the corner of the doctor's office. When the doctor asked Sam's mother to describe any ritualistic behaviors that her daughter engaged in, she said that Sam liked to line up her six favorite dinosaur books on the floor in front of her bed every night before bedtime. She was very particular about having her books in a specific order, spaced evenly apart in a perfectly straight line. She insisted on putting each book face-up first, then flipping each over one by one so that the back covers showed. This behavior, her mother rationalized, grew out of her love of dinosaurs. Sam even slept with her Tyrannosaurus rex statue (not stuffed animal) that her parents bought her at the Museum of Natural History. All of these behaviors, coupled with Sam's fleeting eye contact, hand flapping, and obsession with trains, led to the conclusion that Sam had Autistic Disorder.

Nathan and Sam represent the difference between *low-functioning* and *high-functioning* Autistic Disorder. While these are not diagnostic terms, they are terms that parents may hear. Functioning levels relate to whether or not the child has mental retardation and is verbal and the degree of complex, difficult, and/or idiosyncratic behaviors that the child exhibits. A child who is mentally retarded, nonverbal, and engages in significantly problematic and disruptive behaviors may be considered to be *low-functioning*. A child who has an IQ within average range, has speech/language skills, is rather cooperative, and does not exhibit a range of significantly problematic behaviors may be considered to be *high-functioning*.

Clinicians who are not familiar with symptoms of Autistic Disorder, like Sam's pediatrician, tend to diagnose children like Sam with ADHD. The DSM-IV-TR prohibits diagnosing ADHD when Autistic Disorder is present because all ADHD symptoms can be attributed to Autistic Disorder.

2. Asperger's Disorder

Asperger's Disorder is named after Hans Asperger, the Viennese physician who, in the 1940s, studied a group of children similar to the group that Leo Kanner had described as autistic. Because Asperger's research was not translated into English until many years later, Asperger's Disorder is a relatively new diagnosis in the United States and was not added to the DSM-IV until its 1994 revision.

Asperger's Disorder is also referred to as *Asperger's Syndrome* or simply *Asperger's*. Asperger's is sometimes mistakenly referred to as high-functioning autism because children with this diagnosis tend to have average or above average intelligence and typical or advanced language skills. But in reality, Asperger's is not high-functioning autism. The difference between a diagnosis of Asperger's and high-functioning Autistic Disorder lies in the realm of communication. Because children with Asperger's develop communication skills within the typical range for the first few years of life, they usually present strong verbal skills, which is not a component of Autistic Disorder.

Asperger's is often more difficult to recognize at an early age because children with Asperger's are quite bright, and there is no major warning sign like language impairment. In hindsight, however, parents have identified certain quirky behaviors, awkward motor skills, repetitive behavior, or difficulty relating to others. In fact, Asperger's is often viewed as a social disability.

Unlike other autism spectrum disorders where a child is diagnosed at a very young age, usually by age three, Asperger's is often not diagnosed until the child is school-age, usually five years or older. Like other ASDs, Asperger's is more common in boys than girls, with a ratio of 15:1.

Early signs of Asperger's can include an obsessive interest in a specific topic and memorization of facts related to the topic, often in a rote-like fashion without any actual understanding (such as memorizing train schedules or all of the U.S. presidents); no show of empathy; monotonous, pedantic, inappropriate, or unusual use of speech and language; little or no interest in playing with other children; an inability to engage in a two-way conversation; uncoordinated motor movements and odd posture; and difficulty understanding nonliteral expressions.

Michael's Story

Michael's first grade teacher told Michael's father that, while she acknowledged his son's advanced linguistic skills, Michael's vocabulary and intonation were not typical for his age. While most six-year-olds would simply insist, "I don't wanna play with you!", Michael would say in a monotone, "My preference is to remain alone." In fact, all of Michael's vocal interactions were delivered in an affectless, almost pedantic, tone with limited facial expressions.

Michael loved memorizing facts. Since he was particularly fond of animals, he would memorize everything he could find about a certain species, from their original habitats to their mating rituals. He did not understand all of the information he collected, but this did not prohibit him from sharing these facts. When he went out with his parents, he would often approach strangers and recite animal facts to them. He'd go on and on about *Danaus plexippus* (the Latin name for monarch butterflies) or other obscure animal facts, much to the listener's dismay. Michael did not read facial expressions or affect and was socially unaware; he did not pick up on the listeners' impatient or quizzical looks. Michael would also tell strangers, "You're fat" or, "That's an ugly dress," with no sense of social consciousness or remorse. At his aunt's funeral, while his mother was crying, Michael kept tugging on his mother's jacket, telling her that he was the elf from *The Lord of the Rings*.

Michael likes to pick up every rock he sees. His mother has to drive him to school early so that she can get a parking space near the entrance for Michael to make it to his classroom on time. Sometimes, it can take Michael thirty minutes to navigate the short distance between the car door and the school door. His mother generally leaves school with her pockets full of rocks, which she keeps in a pile in back of the garage because she knows Michael checks to make sure she's saved them.

Michael has no real friends but seems unaware of this fact. At the playground, he will jump on the other children, unaware of his physical strength as he knocks them down. Michael demonstrates awkward motor coordination and is unaware when he hurts another child. Once, in a swimming pool, he almost drowned another boy by accident: Michael dunked the boy's head under the water and did not let go.

Michael enjoys when his mother reads to him, especially nonfiction stories filled with factual information about animals.

3. Childhood Disintegrative Disorder (CDD)

CDD was actually identified many years before Autistic Disorder. Special educator Theodore Heller described the condition in 1908, and it is still sometimes referred to as *Heller's Syndrome*. Occurring more often in boys than girls, CDD is very rare; it is 100 times less common than Autistic Disorder. The usual onset of CDD is later than that of Autistic Disorder—between three and five years old. Children generally develop typically and then experience marked regression in communication (loss of speech and receptive language/inability to hold a conversation), social interactions (including play skills), and everyday functioning (dressing and feeding themselves). Other traits of Autistic Disorder can be present, such as hand flapping or other repetitive behaviors. Bowel and bladder control are lost. There is a high frequency of seizure disorder associated with CDD, and CDD is usually accompanied by profound mental retardation. To meet the criteria for CDD, regression must be preceded by a period of at least two years of apparently typical development, and the onset of decline must occur prior to age ten.

Teddy's Story

As a toddler, Teddy was always trying to be like his big brother, Doug. If Doug wore his red T-shirt and jeans, so did Teddy. If Doug ate his broccoli with dinner, Teddy scrunched up his face and ate his, too. "Me, too!" was Teddy's favorite expression. When he realized that his brother didn't wear diapers, Teddy insisted on being a big boy and was quickly potty trained by the age of eighteen months. He allowed Doug to boss him around and always did whatever Doug asked.

Teddy's parents became worried when, at age four, Teddy experienced a sudden regression. Over a period of weeks, Teddy stopped speaking. He wouldn't look up or answer when his name was called. He couldn't even follow simple directions such as getting dressed or bringing his cup to the table. He became extremely anxious every time his parents took him out of the house, even when going to his favorite place—the local toy store. Instead of playing with his trains on the track that his father had put together for him, he now flipped them over and hurled them across the room.

Teddy had prided himself on being a "big boy" like his brother, but his behaviors became anything but. Having once been able to walk up the stairs one foot in front of the other to get to his bedroom, Teddy now crawled up the stairs. The boy who had prided himself on early potty training was having so many "accidents" that his parents had to put him in diapers again. Teddy didn't even seem to notice. He regressed to eating with his fingers and stopped playing with everyone, including his big brother. He actually became physically aggressive toward his brother—biting, hitting, and scratching him—and began to experience dramatic tantrums that included throwing himself off furniture and banging his head on the floor. His parents and brother couldn't seem to calm him down.

Alarmed by how quickly Teddy seemed to deteriorate, his parents took him to their pediatrician, who ran thyroid and blood tests and ultimately referred them to a pediatric neurologist who diagnosed him with CDD.

4. Rett's Disorder

Rett's Disorder was named after Dr. Andreas Rett, who described the condition in 1966. Rett's is a rare genetic disorder that occurs in 1:10,000 to 1:23,000 female births worldwide. Unlike most of the other disorders on the autism spectrum, Rett's is seen almost exclusively in girls. Girls diagnosed with Rett's generally develop normally until six to eighteen months of age, after which their development either stagnates or regresses. Symptoms of Rett's include lack of communication skills, loss of purposeful hand skills, stereotyped hand movements (such as hand-wringing), difficulty walking and poor coordination, slower head and body growth, sleep disturbances, seizures, and difficulty breathing. Severe mental retardation may also be present.

To receive a diagnosis for the other ASDs, a child is required to meet only some of the criteria. For Rett's, a child must demonstrate all of the criteria.

Maria's Story

Maria's mother had a typical pregnancy and gave birth to Maria just three days short of her due date, on Thanksgiving Day. As her parents celebrated with lukewarm hospital turkey dinners, Maria seemed content lying across her mother's chest and nursing.

Maria's first year and a half of life were quite typical. She walked at ten months of age, and said "Mama," "Dadda," and lots of basic words at twelve months old. She was a social and active little girl. One of her favorite games was playing patty-cake with her dad; she loved to clap her hands and slap his, while they both sang along. At around eighteen months old, Maria's parents noticed that she didn't like playing this game anymore. In fact, she seemed to lose interest in playing altogether. They tried to engage her in other activities like blowing bubbles and banging on her little drum, but then concluded that maybe she was just quiet and passive.

Maria had once loved being chased around the house, but she stopped running and her walk seemed unstable, especially compared with the way other children at the day care center walked. At age three, Maria's parents noticed that she began using her hands in unusual ways. They nicknamed her Lady M (a reference to Lady Macbeth) because she looked as if she were constantly washing her hands. She did this all the time, which became more worrisome than cute when Maria stopped using her hands to indicate what she wanted. Her mother had to focus on Maria's eyes and facial expressions to try to figure out what she wanted. Maria had trouble feeding herself and couldn't even hold a crayon anymore. She began to have a hard time sleeping and would grind her teeth. Often, she would wake up in the middle of the night with terrible nightmares, which would leave her awake for hours. At age four, she developed seizures. Her parents brought her to a pediatric neurologist to have an electroencephalogram (EEG)—a brain wave measurement.

At first, the pediatric neurologist suspected that Maria had cerebral palsy because of her extremely poor coordination, scoliosis, and spastic movements. But upon further examination and extensive interviews with her parents, classic symptoms of Rett's began to emerge. In addition to Maria's motor difficulties and hand-wringing, she engaged in idiosyncratic hand-to-mouth movements, such as pulling on her tongue, and had breathing difficulties, sometimes holding her breath for so long that she'd pass out. Maria was officially diagnosed with Rett's when she was three-and-a-half years old.

5. Pervasive Developmental Disorder–Not Otherwise Specified (PDD-NOS)

PDD-NOS is sometimes referred to as *atypical PDD* or *atypical autism*. A diagnosis of PDD-NOS means that children show *some* but not all of the criteria for Autistic Disorder, Asperger's Disorder, Rett's Disorder, or CDD.

PDD-NOS can be one of the most confusing diagnoses of all of the ASDs. While there is more detailed criteria for the other four ASDs, there is only a short paragraph in the DSM-IV-TR describing PDD-NOS. It's true that a diagnosis anywhere on the autism spectrum is somewhat subjective, based on the evaluator's interpretation of the test results, but it is even more so when it comes to PDD-NOS. This is why it's possible for one doctor to diagnose a child with PDD-NOS and for another to diagnose that same child with Autistic Disorder. There is a theory that some doctors prefer giving a diagnosis of PDD-NOS to ease parents into the world of ASDs, as it can seem like a kinder, gentler diagnosis.

Jake's Story

Jake was our first child and our family's first grandchild, so it was difficult for me to argue with our family pediatrician about my concerns. "You're a first-time mother," he told me repeatedly. "Stop worrying so much."

But I was worried. Jake had been a talkative, happy, and energetic toddler, but something wasn't right. He wasn't talking much anymore. He didn't run and play the way he once did. Often, he would just lie on his back and stare—light fixtures and ceiling fans were his favorites. When he walked, he would walk on his tiptoes. If I attempted to bring him to the swings or the slide, his former favorite playground activities, he began shrieking. He didn't even respond when I called his name.

I thought Jake had a hearing problem. But the audiology reports indicated that Jake's hearing was fine.

Jake's behavior became more obsessive and odd; he clenched and unclenched his fists when he was excited or agitated, constantly covered and uncovered his ears with his hands, made odd facial expressions, and grunted and lifted up his leg for no reason. Wherever he was—in his high chair, car seat, bathtub, or simply sitting on the floor—he strained to peer out of the corners of his eyes while turning his head back and forth as if indicating "No." He stopped clapping and waving—things that he'd done as a baby. He now communicated mainly by grunting.

Eating also became a struggle. Jake would only eat certain foods and would no longer feed himself. One week he ate only Cheerios in a yellow bowl for every meal. I spoon-fed him like an infant. If the milk accidentally trickled inside his shirt, he screamed as if he were being tortured. Another week he ate only hotdogs cut into nine even pieces. But hotdogs could not touch ketchup. One night, as his father smothered ketchup on the hotdog (Franklin didn't know the rule yet), Jake had another one of his hysterical outbursts. On pasta week, a bowtie accidentally touched his skin; Jake screamed, grabbed the tray of his high chair, and shook it so hard he tipped himself over.

I took Jake to see a developmental pediatrician, who took each and every one of Jake's symptoms quite seriously—so seriously, in fact, that she diagnosed him with PDD-NOS. Even with all of Jake's early warning signs, and even though I knew in my heart that something was wrong, the diagnosis still came as a shock. It was too much for me to absorb, so my denial took over. I took Jake to a child psychiatrist for a second opinion to ensure that he did not have autism.

"Your son has autism," he said bluntly. When I protested, now defending the PDD-NOS diagnosis that I had so desperately wanted to reject, he said, "It's all the same. PDD-NOS is just a way of sugarcoating a diagnosis of autism. You can call it what you want, but your son has autism."

The news of an ASD diagnosis can be devastating. During my own journey with Jake, I found that his diagnosis seemed to raise more questions than it answered. Since then, as a consultant, I've spoken with countless parents who have had similar questions after their children have been diagnosed with ASDs—questions that range from "How do I know if the right doctor diagnosed my child?" to "What exactly does the diagnosis mean?" to "Why doesn't my child look at me?" to "Why does my child spin or flap or stare at nothing at all?" In the next chapter, you will find the answers to these questions and many more of the most frequently asked ASD-related questions.

2

WHO DIAGNOSES MY CHILD? GOING BEYOND YOUR PEDIATRICIAN

Who will diagnose my child?

Usually, most parents will seek out the advice of their family pediatricians when they suspect a developmental delay or an ASD in their children. Your pediatrician may suggest medical testing to rule out other conditions. This testing may include special hearing tests such as audiograms or tympanograms (done by audiologists), blood tests for genetic testing, an EEG (electroencephalogram), an MRI (magnetic resonance imaging), blood and urine tests (metabolic screening), or a CAT scan (computerized axial tomography) for the brain.

Even if your family pediatrician suspects an ASD, it's a good idea to bring your child to a professional who specializes in diagnosing ASDs. Your pediatrician can recommend a specialist or you can find one through your local hospital, school district, university, or state agency that specializes in ASDs.

Developmental pediatricians are an excellent choice because most have broad experience in diagnosing ASDs and are trained to assess your child's overall development—including physical, cognitive, behavioral, and emotional development. Other excellent choices of diagnosticians include pediatric neurologists, child psychologists, and child psychiatrists. Some parents take a multidisciplinary approach to diagnosis and also bring their children to evaluators who specialize in specific areas of development, such as speech and language pathologists, occupational therapists, and physical therapists. Sometimes a team of evaluators is located under one roof, such as at hospital or university clinics. Other times, parents will have to bring their children for individual appointments at various doctors' and specialists' offices.

No matter who evaluates your child, make sure they have experience in diagnosing children with ASDs. It's also important that you be 100 percent honest when you describe your child's behaviors. While this may seem like obvious advice, some parents try to hide symptoms because they fear a devastating diagnosis or they mistakenly believe that their child's symptoms are a reflection of bad parenting.

Diagnosticians will review the tests results with you and recommend a treatment plan for your child.

Can evaluations for my child be done through my school district?

From birth to age three, your child can be evaluated by a state agency through their Early Intervention program—at no cost to you. Each state has a lead agency in charge of early intervention services for infants and toddlers with special needs. They will provide you with a list of approved evaluation sites where you can bring your child. In some cases, the evaluators will come to your home to administer the evaluations. If your child is between the ages of three and five years old, the state agency will still pay for your child's evaluations, which will be administered by the preschool evaluators. When your child turns five, he or she can be evaluated by the school district—again, at no cost to you. These evaluations often involve a multidisciplinary team to assess your child, using parent information and comprehensive cognitive, language, and learning evaluations. The team may include a psychologist, speech and language pathologist, occupational therapist, physical therapist, and other professionals. The focus of the evaluations is to determine how your child's disability will impact his or her classroom performance—or, in the case of a preschool child, participation in appropriate activities.

Unlike a doctor or specialist, the team evaluating your child will not give you a medical/clinical diagnosis or recommend a treatment plan. Instead, the evaluators will decide upon a classification for your child (one of which is the general category *autism*—you can think of this as the educational equivalent of a medical diagnosis). They will also discuss the tests results with you, and inform you about your child's strengths and delays.

These evaluations are very important because they are key components in helping to get your child treatment services through the state or school district. The evaluators will discuss the results of your child's testing in a committee meeting to determine which services are best suited for your child's needs. You'll learn all about these meetings in Part II: Treatment.

When you call to request an evaluation for your child, you can simply explain that you are concerned about your child's development and think that he or she may require special services. If you're not sure where to call, you can always contact your local elementary school to help you locate the local early intervention agency or the special education office in your area.

To locate an agency in your state that provides evaluations for your infant, toddler, or preschooler up to age five, you can call 1-800-695-0285 or log onto the National Dissemination Center for Children with Disabilities at www.nichcy.org/.

What's better—taking my child to a medical specialist, the school district, or an early intervention evaluator?

In an ideal situation, you want your child to be diagnosed by a medical expert *and* a school or early intervention evaluator. They use different assessment tools that can give you a well-rounded picture of your child and his or her specific needs. Plus, the school district or early intervention agency is ultimately responsible for giving your child treatment services.

If you are able to obtain both a medical and school/early intervention evaluation for your child, go to the medical/clinical expert first. Getting that diagnosis—actually knowing the name of your child's condition—can help you in many ways. On an emotional and psychological level, the diagnosis can help you make sense of why your child isn't speaking or why he or she is behaving in a certain way. On a practical level, the diagnosis can provide you with treatment recommendations that can direct you to the services your child will need. For example, Jake was diagnosed PDD-NOS by a developmental pediatrician, who recommended a treatment plan that included Applied Behavior Analysis (ABA), speech therapy, and occupational therapy. The child psychiatrist who offered a second opinion also recommended this treatment plan. That served as a guideline for me when I called to request evaluations from our early intervention state agency. I knew what to call my son's condition and what symptoms to point out so that the agency had an idea of what evaluations to use. Ultimately, the committee that determines your child services will take all reports into consideration when making its decision about your child's educational needs.

Who pays for my child to be evaluated or diagnosed?

According to the Individuals with Disabilities Education Act (IDEA), your child is legally entitled to evaluations at *no cost to you* from either your state agency or Department of Education if your child is twenty-one years old or younger.

If you choose to bring your child to a private specialist, such as a developmental pediatrician, pediatric neurologist, child psychiatrist, child psychologist, any other medical professional, or an ASD specialist, you need to check with your health insurance company about what coverage you are entitled to. If you plan on paying out-of-pocket, make sure to ask what the cost of the appointment is when you book it. Some medical/clinical assessments can cost thousands of dollars.

Which assessments are used to evaluate my child?

Most evaluators will begin the evaluation process by interviewing you to find out about your child's developmental history. They may ask when your child first walked and talked and about your child's current behaviors and skills. Depending on your child's age, evaluators may use a standardized list of interview questions known as the Autism Diagnostic Interview-Revised (ADI-R), or questionnaires such as the Childhood Autism Rating Scale (CARS) or the Parent Interview for Autism (PIA) to assess your child's communication skills, social skills, and overall behavior. You may be asked to fill out a checklist called the Gilliam Autism Rating Scale (GARS). Evaluators may also interview your child's caretakers and/or teachers to get an overall picture of him.

If evaluators suspect an ASD, they will use interviews, observations, and specific testing to see if your child meets the diagnostic criteria for an ASD in the DSM-IV-TR. Sometimes during the evaluation, evaluators will play games and interact with your child; other times, they will simply observe your child's behavior while your child is playing or interacting with you. With younger children, parents usually remain in the assessment room. Many times, there is a two-way mirror on one wall that allows another assessor to observe and/or videotape the evaluation.

Typical assessments for ASDs may include physical and neurological examinations, such as the Bayley Scales of Infant Development-II (measures mental and motor scales), Vineland Adaptive Behavior Scales (measures behavior, communication, daily living skills, socialization, and gross/fine motor skills), Stanford-Binet Intellegence Scale, Beery-Buketnica Test of Visual-Motor Integrations, and Autism Diagnostic Observation Schedule (ADOS). Other assessments may be used depending on your child's specific needs.

If your child is being evaluated by the state agency or the school district, it is certain that your child will be given a core evaluation that consists of a social history, observation, psychological testing, and educational testing. Speech and language skills may also be included in the core evaluation. If scores reveal that there are other factors involved in your child's condition, occupational therapy, physical therapy, or other kinds of measures will be added. The tests must be up-to-date and standardized. Often, the type of psychological or educational test will be determined by the evaluators at the time of evaluation, depending on what is being observed.

In all cases, you will receive written evaluations that include test results and notes on observations. Clinical evaluations will usually include treatment recommendations in the written reports; agency and district evaluations will not.

How can my child be assessed if he or she cannot speak?

Because many children with ASDs have little or no speech, special assessments have been developed to test whether or not a nonverbal (or mostly nonverbal) child has an ASD. Parents play an integral part in the process by answering specific questions about their children's behaviors. A diagnostician can also observe and assess your child's nonverbal behaviors to focus on communication and cognitive abilities and deficits.

One assessment tool that is especially valuable for nonverbal children is the Vineland Adaptive Behavior Scales, which compares your child's communication, social, daily living, and motor skills with those of children who have developed typically and with those who have other developmental disabilities.

Cognitive tests can be given by a licensed psychologist. In some cognitive tests that measure problem-solving skills, expressive language is not required on the part of your child. Your child may be asked to stack blocks or match pictures and shapes—tasks that may require receptive language (understanding the instructions) or imitation skills (stacking the blocks in the same pattern as the tester) but that would not require your child to speak the answers.

A certified speech and language pathologist (SLP) can test a nonverbal child using the Communication and Symbolic Behavior Scales and/or by engaging the child in games and play activities to see how the child responds. An SLP will observe to see if your child communicates nonverbally by gesturing, pointing, or waving. The SLP may encourage communication by holding a desired object just out of your child's reach to see if your child extends his arms toward it or by playing a tape of your child's favorite music and then stopping the music to see if your child can indicate that he wants to hear more.

Does a diagnosis of an ASD mean that my child is mentally retarded?

Some children with ASDs also have mental retardation, with the exception of children who are diagnosed with Asperger's. Others function in the mental retardation IQ range (which is considered to be a score of 70 or below on the IQ test), without actually meeting the criteria for mental retardation.

IQ is not the sole determinant of whether or not a child is mentally retarded. The onset of mental retardation must occur before age eighteen, and a child must also show significant delays or deficits in conceptual skills (such as communication skills), social skills, and practical adaptive functioning skills. Adaptive functioning refers to the ability to meet the demands of the real world, such as eating or getting dressed. There are four different degrees of mental retardation: mild, moderate, severe, and profound. If there is a question of whether or not a toddler has mental retardation, it can usually be determined by the time the child is at or near school age.

One of the problems of measuring IQ in children with ASDs is that standard intelligence tests are not always accurate measurement tools. These tests require a child to interact, imitate, and use both receptive and expressive language skills, such as following instructions or verbally responding to answers—all skills that may be missing or delayed in children with ASDs. It has been shown that the IQ of a child with an ASD can rise an average of 20 to 30 points following an intensive ABA treatment program.[1] This is what happened with our son, Jake. When he was tested at age two, his IQ was 58. At age four, after intensive ABA treatment, his IQ jumped to 110.

Children who meet the criteria for both mental retardation and an ASD can benefit from the same treatment as children who meet the criteria only for an ASD.

Does a diagnosis of an ASD mean that my child will experience seizures?

Although the majority of them do not, some children with ASDs do experience seizures. The risk of seizures among children with ASDs is higher than among typical children, and approximately 25 percent of children with ASDs develop epilepsy, which is a chronic brain disorder characterized by recurrent seizures. Seizures are generally seen in children with ASDs who are also mentally retarded.

According to the National Society for Epilepsy, "the word 'seizure' describes a sudden, short event where there is a change in a person's awareness of where they are or what they are doing, their behaviour or their feelings."[2] Seizures are episodes of disturbed brain function that are caused by abnormal electrical excitation in the brain. Sometimes seizures can seem to be merely odd or idiosyncratic behavior in children, which is why they may initially be confused with symptoms of ASDs. But unlike self-stimulatory behavior that may be triggered by overstimulation or anxiety, seizures come on suddenly with no apparent trigger.

There are two main categories of seizures: generalized and partial. Generalized seizures affect both sides of the brain simultaneously and include petit and grand mal seizures. In a petit mal (or "small and bad") seizure, a child may have a blank stare and then experience a sudden loss of awareness or conscious activity for seconds. In a grand mal (or "big and bad") seizure, a child's whole body may go into violent muscle contractions or else become totally rigid. Partial seizures affect only a part of the brain and can include nausea, body jerking, skin flushing, and dilated pupils. Depending on the severity of the partial seizure, a person may or may not lose consciousness.

If you are concerned that your child may be having seizures, make sure to bring your child to a neurologist or pediatric neurologist (who specializes in the brain and diseases of the nervous system) to perform an EEG. Your pediatrician may send your child for an EEG even before you go for an official neurological exam. In an EEG, electrodes (metal discs) are placed on the scalp over various areas of the brain to measure its electrical activity. The test isn't painful; the only discomfort children may experience is from the stickiness of the paste used to keep the electrodes in place. EEG tests are performed by a special technician and may take place in your doctor's office or at a hospital. In some cases, the doctor may recommend a twenty-four-hour EEG, which requires hospital stay. In addition to the EEG, the neurologist will also perform a physical examination and an examination of the central nervous system.

Seizure disorders can be treated with a number of different kinds of medications known as anticonvulsants. In some cases, special dietary treatments or surgery are recommended.

Are there disorders that resemble ASDs but are not?

There are some disorders that resemble ASDs but are not ASDs. The following information is adapted from Carolyn Thorwarth Bruey's book *Demystifying Autism Spectrum Disorders: A Guide for Parents and Professionals*:[3]

- Aphasia: A speech and language disorder caused by brain injury such as a stroke. A child with aphasia has difficulty communicating with words but does not have other symptoms of ASDs such as ritualistic and repetitive behaviors.

- Fragile X Syndrome: The most common genetic cause of mental retardation, fragile X syndrome can be detected through a DNA blood test. Children with this syndrome have similar behaviors to children with ASDs (e.g., self-stimulatory behaviors and sensory issues), but socially, they are shy rather than aloof.

- Landau-Kleffner Syndrome (LKS): A rare condition often confused with CDD because children experience typical development followed by significant regression. Unlike CDD, LKS can be detected through an EEG.

- Mental Retardation (MR): A child may have a dual diagnosis of mental retardation and an ASD. But a sole diagnosis of mental retardation means a child has pervasive delays across *all* developmental areas rather than a pervasive disordered developmental delay. (For example, a ten-year-old child with severe mental retardation without an ASD may display the skills of a two-year-old across all skill areas, such as social skills and language, whereas a child with an ASD might have some skills in the ten-year-old area and other skills in the four-year-old area).

- Nonverbal Learning Disorders (NLD): Children with NLD are often confused with having Asperger's because they have above average intelligence and strong verbal skills. They also have difficulty with social skills and often display a hypersensitivity to sensory input. But these children do not display ritualistic and repetitive behaviors or other characteristics indicative of ASDs.

– Obsessive-Compulsive Disorder (OCD): While children with OCD and children with ASDs both demonstrate obsessive, ritualistic behaviors, the biggest difference lies in their levels of awareness. Children with OCD are aware that their repetitive actions are irrational and have no meaningful purpose, whereas children with ASDs are not. Children with OCD do not have social or communication skills problems indicative of an ASD.

– Schizophrenia: The word autistic was originally used to describe schizophrenics. While children with ASDs and schizophrenics may both have speech and language problems, the conditions are quite different. Unlike ASDs, the onset of schizophrenia occurs when a child is an adolescent or young adult and is marked by hallucinations or delusions.

– Reactive Attachment Disorder (RAD): Children with RAD have difficulties relating to others, but these difficulties are usually a result of a history of abuse and don't have a physiological basis as seen with ASDs.

– Speech and Language Disorders: While children with ASDs may have speech and language difficulties, children with speech and language disorders are more motivated to communicate and develop nonverbal communication skills, such as pointing and gesturing.

– Sensory Impairments: Deaf and blind children may appear to show symptoms of ASDs; deaf children may be less responsive initially to social interactions, and blind children may rock back and forth or weave their heads (roll their head in a figure-eight motion) as if they are engaged in self-stimulatory behaviors. But these symptoms are greatly reduced or disappear as children get older, and their social and communication skills increase. (Blind and deaf children can have ASDs; their incident rate is the same as for the general population.)

– Social Phobia: The largest similarity between a social phobia and an ASD is in the area of limited social skills, but a child with social phobia does not exhibit the same problems in communication or the repetitive or ritualistic behaviors that are characteristic in children with ASDs.

If your child receives a diagnosis that only resembles an ASD and you're still feeling unsure, make sure you bring your child to a professional who specializes in diagnosing ASDs for a second opinion.

Is it possible that my child was misdiagnosed with an ASD?

There is the possibility that a child diagnosed with an ASD may actually have one of the previously described disorders instead. While the criteria for ASDs are quite detailed, there can still be some confusion and disagreement about a specific diagnosis, even among professionals. This is because, even though the specific criteria for ASDs are outlined in the DSM-IV-TR, the diagnosis is ultimately a professional's interpretation of your child's behaviors according to the criteria. There may also be confusion because there are no clearly established guidelines for measuring the severity of a child's symptoms. This is why the same child can receive two different diagnoses on the autism spectrum. For example, a child may receive a diagnosis of Autistic Disorder from one doctor and a diagnosis of PDD-NOS from another doctor.

There's a theory that the radical rise in cases of ASDs is due to developmental pediatricians handing out diagnoses of ASDs the way they used to hand out lollipops. In fact, when Jake was initially diagnosed with PDD-NOS, a pediatrician friend commented, "PDD-NOS is a popular diagnosis that doctors give out when they really don't know what's wrong with your child." As well-educated as she was, this pediatrician did not recognize that Jake's symptoms were in fact classic signs of an ASD.

On the off chance that your child receives a false positive diagnosis of an ASD, there's a good possibility that your child has developmental delays that would require the same treatments used for treating ASDs.

UNDERSTANDING YOUR CHILD'S BEHAVIORS

My friend's child has some of the behaviors listed as symptoms for ASDs, and he's considered to be typical. Why is this?

Before Jake's diagnosis, I bragged to a friend about how neat he was because he lined up his toy trains. My friend, whose typical son was Jake's age, commented that her son did the same thing. I later learned that Jake's aligning of his trains was considered perseverative behavior in the world of ASDs. Why? Perseverative comes from the word persevere, and Jake would obsessively and relentlessly repeat this behavior for hours on end. If anyone dared to disrupt him, he would throw a monumental tantrum that could last for hours. Other behaviors of Jake's—such as turning light switches on and off, opening and closing doors, and staring at ceiling fans—didn't seem out of the ordinary to Franklin and me, but were also subsequently identified as classic perseverative behaviors.

Behaviors that appear typical in most children can be atypical in children with ASDs. What distinguishes these children's behaviors is often a matter of severity. For example, many children, both typical and with ASDs, engage in spinning. A typical child may spin around and fall to the ground laughing before switching to another form of play. A child with an ASD may spin for hours. Typical children who eat only chicken nuggets for every meal are considered to be picky eaters. Children with ASDs who eat chicken nuggets for every meal are considered to be engaging in an idiosyncratic behavior characteristic of an ASD. Why the distinction? The crucial difference lies in the intensity, frequency, duration, and nature of the behavior; children with ASDs exhibit these behaviors along with a cluster of other behaviors that are symptomatic of ASDs.

Other seemingly typical behaviors can be observed and misinterpreted in children who should have a diagnosis of an ASD. An unresponsive child may be seen as obstinate, an unsocial child as simply shy, and a child engaged in repetitive behaviors as anxious. Even a nonverbal child can be seen merely as a late talker. (Parents often hear that they needn't worry because Albert Einstein didn't speak until he was four or five. However, in some circles, it's speculated that Einstein had an ASD). Sometimes parents may miss early symptoms of ASDs because their children don't display common stereotypical behaviors. Parents will say, "But my child makes eye contact!" or, "My child likes affection!" and dismiss other early warning signs. Also, since much of the focus of ASDs is on developmental delays, parents can miss symptoms if their children are demonstrating advanced skills in certain areas. Early precocious behavior can be deceptive. One mother of a child who was later diagnosed with an ASD assumed that her son was gifted because he was speaking in full sentences by age one and was explaining the solar system by age three. Parents who have the misconception that all children with ASDs have low IQs or exhibit obvious autistic behaviors may mistakenly ignore other symptoms if their children display some typical behaviors.

My child used to speak. He seemed to develop normally until he was about two years old but then seemed to regress. What happened?

Approximately 20 to 40 percent of children who are diagnosed with ASDs seem to develop communication skills, then experience a regression, losing most or all of their communication skills at around the age of nineteen months. Like many parents, we noticed this phenomenon in Jake. At the time of his diagnosis, the doctors had little explanation for why he stopped speaking and gesturing, and very few studies concerning this type of behavior were being conducted.

But now, researchers are looking into why some children develop, then regress. The largest known study on regression is being conducted at the University of Michigan as part of the U-M Autism & Communication Disorders Center under the direction of Catherine Lord, Ph.D., a pioneer in research on ASDs. Using data on preschool children, collected from thirteen sites across the United States over a five-year period, the study is part of a larger project within the Collaborative Program for Excellence in Autism.

Even though most parents recognize the loss of speech and language as the most obvious warning sign of regression, this study shows that most of these children also have other communication delays that may not be as obvious to parents. Researchers found that almost 77 percent of children who experienced language loss also lost communication skills in nonverbal areas. Children not only stopped speaking but also stopped gesturing to indicate what they wanted, responding to their name, imitating, understanding simple requests, and playing with other children.

The researchers in this study are looking at potential causes for this pattern of regression. One theory points to a possible regressive phenotype of autism. But this theory is inconclusive because children with ASDs who experience regression have overlapping symptoms with children with ASDs who had never experienced regression. Other theories have looked at a link between regression and gastrointestinal symptoms and a family history of autoimmune thyroid disease, but again, there is no conclusive evidence. There was also speculation that the measles-mumps-rubella (MMR) vaccine might be to blame, since most children receive the vaccine between the ages of fifteen and eighteen months, right around the time that parents notice a regression. But the University of Michigan study showed that even when children receive the vaccination at different times, there is no variation in the timing of regression. Children who receive the MMR before parents report concerns are just as likely to have already developed symptoms of ASDs (which parents haven't necessarily noticed) as those who receive vaccinations after the onset of an ASD.[1]

Researchers are also looking at whether or not there is a difference in progress between children who experience regression and those who do not. But one thing remains clear: Children with ASDs, with or without regression, require intensive early intervention.

Why won't my child make eye contact with me?

Typical newborns will turn their heads in the direction of their mothers' voices and, as they develop, their eyes will be drawn to their mothers' faces. Later on, faces in general will continue to hold a special fascination for them. Typical children perceive a face as a whole. Our brains are not wired to register features discretely—eyes, nose, mouth, chin, and forehead—then piece them together as if they were objects. When tested, typical children perceive faces more quickly than objects, whereas children with ASDs see faces feature by feature without compiling them into a whole.

Eye contact can be particularly difficult for children with ASDs because faces are rarely static: Our eyebrows rise when we show surprise, our eyes look up or to the side when we're thinking, and the corners of our mouths curl up or down to connote happiness or disappointment. There's a lot of facial activity taking place at any given time, and for children with ASDs who view faces as components rather than as a whole, looking at a face may be overwhelming.

A fascinating experiment on tracking the eye movements of people with ASDs was conducted at the Yale Child Study Center by Ami J. Klin, Ph.D., in collaboration with Warren R. Jones, a research associate, using excerpts from the 1966 film *Who's Afraid of Virginia Woolf?* A group of typical subjects and subjects with ASDs were given special eye tracking equipment that measured what they focused on while watching the film. During emotionally charged scenes, typical subjects zeroed in on the actors' eyes. Subjects with ASDs stared at the actors' mouths, primarily at the mouth of the actor who was speaking. In scenes with two actors, where one was not speaking but displaying an intense emotional reaction through his face and body language, subjects with ASDs remained focused on the speaker's mouth. They would miss the silent actor's reaction, and therefore not take in the true significance of the scene. Sometimes, individuals with ASDs didn't focus on the actors at all but rather on objects in the background of the screen. In a passionate love scene between Elizabeth Taylor and Richard Burton, one subject with an ASD peered intently at a light switch located on the back wall of the set.[2]

Neuroscientists now believe that a specific part of our brain is responsible for recognizing faces—a tiny patch of the cerebral cortex that is activated when people look at pictures of faces but not objects. They refer to this part of the brain as the fusiform face area (FFA). A fascinating study using functional magnetic resonance imaging (fMRI) was conducted by Robert T. Schultz, Ph.D., at the Yale Child Study Center. When typical subjects were shown pictures of faces, there was a high level of activity in the FFA. When subjects with ASDs were shown pictures of faces, there was little activity in the FFA; but the researchers did note a high activation level in nearby brain regions—the ones used for recognizing objects.

Why does my child prefer to play alone? He won't interact with other children. It's as if they're not even there. He used to be social and loved attention.

It's not clear whether children with ASDs prefer to play alone or if playing alone is all they can handle. Studies show that aloneness for children with ASDs is not the result of innate fear or an act of deliberate defiance. Children with ASDs may be overstimulated by the presence of too many people, which causes them to retreat. Some may not have the capacity to read and understand other people's feelings and consequently lack the skills to know how to behave with others.

Dr. Leo Kanner was one of the first researchers to identify this trend of aloneness in children with autism. The word autism, which implies self, was used to describe these children because it was originally thought that they had a genuine proclivity toward being alone.

We now know from anecdotal experiences described by subjects who have ASDs and from scientific studies of the social brain that aloneness may not be a preference. In fact, it's possible that parts of the social brain in people with ASDs may be weak as a result of lifelong social deprivation. This is why social skills training can play an integral role in a child's treatment.

My child doesn't point out things to me like I've seen other children do. She doesn't really seem interested in sharing anything with me. Why?

This relates to the phenomenon called *joint attention,* which refers to the parent and child coordinating their attention so that they are looking at the same object or sharing in an activity. Joint attention between a parent and a typically developing baby becomes evident when the baby is around eight months old. At this time, babies check in with their mothers to make sure it's okay for them to touch something, such as a new toy or a wall outlet. Babies will look at their mothers' faces to gauge their expressions: A smile means "okay" whereas a furrowed brow means "stay away." At ten months, joint attention is usually seen in children as they begin to point to things in their environments. But typical babies aren't simply interested in the objects they're pointing to; they're interested in their parents' responses to those objects. And they don't necessarily want the objects they're pointing to; they may just want to share the experience of looking at the objects with their parents. For example, a baby who points outside to a sunset or to a bug on the window wants Mom or Dad to look at it with him. That's what makes joint attention so special. Babies begin to have an awareness of other people's feelings and attitudes.

One of the first warning signs of a lack of joint attention in children with ASDs appears in infancy, when children don't look for their parents' facial reactions and don't have (or have lost) the ability to physically point out things in their environments. Children with ASDs who can point use pointing to get something they want rather than sharing the experience with someone else. This kind of behavior is known as instrumental pointing.

An experiment involving joint attention was conducted by Marian Sigman, Peter Mundy, and their colleagues at UCLA, and Katherine Loveland and Susan Landry at the University of Texas. Both typical children and children with ASDs were put in a room full of toys. The observers wanted to see which group of children would show the toys to their mothers more often. As predicted, typical children showed the toys to their mothers far more often than children with ASDs. In these types of situations, children with ASDs tend to focus more on the objects themselves than on sharing the experience with another person. The experimenters learned that joint attention is missing in children with ASDs, not only through pointing and showing but also through speech.[3]

The speech component of joint attention becomes more evident by preschool age, when typical children use both speech and pointing to share experiences. "Look at the bird!" a typical child will say, tugging on her mother's jacket. A child with an ASD may notice the bird but not point it out. In addition to initiating engagement, joint attention also involves attempts at receiving joint attention from others. For example, a mother will say, "Look at the funny clown!" If her child is unresponsive, it indicates a lack of joint attention.

As children with ASDs grow older, the lack of joint attention can be evident in those who have more fully developed speech and language skills. These individuals often have trouble carrying on two-way conversations because they don't have an awareness of the other person's intention or mental state. Many people with ASDs will dominate the conversation, engaging in one-way communication and expressing little interest in the other person.

Why does my child seem oblivious to everyone's feelings?

In his work with children with ASDs, Kanner noted an apparent lack of attention that extended far beyond facial recognition—that is, he noted an indifference to people in general, including parents and siblings. When he placed both typical children and children with ASDs in a room that contained both toys and people, children with ASDs gravitated to the toys more than to the people, while typical children gravitated more to the people. In this study, we can trace the roots of what Simon Baron-Cohen, Professor of Developmental Psychopathology at the University of Cambridge in the Departments of Experimental Psychology and Psychiatry, would later call Theory of Mind.[4]

Theory of Mind is the concept that individuals with ASDs have difficulty understanding another person's thoughts, affects, emotions, or points of view because they are mindblind. *Mindblindness* is the inability of a person to empathize or understand that people think or feel differently. Mindblindness has nothing to do with intelligence; individuals with high IQs and Asperger's can be mindblind. Because mindblind people with ASDs do not show empathy, they can be mistakenly judged as egocentric or uncaring.

Believe it or not, most of us are mind readers. We observe an elderly homeless man slumped on a park bench and sense his despair. We look at a photograph of a mother and father smiling at their newborn and partake of their happiness. By merely hearing someone's tone of voice on the phone, we can identify the caller's emotional state. This is possible because our unconscious is constantly piecing together cues from our environment that allow us to make inferences about people, whether or not we know them. The homeless man on the bench is a stranger, and yet we are able to make certain assumptions—that he is sad and lonely—based on his appearance and his posture. We assume the new parents are joyous and proud. We can tell by our friend's stern tone of voice over the phone that she is angry about something. Mind reading comes naturally to most of us, but not if we have an ASD. It's not that people with ASDs don't see the same things other people do; they just see them extremely differently.

For example, a typical child and a child with an ASD may be shown the same black-and-white photograph of a group of children waiting in line in front of an ice cream truck. In the photograph, one boy in line looks at a little girl who is standing off to the side, holding an empty cone while looking down on the sidewalk at a scoop of ice cream. A dog is running toward the little girl. When asked to talk about the photograph, a typical child may describe the girl's disappointment at dropping her ice cream and the dog's joyful anticipation of getting an afternoon treat. The child may wonder if the boy who has noticed the girl will leave his place in line to console her and wonder if he or she would do the same if placed in that situation.

A child with an ASD, in contrast, may state that in the photo there are seven boys, two girls, and a dog, without referring to the story that has unfolded. Another child with an ASD may not talk about the contents of the photo at all, but comment instead on the tones of black and gray in the picture and the shininess of the processing paper as if there were no storyline at all. The child with an ASD is simply not picking up on the same cues as the typical child.

We can see similarities between mindblindness and a lack of facial recognition; just as children with ASDs see faces as component parts rather than wholes, they regard the scene described above as component parts, often unable to see the larger picture, and thereby miss what's going on emotionally. This explains why many adults with ASDs report that they don't understand other people's feelings, and perhaps why many children with ASDs seem oblivious to other people's emotional states.

There are many children with ASDs who appear to be mindblind. Michael, the child diagnosed with Asperger's in the case study, represents a clear example of what mindblindness can look like. One afternoon, he was in the kitchen with his mother when she received an upsetting phone call from her soon-to-be ex-husband. She tried to remain composed, but after hanging up the phone, she broke down and started sobbing. Michael seemed oblivious. He sat at the table and continued his one-way conversation about the life cycle of the monarch butterfly. His mother cried, and Michael talked. It was as if they were not even in the same room.

Michael's reaction is typical of children with ASDs who have trouble considering another person's point of view. Most of us consider other people's feelings naturally. We know what birthday present to buy for friends because we can imagine ourselves in their shoes. We know when to stop talking and just listen because we see friends in tears and recognize their distress. In typical children, we can observe this ability in the way they play hide-and-seek. Children have to think of a hiding place where the seeker will not look; they are making the leap into the other person's head to figure out how to outsmart him or her.

In an experiment conducted at our own kitchen table, three-year-old Jake was seated across from his ABA therapist. She placed a quarter under a teacup. Then she asked me to leave the room. After I left, she showed Jake that she was moving the quarter from underneath the teacup and into her pocket. Then she called me back into the kitchen. She asked Jake, "Where do you think Mommy will look for the quarter?" He responded, "In your pocket."

It turns out that our little experiment in the kitchen is actually based on a method created by developmental psychologists Heinz Wimmer and Josef Perner and adapted by Baron-Cohen. It's called the Sally-Anne experiment and involves a scenario between two dolls and hidden marbles. Again, the point of the experiment is to see if a child can identify where one of the dolls will look for the marble after it has been moved without her knowledge. In almost every case of this experiment, typical children and children with Down syndrome got the right answer, whereas children with ASDs got it wrong.[5]

The fact that Jake did not think to take my perspective into consideration and assume that I would look for the quarter under the teacup is typical of many children with ASDs. However, through ABA treatment, Jake was able to learn how to consider another person's point of view, which ultimately translated into his ability to show empathy.

Mindblindness can also be tied to lack of eye contact. By avoiding looking at people's faces, particularly the eyes, children with ASDs are missing out on being able to read affect or emotional states. Since our words don't necessarily convey our true emotional states, the expression, "I can see it on your face" is a perfect example of how much we rely on intuition and nonverbal cues to identify another person's mood. How many times have we responded with "Fine" to the greeting "How are you?" when we're really not feeling so great? Chances are, our listener will glean insight into how we're really feeling by reading our facial expression. To the person with an ASD, someone's facial expression may give absolutely nothing away because he can't read it. Baron-Cohen tested this theory by showing to his subjects with ASDs a set of thirty-six photographs of the eye regions of male and female actors. The test was called Reading the Mind in the Eyes Test. Subjects were required to distinguish between subtle emotional states that could be detected in the eyes. They evaluated the expressions by labeling them serious, ashamed, alarmed, or bewildered. This was extremely difficult for the subjects with ASDs. In fact, most subjects with ASDs consistently failed the test.

Because many children with ASDs experience mindblindness, they may unconsciously alienate others through their behaviors. This can be especially difficult at home or school. Family members or peers may feel ignored or dismissed. But research and anecdotal evidence show that some children with ASDs can learn to consider other people's perspectives and learn empathy skills, as Jake eventually did. There are treatments specifically designed to help children understand other people's points of view and facial expressions and modify their behaviors in social situations.

Why does my child stare at nothing at all, like a wall or a ceiling fan, for hours? It's as if he's in a hypnotic state. He also likes to spin and rock back and forth. What's going on?

Many children with ASDs engage in what's called *stereotypy*, or self-stimulatory behavior, commonly referred to by parents and professionals as *stimming*. Stimming can involve gazing at a wall or fixating on an object; repetitive body movements, such as rocking back and forth; or the repetitive movement of objects, such as turning light switches on and off.

Stimming can occur in different ways and involve any or all of the senses. Here are some stereotypical stimming behaviors. You may recognize some of these behaviors in your child. This is not a complete list, but it describes some of the most commonly observed types of stimming among children with ASDs.

SENSE	SELF-STIMULATORY BEHAVIOR
AUDITORY:	Vocalizing in the form of humming, grunting, or high-pitched shrieking; tapping ears or objects; covering and uncovering ears; snapping fingers; repeating vocal sequences; imitating vocal sequences (echolalia); repeating portions of videos, books, or songs at inappropriate times
VISUAL:	Staring at lights or ceiling fans or gazing at nothing in particular; tracking eyes; peering out of the corners of eyes; flicking fingers in front of face; lining up objects; turning light switches on and off
TACTILE:	Scratching or rubbing skin with hands or objects; opening and closing fists; tapping surfaces with fingers
VESTIBULAR:	Rocking back and forth or side to side; spinning; jumping; pacing
TASTE:	Sucking or licking body parts or objects
SMELL:	Sniffing or smelling people or objects

While stimming is seen in children with other forms of developmental disabilities, it is most common in children with ASDs—to the point where children with other diagnoses may be said to have autistic characteristics if they engage in similar actions.

Scanning this list of stimming behaviors (as with the list of symptoms for ASDs), a parent with a typical child may remark that her son also likes to jump and spin. Again, it's a matter of severity. A typical child may like to jump or spin, but not with the same repetition and intensity as a child with an ASD. A child with an ASD will spin for hours on end or engage in strict ritualistic behavior that may involve compulsively lining up toy cars in specific arrangements before bedtime every night. If deprived of these behaviors, a child with an ASD will most likely have an extreme tantrum or engage in out-of-control behavior.

Some stimming behaviors that are ritualistic in nature seem to have an obsessive-compulsive component. Picking up every loose piece of thread and rubbing it between the fingers or lining up paper clips from one end of the room to another every night seem like obsessive-compulsive behaviors. As mentioned on page 36, people with obsessive-compulsive disorder know that they are engaging in a purposeless, nonfunctional behavior; people with ASDs do not. This characteristic of ASDs can also be related to what Kanner described as "insistence on sameness."

Why do children with ASDs engage in stimming? One explanation is that it releases opiate-like substances in the brain called beta-endorphins, which can produce either a euphoric or anesthetic effect. Researchers hypothesize that stimming could be the mechanism that provides an extra dose of internal stimulation for children with ASDs who are feeling understimulated or a feeling of tranquility for children who are feeling overstimulated.

Children who are hypersensitive, or overly sensitive to stimuli, may engage in stimming because they want to reduce their current level of stimulation—whether they perceive their environments as too loud, bright, or crowded. For this reason, many children with ASDs seem to disconnect from the outside world by engaging in repetitive, often mesmerizing activities such as staring fixedly at an object or repeating a line from a movie or book.

Jake, overwhelmed by the presence of more than two people in the room, would immediately lie down on the floor and stare at whatever was in front of him. If he happened to have a toy car in his hand, he would push it back and forth in front of his face. His eyes would follow the car's wheels, a stimming behavior known as eye tracking. Jake engaged in eye tracking even if objects weren't present. Sitting in his high chair, car seat, or the bathtub, Jake would move his head from right to left and peer out of the corners of his eyes. Jake would eye track when he was either bored or anxious, and sometimes I could tell how he was feeling by the intensity of his stimming. When he was bored, his eye tracking occurred as if in slow motion; when he was stressed, he moved his head and eyes quickly.

Sam, the excitable girl diagnosed with Autistic Disorder, engaged in stimming that involved auditory stimuli; she liked to repeat the same nursery rhyme over and over to calm herself when she was feeling inundated by sensory stimuli. She would repeat the line "Twinkle, twinkle little star" in a mantra-like voice fifty times in one sitting. For both Jake and Sam, as for many children with hypersensitivity, stimming seems to be a way to block out the intensity of their environments.

In some cases, however, stimming may have the opposite effect and actually increase arousal.[6] For children who are hyposensitive, or under-responsive to stimuli, stimming may provide that extra dose of sensory excitement; flapping or spinning may flip the "on" switch in an otherwise dormant nervous system. Some hyposensitive children will lick toys, suck on household objects (such as the TV remote control), or stand at the sink and run their hands under very hot or very cold water.

In some extreme instances, stimming takes the form of self-injurious behavior such as persistent head banging, eye poking, or hand biting. It should be noted that not all self-injurious behaviors are considered to be self-stimulatory. Self-injurious behaviors can also be communicative; children may hit their heads because they are frustrated and unable to tell parents what they want.

Nathan, the silent boy diagnosed with Autistic Disorder, stims by tapping his knuckles repeatedly on window panes. His parents report that he does this when he's feeling either frustrated and overwhelmed or bored. If he is frustrated, his tapping becomes so aggressive that he breaks the window. If he is bored, his tapping is soft and rhythmic, and he smiles at the sound that he creates. Behavior theorists state that the sensory experience of a stimming behavior may reinforce the behavior itself. In other words, Nathan may repeatedly tap on the windows simply because it feels and sounds good to him.

Stimming can prevent children from learning and building social relationships. In some cases, self-stimulatory behavior, such as eye tracking or rocking, can be off-putting to typical peers, making children with ASDs seem odd. But don't lose hope. If you're the parent of a child who is stimming, you can find treatments to help reduce or eliminate your child's stimming behaviors. These will be discussed in Part II: Treatment.

Our daughter with Autistic Disorder has a very specific and complex bedtime ritual that involves tapping the headboard and lining up her dolls in a certain order on the bed. It can take up to an hour. Her brother gets ready for bed in ten minutes. What's going on?

The repetitive stimming activities and behaviors that we just discussed are related to the routines and rituals exhibited by children with ASDs. Again, this goes back to what Kanner wrote about their insistence on sameness. Even though typical people also like their routines (buying their newspaper at the same newsstand or going to the same coffee shop every morning) and may engage in certain rituals (walking the same route to work every day or riding in the same elevator), these routines and rituals are different from those of people with ASDs.

The difference lies in two key words within the criteria for ASDs, as defined in the DSM-IV-TR: "apparently inflexible adherence to specific, nonfuctional routines or rituals." *Nonfuctional* means that children's routines and rituals have no specific purpose. *Inflexible* means that any kind of change can cause a major upset. The routines and rituals involved in your morning commute have a purpose—they get you to work. And if you had to, you would buy your newspaper at a different stand or walk a different route to work. While making these adjustments may cause you some minor discomfort, they would be nothing compared with the turmoil that children with ASDs may experience if they had to make the same minor adjustments to an everyday routine.

Not all children with ASDs have routines or rituals, but for those who do, they can range from simple to elaborate. As already discussed, simple routines can involve activities such as lining up cars or trains in a particular way. Elaborate routines have a ritualistic quality. For example, a child will tap the sofa three times and spin around when she passes through the living room or arrange toys in a very specific way on a special shelf in her bedroom and insist on touching them once every morning. If someone accidentally moves one of the toys, the child will likely become distressed. If someone or something accidentally disrupts a ritual halfway through, the child will insist on starting it again from the beginning. One boy I work with has to watch the same video from beginning to end in one sitting. He will only watch this one particular video. If someone accidentally interrupts his viewing, he must start the tape over from the very beginning—FBI warning and all.

In the case study of Sam, diagnosed with Autistic Disorder, her father reported that the entire family spent a sleepless night because, while Sam was carrying out her elaborate bedtime ritual—making sure each of the six dinosaur books was exactly the same distance from the next one and alphabetized from left to right (Allosaurus, Brontosaurus, and so on), she discovered that her Triceratops book was missing. Sam shrieked and sobbed while her family searched the house. Her father promised her that he would buy her another book the next day, but she would not have it. Sam screamed, cried, and paced in her bedroom all night.

Indeed, a slight change in a child's routine, even simple everyday routines like taking a bath, can cause problems. One mother knew that her daughter's bath time had to occur the same way every evening, in the same sequence, at the same time. When she introduced a new bar of bath soap that looked almost identical to her usual soap, her daughter had an outburst that included so much splashing she practically flooded the bathroom.

Some children have an inappropriate attachment to certain objects that become part of their routines. Sometimes they are objects that are commonly loved by typical children as well (such as stuffed animals); but in most cases, the objects are rather unusual. In the case study of Nathan, diagnosed with Autistic Disorder, we saw that he liked collecting thread—he'd pull thread from his mother's blouses, from the corners of the area rug, and from any place else he could find it. He would run the thread through his fingers while he walked around the house. He even slept with his thread. Some children collect dust balls, pieces of wax, lint, spray bottles, or brightly colored scraps of paper, which they either keep arranged in a special place or insist on carrying with them at all times.

Children can also develop intense preoccupations with numbers, symbols, the weather, animals, vacuum cleaners, or specific topics of interest. They will collect, memorize, and repeat facts related to these topics. One girl with Asperger's collects and researches tiny paper dolls from Asia, which she keeps pasted all over the walls of her bedroom. Her mother reports that she has also thoroughly researched every fact and collected books and objects related to astronomy, rocks, LEGO blocks, and the cartoon characters Transformers, Ninja Turtles, Digimon, and Pokemon. Her daughter's latest project, in addition to the dolls, involves cutting out and learning all of the elements from the periodic table. (She is ten years old and years away from taking chemistry class!)

Sometimes children with ASDs become obsessed with the routines of others. For instance, children may insist that their moms make their beds exactly the same way every day, that their dads make the pasta dinner using the same pot, and that the parents drop them off at school in exactly the same place every day.

Order and sameness seem to provide a level of comfort and stability in children with ASDs. Some parents will accommodate their children's needs to avoid undue anxiety. But sometimes a child's routines and rituals can impact the life of the entire family and cause stress. Parents can try treatment strategies such as behavioral techniques to help reduce or eliminate ritualistic behaviors. Some of these treatment strategies are discussed in Part III: Coping.

My son seems overly sensitive to even the slightest sounds. The doorbell can drive him into a tantrum. What's going on?

Every second of every day, we are bombarded with sensory information. Right now as you read this book, on some level, you are aware of background noise (the sound of voices in the next room, noise of distant traffic, or whoosh of a radiator). You are also conscious of a field of visual stimuli extending beyond the words on this page: Is the book on a table or a desk? Are you holding the book in your hands? Is there a reading lamp nearby? You are also experiencing tactile stimuli, such as the feel of paper in your hands. We constantly register all of this data and more, yet we do not feel bombarded because our brains allow us to sort out information so that we can focus on a single task—in this case, reading a book.

Now imagine that, while you are trying to read this book, you become overwhelmed by all the existing stimuli around you—the sounds, sights, and textures. This sensory overload makes ordinary conversation sound like screaming, the distant ringing of a phone becomes cacophonous, the lamp emits a blinding glare, and the paper beneath your fingers feels so rough it's difficult to turn the page, much less focus on reading the words. If you are able to imagine yourself in this state, perhaps you have some idea of what hypersensitive children with ASDs may experience.

Hypersensitive children register and process sensations to the extreme. Not all children with ASDs are hypersensitive, and those who are don't necessarily have sensitivities to every category of stimuli or even to all stimuli within the same category. For example, one child may be overstimulated by certain sounds but not experience any distress in the presence of bright lights. Another child may be overly sensitive to high-pitched sounds but not to low-pitched sounds.

In the case of auditory sensory issues, children may be under-responsive to some sounds and over-responsive to others. For example, while a child may not respond to his mother's loud voice, he may be sent into a screaming tantrum at the sound of a bird chirping. This trend was documented by Dr. Edward Ornitz, who found that people with autism either underreacted or overreacted to different stimuli. What caused these diverse reactions? Dr. Ornitz suggested that they were a result of distorted sensory input.[7]

Auditory sensory issues may account for why many parents report that their children with ASDs seem to be deaf. In her book *News from the Border,* Jane Taylor McDonnell writes that her son responds to some (not all) pitches and frequencies when certain musical instruments are played.[8] Jake seemed to have a similar experience to sounds. Sometimes he appeared to ignore sounds completely, such as the sound of my voice or Franklin's when we called his name. In fact, that was what made us think that Jake was possibly deaf. To get his attention, we couldn't call him from another room or even stand behind or beside him in the same room. We'd have to face Jake directly, crouch down to his level, make big gestures, and talk loudly.

When I took Jake to a special auditory clinic for testing, it seemed clear to me that he couldn't hear some sounds. He sat perfectly still on my lap in a soundproof booth while tones were piped into the booth. The only time he responded was when the tones were high-pitched—and those sounds made him scream or cry. But I was wrong. It wasn't that Jake *couldn't* hear certain sounds; he just didn't respond to them. Or at least he didn't respond to them in a way that I could notice. The testing results revealed that Jake's hearing was within normal range. So, even though I didn't observe Jake's responses to the tones, the doctors did. Since Jake wasn't speaking at the time (which, it turns out, is fairly common among children who go in for auditory testing), the doctors watched his body language closely—especially his eyes—to measure responsiveness. Sure enough, somewhere in Jake's eyes, they were able to see what I could not: My son could hear me.

Auditory stimulation had two different effects on Jake; he would be either under-responsive, appearing to ignore certain sounds, or over-responsive, having shrieking tantrums. Most two-year-olds raise their faces to the sky and point when an airplane flies by. A fleet of planes could have flown by, and Jake wouldn't have noticed. However, the beeping of the microwave oven would send him into a screaming fit. Certain high-pitched voices also sent him over the top. We often had to ask houseguests to lower their voices to practically a whisper. Once, at a family reunion, we had to take Jake out to the car because he couldn't calm down after hearing a group of female cousins burst into laughter.

I have observed auditory sensitivity in some of the children I consult with. One mother reports that when her son hears the sound of rain, he puts his hands over his ears and rocks back and forth, often for as long as an hour. Another little girl can't tolerate usual household sounds, including the flush of the toilet, the vacuum cleaner, or the blender.

If your child experiences auditory sensitivities, effective treatments are available. Some of them involve sensory integration techniques, which can be incorporated into your child's occupational or speech therapy sessions. Some parents find that Auditory Integration Training (AIT), described in Appendix C, helps to reduce their children's auditory sensitivities.

Children with ASDs may also experience auditory processing issues. A child may have problems identifying different sounds (auditory discrimination), differentiating between sounds in the foreground and background (auditory figure-ground), or processing receptive (what we take in) and expressive (what we put out) language. If children have trouble following directions, their receptive language may be affected. It's possible that either they don't understand the words or are distracted by background noise (or both). If children have trouble answering questions or telling a story, they may have problems with expressive language.

When Jake started to regain his speech, he still experienced slower auditory processing. For example, when asked "How are you?" there was a hesitation before he answered, "Okay." Even though this was a frequently asked question, it would seem to the casual observer that he was being asked this for the first time and had to think about his answer. To help Jake process more quickly, we used computer-based programs called Fast ForWord and Fast ForWord Two (by Scientific Learning Corporation) and Earobics (by Cognitive Concepts). We were able to use them right in our home with the aid of a speech and language pathologist. However, we didn't use these programs until Jake was five years old and had acquired a foundation of speech and language skills through intensive ABA sessions coupled with speech therapy and occupational therapy sessions. At the same time, we worked collaboratively with his entire treatment team to help his auditory processing. His ABA therapists incorporated audiotapes with the sounds of schoolchildren talking and play-ing (which I tape-recorded at his preschool) into his sessions so that Jake could learn to focus on tasks in the presence of background noise. During his speech therapy sessions, the therapist had conversations with Jake while playing games to encourage multitasking. We also added music therapy to Jake's treat-ments to enhance his auditory processing.

You can consult with your child's speech and language therapist and other treatment providers to determine ways to help your child with auditory sen-sory and processing issues.

My daughter doesn't hug me anymore, and she doesn't like it when I hug her. What's happening?

In addition to having auditory sensitivities, children with ASDs may be hyper-sensitive to touch. Some children can't tolerate the feeling of certain fabrics. One boy I know can't stand to have wool touch his skin, so his parents make sure all of his clothes and blankets are 100 percent cotton. Other children don't like to be touched by anybody. As Jake's typical behavior declined, he no longer accepted our gentle hugs. His body stiffened when we embraced him, yet he welcomed big bear hugs or being playfully thrown on a bed.

Temple Grandin's book *Thinking in Pictures: And Other Reports from My Life with Autism,* offered me insight into what Jake may have been experienc-ing: "From as far back as I can remember, I always hated to be hugged. I wanted to experience the good feeling of being hugged, but it was just too overwhelming. It was like a great all-engulfing tidal wave of stimulation, and I reacted like a wild animal. Being touched triggered flight; it flipped my circuit breaker. I was overloaded and would have to escape, often by jerking away suddenly."

Temple Grandin is an adult with an ASD who has her Ph.D. in animal sci-ence and is an assistant professor at Colorado State University. According to Grandin in *Thinking in Pictures,* many children with ASDs can tolerate touch only if they initiate it and may prefer pressure stimulation (such as big bear hugs) over gentle stimulation. If children exhibit this type of tactile sensory problem, they may like to bundle up in blankets or wedge themselves into tight spaces, such as under the bed. Jake loved to roll himself up in the living room rug. He also liked being vigorously tossed onto the sofa or bed. Grandin came up with her own treatment, which she called a "squeeze machine." It was inspired by a visit to her aunt's ranch, where she saw cattle being put into a squeeze chute for vaccinations. The cows seemed to relax when the side panels of the chute were pressed against their bodies. After experiencing a panic attack one day, Grandin put her body into the machine and had her aunt adjust the side panels so that they squeezed her body. She experienced a wave of relaxation that she had never felt before. After this, she constructed her own human squeeze machine.[9]

Although we didn't use a squeeze machine for Jake, we did use sensory integration techniques to help reduce his touch sensitivities. Sensory integration was developed by Jean Ayres, an occupational therapist in California. In Jake's case, his occupational therapist had him jumping off a bunk bed onto bean bag chairs to provide him with the deep pressure stimulation that he seemed to crave. Through sensory integration and ABA, Jake learned to get over his food-related tactile sensitivities so that he could use his fingers to feed himself. Jake not only learned how to tolerate our hugs, but also began to actually like giving and receiving them again.

Our son goes beyond the definition of a picky eater. In addition to eating a limited selection of foods, he will only eat soft foods. Why?

In addition to experiencing auditory and tactile sensitivities, a smaller percentage of children with ASDs may be overly sensitive to taste and smell. In a survey of sensory problems in children and adults with autism, Neil Walker and Margaret Whelan of the Geneva Center in Toronto found that 80 to 87 percent of the subjects had hypersensitivity to touch or sound, while only 30 percent had hypersensitivity to taste and smell.[10]

Children with smell or taste sensitivities may not like crunchy foods (which may also relate to texture and auditory sensitivities). Some children will eat only Jell-O, yogurt, and mashed potatoes. Additionally, the smell of certain foods, such as cheese, cause nausea or vomiting. Other children will eat only hot foods. One mother had to heat up her son's cold cereal and peanut butter and jelly sandwiches in the microwave oven.

Eating the same food for every meal may not be a sensory problem but a manifestation of routine behavior, relating to Kanner's definition of insistence on sameness. Some children go through phases in which they'll eat only specific foods in specific ways. One boy had to have all of his foods on different plates—peas on one plate, corn on a second plate, and grilled cheese on a third. It's also possible that children will eat only certain foods because of food allergies. There are some children who refuse food altogether; parents have reported excessive drinking of water, juices, or other fluids.

In her book *The Autism Spectrum: A Parent's Guide to Understanding and Helping Your Child,* Dr. Lorna Wing explains that eating problems may stem from feeding problems because some children have trouble controlling the muscles used for chewing and swallowing.[11] Many children with ASDs are difficult to wean because they don't know how to eat lumpy food or food that requires chewing.

Speech therapists can work with children to overcome chewing and swallowing problems, behavioral therapists can work with children to overcome specific eating rituals, and occupational therapists can use sensory integration techniques to work with children to overcome food sensitivities.

Our daughter seems to feel no pain. She sticks pins in her feet and likes to dig my fingernails into her hand. What's going on?

In contrast to hypersensitive children, hyposensitive children don't seem to be disturbed by an overload of environmental stimuli. Many hyposensitive children seem to seek out additional stimulation. Sam is one of these children. As a toddler, she put anything that was within reach in her mouth; she sucked on electrical cords and dolls' heads and chewed string. She was also prone to self-injury because she did not register pain the way typical children do. She would slide down a flight of stairs head-first or place her hand on a hot toaster oven without so much as an "ouch." She also engaged in hand biting and has even drawn blood with no reaction to the pain. There are stories of children with broken bones and appendicitis who don't complain—and don't even seek out their parents for comfort.

Why do children with hyposensitivity seem to seek out extra environmental stimuli? One adult with an ASD recounted the feeling of being "wrapped in a layer of insulation" as a child. To "feel" or have a sense of what was happening in the world around her, she needed extra stimulation. Why did she not experience the appropriate reaction of pain after injury? Again, the beta-endorphins released in the brain can produce an anesthetic effect, which would account for her indifference to pain.

In addition to being either hypersensitive or hyposensitive, some children are a combination of both. Some are overly sensitive to gentle touch (a feather brushing lightly on their skin may send them into a screaming fit), yet can accept being hit over the head with a block by another child. Nathan is a combination of hypersensitive and hyposensitive. He is extremely sensitive to noise (he can't tolerate the sound of the car radio), but when he cuts himself on a broken window and is bleeding, he shows no reaction to the pain.

Why does my son bang his head and bite his hand?

Children with ASDs may engage in self-injurious behaviors that range from mild to severe. Self-injurious behaviors are behaviors that cause tissue damage in the form of redness, bruises, scratches, or open wounds. Head banging, hand biting, and excessive scratching or rubbing are the most frequent forms of self-injurious behaviors. More severe self-injurious behaviors include poking fingers into their eyes or other orifices and self-induced vomiting.

There are two sets of theories about why children engage in self-injury: physiological and social.[12] According to the physiological theory, and as already mentioned, self-injurious behaviors release beta-endorphins in the brain, which can provide an opiate effect and thus give a child an internal sense of pleasure. Self-injurious behavior may also be an extreme form of stimming—either to induce a state of arousal or to lower a state of arousal, depending on whether a child is under- or overstimulated. For instance, a child who doesn't experience typical levels of physical stimulation may engage in excessive self-rubbing to receive stimulation or an increased arousal state.

Some children engage in self-injurious behavior because they are suffering from a medical condition that they cannot explain to you. Dr. Margaret Bauman, pediatric neurologist and director of Massachusetts General's Ladders Program, has noticed this in her clients and, therefore, urges other practitioners to assess overall health in addition to offering treatments such as behavioral interventions and physical therapy. She worked with a teenager who cried while twisting and contorting her body, symptoms that other doctors had attributed to a tantrum or other autistic behaviors. Dr. Bauman sent the girl to a gastroenterologist, who discovered that the girl had ulcers in her esophagus and had actually been writhing in pain.[13] In another example, a child who bangs his head or swats at his ears may be trying to tell you that he has an ear infection, and he may be trying to tell you that he is overly sensitive to a certain sound. If sudden episodes of self-injurious behaviors occur, they could be an indication of subclinical seizures (smaller seizures that are not typically detected by parents because they look like stimming or self-injurious behavior).

According to the social theory of self-injurious behavior, children with

ASDs may engage in self-injurious behaviors for the same reasons that a typical child or a child with an ASD throws tantrums. Like tantrums, self-injurious behaviors may be a cry for attention or a ploy to avoid a demanding task or an uncomfortable situation. For example, a child who doesn't want to go to sleep may bang his head against the headboard of his bed.

Dr. Lorna Wing states that self-injurious behavior is most often seen in children who have little or no communication skills. She suggests doing a functional analysis of children to determine why they may be engaging in self-injurious behavior. This involves observing when these behaviors occur and what happens right before and after each episode. The goal is to identify the function of the self-injury so parents can anticipate situations that may trigger these behaviors and teach their children more appropriate behaviors.[14]

Techniques for treating, reducing, and eliminating self-injurious behaviors are discussed in Part III: Coping.

My daughter becomes overexcited if there is too much to look at, but she loves staring at lights. Why?

Children with ASDs have different responses to visual stimuli. Some children are fascinated by visual stimuli such as bright lights, while others are distressed by them. Children may also be fascinated by an object while it's moving, but lose interest when it stops moving. For example, Jake used to like to watch the automatic doors of the supermarket slide back and forth, but when people stopped coming through and the doors were static, he'd lose interest and stop looking. Yet in situations where he could control the visual stimuli, there often would be no stopping point. As I mentioned before, Jake could turn the light switch in our foyer on and off for hours, staring fixedly at the light fixture that hung above his head.

One theory suggests that children identify people and objects by their overall shapes rather than by the details of their appearances. While people typically use their central vision for identifying details, it's possible that children with ASDs instead favor the peripheral part of the retina that focuses on shape and movement. This may explain why some children with ASDs are so comfortable moving about in the dark or running aimlessly without looking where they're going. It turns out that the motion-sensing part of the eye is engaged mostly when we're in near-darkness, when we can't make out details. Like Jake, many children I work with demonstrate a preference for peripheral vision—you can observe it through their stimming behaviors. They will peer out of the corners of their eyes while moving their heads back and forth, as if watching a tennis match in slow motion. One adult with an ASD reported that he felt more comfortable looking at people and objects from the side rather than straight on.

Many of the visual problems seen in children with ASDs fade as they get older or can be reduced or eliminated through sensory integration therapy or through behavioral treatments that focus on decreasing or eliminating stimming behaviors.

Why does my son constantly seem aloof? Most of the time, he acts as if I'm not even there.

As discussed earlier, one of the criteria for ASDs is impairment of social interaction. Dr. Lorna Wing describes four main types of children with ASDs who display symptoms of social impairment:[15]

– *The aloof group* is the most common type. These children act as if you're not even there, don't come when you call them, and don't reveal any emotional expression on their faces unless they are experiencing extreme rage or joy. Jake, like many children with ASDs, would have been considered part of the aloof group. He would lie on his belly on the floor and stare at what seemed to be nothing at all. It was as if he had checked out and unplugged himself from present reality—unaware of anything that was going on around him and unresponsive to any sort of interaction. Children in the aloof group generally make little eye contact and show little interest in others, except to use them to get what they want. One little boy with an ASD will grab his mother's hand if he can't reach his favorite green yo-yo, and as soon as she hands it to him, his focus is completely on the yo-yo. Even if his mother is sitting right next to him, it's as if she's invisible. Children in this group seem to have no empathy for others; if someone around them is sad or upset, they will remain emotionally neutral, as if nothing out of the ordinary is happening. They show little interest in other children as well. Before their children are diagnosed, some parents may be mistakenly told by teachers or day care workers that their socially impaired children are simply shy.

– *The passive group* is the least common type of social impairment. Children in this group seem more open to being approached socially and may establish some eye contact, but they don't initiate social interaction. They are good at being told what to do and, therefore, can engage in activities when led by others.

– The "active but odd" group was first described in 1979 (since then, Dr. Wing has tried to come up with a name that sounds better). This group tends to be more assertive in social situations—sometimes to the point of being aggressive. You saw this in the case study of Michael, the boy with Asperger's, who became aggressive in the swimming pool and almost drowned another child. His mother explained that his intention was to hug the other child, but his hug was inappropriately tight. Children in this group will also initiate verbal interactions, but often their interactions involve a one-way dissertation on their favorite topic with no concern for the other person's interests. Again, Michael would often alienate other children by lecturing to them in a pedantic tone about monarch butterflies.

– The over-formal, stilted group isn't generally noticed until children reach late adolescence or adulthood. Individuals in this group are unusually and inappropriately polite, formal, and extremely rule-driven. They interpret the world in black and white, not acknowledging gray areas. Even though these behaviors usually emerge when the child is older, early signs of these behaviors may be seen in younger children. Social skills behavioral therapist Terese Dana relates stories of young children who cannot relax the rules at school. One boy who went on an apple-picking field trip was told by the teacher that every child needed to hold hands with his buddy. The other typical children intuitively knew that once they reached the apple orchard they could stop holding hands. The boy with an ASD insisted upon tightly holding onto his buddy's hand even when the other child tried to wrestle free from his grip. It wasn't until his buddy began to cry that the teacher realized there was a problem; the boy with an ASD promptly released his hand when the teacher told him that the new rule was for everyone to let go of their partners' hands.

My son doesn't speak properly and has trouble communicating in general. Why?

Most children with ASDs have delayed speech or an abnormal development of speech. All children with ASDs have some problems with communication. Communication implies more than simply speaking. Their language (grammar, vocabulary, and understanding of words) may or may not be impaired, but the way they use their language may be problematic. For example, children with Asperger's may talk a lot, but in a monotone or robotic voice, lacking any affect ("I have a brand new toy" may sound the same as "My dog died"). They may fixate on specific subjects. Some children seem to speak in entirely different voices. In an interview in *Newsweek* (2005), Ami J. Klin, Ph.D., at the Yale Child Study Center, shared a story of a child who spoke in Shakespearean English, "almost as if I had plucked him from 14th century Verona."[16]

Some children with ASDs have echolalia, which, as the name implies, is like echoing. These children repeat words, phrases, and/or songs that may mean little to them. Some of them will echo words the moment they hear them, whereas those who have delayed echolalia will repeat things they've heard in the past, such as lines from a favorite video. Some children with echolalia have an uncanny way of mimicking people's or video/TV characters' voices with the same intonation and accent. When a mother asks her child, "Do you want a cookie?" instead of hearing, "Yes" or, "I want a cookie," she may hear her own voice and words echoed back to her in her child's response. A child may respond with the exact same phrase or drop the first word and simply say, "You want a cookie?" when he wants a cookie. Children with ASDs often confuse pronouns, reversing *you* and *I,* or leave them out all together, saying, "Want cookie."

Kanner wrote about echolalia in a paper in 1943. He was working with a two-year-old boy who began chanting "Peter eater" repeatedly whenever he saw something that resembled a saucepan. It turned out that his mother had been singing "Peter, Peter, pumpkin eater" to him in the kitchen one day when she accidentally dropped a saucepan. For some reason, her son picked up on this phrase and would not let it go.[17]

Some children with ASDs who do not speak can learn to speak, but usually much later than their typically developing peers. Others who do not speak at all can learn to use alternate forms of communication such as Picture Exchange Communication Systems (PECS) or other forms of augmentative communication, which are described in Appendix C. Children who do learn to speak may experience difficulties along the way. Children with ASDs usually begin by learning how to label people and things in their environment, often first learning how to name "Mommy" and "Daddy," and items that they want, like "juice" or "toy." But confusion can set in when identifying items in the same category. For example, sometimes children will consistently mislabel, saying "sock" instead of "shoe" or "milk" instead of "juice." Other times children end up merging words together that they've heard. When I was trying to teach Jake to label, I pointed to the sky one day and said, "Mama sees plane!" In the following months, Jake identified planes as "mama-manes." I kept trying to say the word "plane" with an emphasis on the "peh" sound. Jake would stare intently at my mouth, then say, "mama-mane!" I felt as if I were teaching him a foreign language. Sometimes, when children with ASDs begin to speak, their expressive language is limited and may sound stilted. For example, when Jake first started speaking, he sounded as if he were reciting lines from a script. But after a while, as his spontaneous language emerged, so did proper voice inflections.

Children with ASDs may also have issues with receptive language, which relates to their abilities to understand. It can be confusing for parents to figure out exactly what their children with ASDs actually understand, especially if their children can't offer verbal responses, don't look up when their own names are called, or seem to ignore simple commands. But not responding isn't the same as not understanding. And while we can't crawl into our children's heads to figure out the difference, research has shown that most children with ASDs have some level of understanding. Children may understand the names of familiar people or objects, or comprehend simple instructions, but not appear to understand. It has been shown that their responses can be taught to them so that they demonstrate behaviors indicative of understanding. For example, Jake was taught through behavioral intervention how to respond to "Go get your cup." Initially, he had to be manually prompted. His behavioral therapist told him, "Go get your cup," as she brought Jake over to the cup and put it in his hand. "That's getting your cup!" she'd say, encouraging his efforts. Jake also learned how to recognize familiar objects and people by being shown pictures of his favorite toys and his family members.

Our son takes everything so literally. The other day when his sister mentioned it was "raining cats and dogs," he hid under the sofa for the rest of the afternoon. We couldn't get him to understand that it was only an expression.

Literal interpretation is common to children with ASDs and is associated with a child's receptive language or how a child understands what is being said.

Idioms, or phrases such as "put all your eggs in one basket," "at this point in time," "a breath of fresh air," "a head start," and "back out" are easy for typical people to understand but nearly impossible for many people with ASDs to grasp. This is because such expressions are open to interpretation and require comprehensive, imaginative strategies that may not be available to people with ASDs. This could explain why some people with ASDs take everything so literally. This explanation ties into Baron-Cohen's theory of mindblindness: Since people with ASDs cannot mind read, they are incapable of interpretation.

One of the mothers I contacted told me about her daughter Anna, who was diagnosed with autism twenty-five years ago. After years of intensive treatment, Anna, who is now thirty years old, went to college and is an MIT graduate. Both Anna and her mother are extremely proud of her accomplishments, but one thing still puzzles them: Despite her high level of intelligence, Anna continues to take things quite literally. She does not understand expressions such as "I almost died laughing" and has trouble interpreting e-mails at work that include phrases like "change for the better" and "bottom line." Her mother recalls Anna's frustration as a little girl when she read nursery rhymes to her. "How can the cup run away with the spoon?" she'd ask, practically in tears. To this day, Anna does not understand all idioms, but she has been taught enough to be able to get by in the world. Through treatment, many children with ASDs can be taught to understand idioms.

My daughter doesn't point or use any gestures, and she's still not speaking, and it takes me a while to figure out what she wants. She also doesn't seem to understand when I use gestures with her, like when I use my hand to motion for her to come to me. Why is this?

Most children with ASDs do not use or understand gestures the same way as typically developing children. They may have difficulty using and understanding other nonverbal communication as well, such as facial expressions or body movements that may or may not accompany speech. They may not understand what it means when you shrug your shoulders to indicate that you don't know something or when you roll your eyes to indicate you are annoyed. They may not be able to use simple gestures themselves, such as waving good-bye when someone leaves or pointing with their index fingers when they want something. Jake used to shake his whole hand in the direction of a box of crackers or a toy that was out of reach, rather than use his index finger. Most typically developing children use gestures to indicate what they want even before their language emerges or while it's in the initial stages of development, such as tugging on a mother's hand and leading her into the kitchen to express hunger.

When looking back at early home videos—especially of birthday parties since those are the childhood events that most parents videotape—many parents notice that their children with ASDs did not use gestures. In 1994, researchers Julie Osterling and Geraldine Dawson reviewed videotapes of the first birthday parties of eleven children diagnosed with ASDs and eleven typically developing children. In addition to finding that children with ASDs made little eye contact, didn't respond to their names, and didn't show objects to others (joint attention), they also found that, at the age of one, children with ASDs did less gesturing—specifically, they didn't use their fingers to point out people or objects of interest as their typical peers did.[18] In a follow-up experiment, they found that infants who had both ASDs and mental retardation used gestures less often than typically developing infants.[19]

Based on this research, it would seem that from a very early age, children with ASDs are unable to access a whole realm of communication that most of us seem to use naturally. This may lead us to another question: If children with ASDs don't naturally gesture, do they understand the gestures of others?

In an interesting experiment done by Tony Attwood as part of his Ph.D. thesis, he found that there are certain gestures that children with ASDs are capable of understanding. These gestures are known as instrumental gestures because they have a purpose. Children with ASDs were shown illustrated images of a man with his index finger over his lips (with the caption "quiet"), a man pointing and looking up to the sky as a boy beside him looks up as well (with the caption "look up"), as well as others. He found that children with ASDs could respond appropriately and spontaneously to these gestures, but took them at face value as an instruction or command, without searching for any meaning behind the gestures. Thus a gesture that indicates "Go away!" or "Leave the room!" would simply prompt a child with an ASD to leave, without questioning an underlying motive or meaning.[20]

In her book *Autism: Explaining the Enigma*, Uta Frith describes Attwood's experiment and its implications. She identifies the concept of "bare communication" in children with ASDs. Bare communication, which is different from ordinary communication, can also be interpreted as "just the facts." In ordinary communication, we look for the message behind the message. For example, if someone both gestures and says, "Leave the room!" we determine in a split second what the person really means. By looking beyond the words and simple gestures and by focusing on subtle cues, such as the speaker's tone of voice and overall body language, we can tell whether the person is angry with us and really wants us to leave or is upset and in need of a friend, and therefore really doesn't want us to leave. But children with ASDs tend to not go that extra step to find meaning that is evident in ordinary communication.[21]

Attwood also looked at expressive gestures in children. Expressive gestures show our feelings or emotional reactions; we put our arms around people to show we like them, hug people to show we love them, or put our hands in front of our faces to show embarrassment. In his research, Attwood found that no child with an ASD demonstrated such gestures.

This research is not meant to imply that children with ASDs can't be taught how to understand gestures and body language and use them appropriately. Rather, many children with ASDs can learn these skills. Jake's behavioral therapists took photographs of me as I gestured with my hands to indicate "hello," "stop," "look," and other common nonverbal cues. The therapists also took photos of me with different facial expressions that indicated different emotions (happy, sad, surprised, angry, and hurt) and taught him how to identify them. Later, Jake learned how to generalize these skills and interact with people in the outside world. He also learned how to gesture to get what he wanted. After learning how to point, Jake was taught how to tap someone on the shoulder to get their attention, how to hug, and other nonverbal gestures. (One of his favorites, which he learned from me, was to put an index finger in the air to indicate "One minute, please.") At first, Jake's gestures were deliberate and rigid, but eventually they became more natural and a part of his everyday communication repertoire.

I was told by the doctor who diagnosed our son that he lacks both "imaginative and purposeful play." What does this mean?

Typical children engage in pretend play. For example, they may use their imaginations to create fortresses out of cardboard boxes or zoom around the house wearing a towel as a cape pretending to be their favorite superhero. Children with ASDs don't do this. Generally, if you watch them play, it's not really playing at all. Children will push a train back and forth rather than push it around the track—or, if they do push it around the track, it becomes a perseverative behavior that they repeat in the same sequence and in the same way. Parents may report that their children with ASDs run around the playground like other typical children; but upon closer examination, it's observed that the children are running aimlessly, without a purpose. Purposeful play is a playful activity with a goal, such as running a race, or chasing another child in a game of tag.

There are other ways that children with ASDs may appear to be engaged in creative play. They may act out one of their favorite TV characters, mimicking their voices and body language. But often they are simply copying the character without being inventive. Some children with ASDs will appear to be interested in fantasy cartoons or movies; yet it's the stimulating music or flashing lights that is capturing their attention. Their lack of imagination may be due in part to their literalness; even a sentence from a nursery rhyme such as "the cow jumped over the moon" requires that we think out of the box and engage our imagination.

Can purposeful play and imaginative skills be taught? Some children with ASDs can learn how to engage in purposeful and pretend play. Some treatments will set up scenarios where a child can learn the steps involved in play sequence to promote purposeful play. For example, a child may be taught to pick up the toy train, put the train on the tracks, push the train around the tracks, stop at the station to pick up the passengers, and so on. Children can also be taught pretend play; a child can be taught how to pretend to be a scary monster or an airplane through imitation. Ultimately, the goal of these treatments is for children to generalize these skills into spontaneous play activities with other children.

My daughter is growing increasingly uncoordinated. At four, she still has trouble climbing up the steps to the slide and looks awkward when she runs. Why is this?

Problems with motor development are commonly seen in children with ASDs. Our motor system is what allows us to respond to external information—whether it's using our legs to run toward or away from something or our mouths to communicate with others.

Hans Asperger noted motor clumsiness in his patients. He observed that many of them had poor handwriting or could not play ball. In the DSM-IV-TR, "clumsy movement" is mentioned as a common feature of Asperger's.

But motor difficulties affect children all across the autism spectrum. Children with low muscle tone may have trouble walking because their muscles can't support their bodies properly. Children with poor motor-planning skills (which involve planning, sequencing, and implementing motor tasks) may have difficulty navigating a flight of stairs because they can't figure out which foot goes first or how to stay balanced. As a result of poor motor planning, young children may have difficulty eating and playing games, while older children may have difficulty greeting people or maintaining a two-way conversation.

After their children have been assessed, parents will usually hear the terms *fine, gross,* and *oral motor skills* when the diagnostician is describing developmental issues. Fine motor skills involve smaller movements, such as writing, drawing, and buttoning a coat. Gross motor skills are movements that require larger muscle groups, such as walking, jumping, and running. Oral motor skills include movements of the mouth, lips, tongue, and jaw, which are used in sucking and chewing.

Parents generally observe that their children display a lack of coordination around the ages of two or three; their children may have awkward gaits or have difficulty holding a crayon. But scientists are discovering that these signs of deficient motor development may be occurring even earlier. Dr. Phillip Teitelbaum, an expert on human movement patterns at the University of Florida, obtained and studied home videos of the first three to six months of life of children who were eventually diagnosed with ASDs. He found that children with ASDs displayed unusual ways to accomplish developmental milestones such as rolling over, sitting up, crawling, and walking. In every child he studied, he saw at least one movement disturbance by the age of six months. For example, many babies had difficulty crawling; they would struggle to pull themselves along, balance on their elbows while lifting their rumps, or leave one arm under their torso while trying to crawl using only the other arm.[22] Franklin and I later recognized this trend in Jake, which we had thought was adorable at the time. At the age of eight months, Jake crawled like a wounded soldier, using his arms to drag himself across the floor. It was only after his diagnosis that we learned that his crawling was an early sign of an ASD.

Why are motor skills affected by ASDs? Teitelbaum points to skewed brain wiring. Parts of the brain that control movements are not connected correctly. Teitelbaum also relates early movement abnormalities to infants who later exhibit difficulties in verbal and social skills. He believes that early movement variations are the result of the same wiring problem in the central nervous system that is responsible for later developmental issues with verbal and social skills.

Dr. Stanley Greenspan, clinical professor of psychiatry, behavioral sciences, and pediatrics at George Washington University Medical School and a practicing child psychiatrist who has also researched infant development, notes that children with ASDs may have motor-planning problems that affect the way they communicate and form relationships with their caretakers. Dr. Ralph Maurer, associate professor of psychiatry at the University of Florida at Gainsville and a director of the Autism National Committee, states, "Autism is a disorder of relationship, and movement is important in relationship. If you watch people with autism in interactions, you will see asynchronies and asymmetries. If a dance is fundamental to relationship, there is something fundamentally wrong with the ability of people with autism to engage in it. . . . Autistic children from an early age fail this dance of relationship. . . ."[23]

Even if children with ASDs "fail this dance" at an early age, it doesn't mean that they will always fail. There are "Fred Astaire" teachers among treatment experts who can help your child. Treatments for motor coordination are discussed in Part II: Treatments.

I thought children with ASDs had unique talents like playing the piano brilliantly at age two or painting masterpieces by age five. My son has been diagnosed with an ASD, and he can barely hold a pencil. Why isn't he gifted in some way?

In the past, individuals with profoundly low IQs who possessed extraordinary talent in a certain area such as math or music were called by the unfortunate term *idiot savant*. Now that it has been linked to ASDs, such a person is known as an *autistic savant*. While the majority of autistic savants have low IQs, there are some autistic savants who are highly intelligent.

Dustin Hoffman's portrayal of an autistic savant in the movie *Rain Man* introduced the notion of autism and savantism to the general public. His character Raymond could memorize phone books and trump the house in Las Vegas. Many people who saw this movie assumed that all people with ASDs are savants. They aren't. As a matter of fact, only 10 percent of people with ASDs have savant abilities (the prevalence in the general non-ASD population is less than 1 percent). Savant syndrome occurs four to six times more frequently in males than females.

There are many forms of savant abilities. The most common type of savant skills are *splinter skills*, as demonstrated by an obsessive hobbyist or compulsive researcher who commits to memory an enormous amount of facts related to his pet subject, such as dates or sports statistics. Dr. Darold Treffert, an expert on savantism, wrote about a boy who had memorized the timetables for the Milwaukee bus system. When given only the route number, the boy could recite the location of a bus at any time of day.[24]

Talented skills are more specialized and proactive skills, such as art or music. There is a dramatic case study of a girl named Nadia who, between the ages of four and seven, produced detailed drawings that resembled cave paintings from 30,000 years ago. (Interestingly, Nadia lost her artistic abilities once she began to speak, which has also been seen in other savants when they make developmental progress that requires other areas of the brain).[25]

Prodigious skills are the rarest form of savantism—as demonstrated, for example, by an individual who can play an entire piano sonata after having heard it only once.

Dr. Beate Hermelin writes in *Bright Splinters of the Mind: A Personal Story of Research with Autistic Savants* that calendar calculations are "probably the most frequently observed ability in savants." These begin with a fascination with dates such as birthdays and holidays.[26] In a lecture by Dr. Fred Volkmar at the Yale Club in New York City (April 2005) that I attended, he noted that one child he works with can actually answer questions like, "What day of the week is May 5, 2040?" or any other random date, in a matter of seconds.

In general, savant skills include extraordinary abilities in mathematics, art, music, language, or memory.

4

AUTISM SPECTRUM DISORDERS—THE FACTS, THEORIES, STUDIES, AND INFORMATION YOU SHOULD KNOW

What caused my child's ASD?

As soon as our children are diagnosed, many of us wonder exactly why they have ASDs in the first place. While extensive research is being done to answer this question, there is still no conclusive evidence that points to a single cause of ASDs.

There are major areas of study that you should know about, and you'll learn about them soon. But before you read this section, I want to issue you a word of caution: Please don't make the mistake of getting so caught up with what caused your child's ASD that you miss out on getting immediate treatment for your child. As much as you may want to find the reason why your child has an ASD, it's important that you attend to what's really important right now. "As soon as children are recognized as having any autism spectrum disorder, they should receive intensive intervention," says Catherine Lord, director of the University of Michigan Autism and Communication Disorders Center and an internationally recognized expert in the field of autism. While it's fine to learn some of the basics about potential causes now, you can always research them in more detail later. You will also be able show your support by being involved with autism organizations and universities that are at the forefront of ASDs research (which you can look up in Appendix D). But now is the time to get your child treatment.

Here are some potential causes of ASDs that are being researched: brain, genetic, environmental, immune system, immunization, and pregnancy components.

THE BRAIN COMPONENT: Research shows that there is a disruption of circuitry in the brains of children with ASDs. Some parts are over-connected; some are under-connected. Studies on brain circuitry have found that people with ASDs process information in different parts of their brains from those in typical people. For example, they recall letters of the alphabet in the part of the brain that normally processes shapes.

There are early developmental cues that point to brain abnormalities: smaller head size at birth followed by a period of excessive head growth between six months and two years of age, where chronic inflammation occurs in the areas of excessive growth. The frontal lobes, where nerve cells are responsible for higher order processing like decision-making and social reasoning, undergo the greatest increase even though they are normally the last brain region to develop. Children with ASDs may have problems in these cognitive areas because even though their frontal lobes are enlarged, their nerve cells are actually much smaller than normal.

The Underconnectivity Theory may help explain why some people with ASDs have typical or even superior skills in some areas, while lacking skills in other areas. Dr. Marcel Just, director of Carnegie Mellon's Center for Cognitive Brain Imaging, uses a sports analogy to explain this concept: In the brain of a typical person, the team members work together to coordinate their efforts, whereas in the brain of someone with an ASD, they don't. This may account for difficulties in complex thinking, social skills, and overall behavior.[1]

The typical brain engages in "spring cleaning." It clears out biological debris so that new connections can form. "Little twigs fall off to leave the really strong branches," explains Catherine Lord. But this doesn't happen in children with ASDs.

Research continues in the area of brain development and ASDs. Other studies are being conducted to determine what gives white matter in the brain of children with ASDs its odd architecture, what genes are involved in innate immunity, and the intricacies of prenatal brain wiring.

THE GENETIC COMPONENT: Researchers have identified a number of genes that may play a role in the onset of ASDs. "There might be six or more genes that have to come together in one individual in the right form to lead to autism," says Dr. Gerard Schellenberg, CHDD (Center on Human Development and Disability) research affiliate, in a study at the University of Washington.[2] Some of these genes may be responsible for inherited traits called endophenotypes, that don't cause ASDs but are associated with them. These traits can be behavioral or biological, and are being identified in family members of children with ASDs. Some of these traits include large head size, abnormal brain processing of faces, and the existence of mindblindness. A study by Daniel Geschwind and colleagues of the UCLA School of Medicine found that using the Social Responsiveness Scale (SRS), which measures the severity of a child's symptoms and social impairments, may help to detect the genetic loci for social impairment caused by ASDs.[3]

Researchers have identified only one specific genetic connection with ASDs—fragile X syndrome, which is also the most common cause of genetically inherited mental retardation. According to the National Fragile X Foundation, between 2 and 6 percent of all children diagnosed with ASDs have a fragile X gene mutation, and approximately one-third of all children with fragile X have an ASD. If a child with an ASD also has fragile X, there is a one-in-two chance that boys born to the same parents will have the syndrome.[4]

Studies of identical twins support the genetic theory. The research of Dr. Edwin Cook of the University of Chicago shows that if one identical twin has an ASD, there is a 90 percent chance that the other will have an ASD as well. Among fraternal twins or siblings, there is only a 3 percent chance.[5]

According to information at the Yale Child Study Center, research has shown that if you have given birth to a child with an ASD, there is a one-in-twenty chance of giving birth to another child with an ASD. This number may even be underestimated because many parents stop having children after having one child with an ASD.[6] Many parents of children with ASDs report that there is a family history of ASDs or related disorders such as depression, obsessive-compulsive disorder, and/or schizophrenia. Other parents report cases of an odd uncle or antisocial grandmother. Because ASDs were defined differently years ago, it's possible that there were family members who had an ASD or autistic tendencies but were either misdiagnosed or never diagnosed at all.

THE ENVIRONMENTAL COMPONENT: Some parents report that their children appeared typical up until a certain age, at which time they developed an ASD. It's possible that these children were born with a genetic predisposition to

ASDs, whose onset was triggered by an environmental factor. Scientists have not yet identified what the trigger may be, but some parents and researchers suggest factors such as viral infections; exposure to environmental chemicals, such as lead and mercury; metabolic imbalances; or childhood immunizations. Recent studies look at the relationship between environmental toxins, such as PCBs (polycholorinated biphenyls), and language development. "There certainly isn't a shortage of environmental suspects that may play a role in autism," says Andy Shih, chief science officer of the National Alliance for Autism Research (NAAR) in Princeton, New Jersey.[7]

THE IMMUNE SYSTEM COMPONENT: Even though ASDs are considered to be brain disorders, there is some evidence that they may also be disorders of the immune system. Studies at the UC Davis Center for Children's Environmental Health and UC Davis M.I.N.D. Institute compared immune cell responses in typical children and children with ASDs, and found a difference in the immune systems' responses to bacteria. It seems that children with ASDs have lower levels of cytokines, which are protein molecules that help mediate the body's immune response and influence both behavior and mood. Further research is being conducted.[8]

THE IMMUNIZATION COMPONENT: There is speculation that immunizations may contribute to the onset of ASDs. Some parents report that they did not notice signs of an ASD in their children until after they were vaccinated. The vaccines in question are the MMR vaccine and vaccines that contain thimerosol, a mercury preservative found in immunizations for hepatitis, whooping cough, tetanus, and diphtheria. In the April 2005 issue of *Molecular Psychiatry,* neuropharmacologist Richard Deth of Northeastern University in Boston and his colleagues described a biochemical pathway by which thimerosal and other compounds may cause neurodevelopmental disorders such as ASDs. To date, no scientific study has discovered beyond a doubt that a link exists between immunization and ASDs, but parent groups and researchers are pursuing this possibility.

THE PREGNANCY COMPONENT: Some research speculates that pregnant women who were given the labor-inducing drug pitocin or who have yeast infections, poor diet, or hormonal or immune system changes during pregnancy have a higher propensity for giving birth to children with ASDs. Dr. Andrew

Zimmerman, pediatric neurologist, believes that environmental influences in utero, such as hormones triggered by a mother's stress, may contribute to ASDs by disrupting normal early development.[9] In the January 1, 2003 *Journal of Neuroscience*, scientists led by Paul H. Patterson of the California Institute of Technology in Pasadena reported that when pregnant mice were infected with a modified human-flu virus, their babies, when grown, exhibited similar behaviors to children with ASDs. Upon further research, Patterson found that the altered brain development in mice wasn't the direct result of the viral infection in the fetus, but in fact was related to the natural immune response in the mother. If the mother couldn't fight off the virus, there was a chance it could cross over into the placenta and affect brain development in the fetus. This finding would indicate that other infections besides the flu virus could lead to the same effect.[10]

The myth of the refrigerator mother: debunking the theory that ASDs are caused by mothers.

While different theories about the cause(s) of ASDs are being proposed, one thing is clear: ASDs are not the mother's fault. Not so long ago, in the 1960s, the once esteemed child psychologist Bruno Bettelheim blamed autism on bad parenting—specifically on the part of mothers, who presumably spent more time with children than fathers did. He claimed that these mothers were responsible for their children's disorders because they did not bond properly with the children, due to a particular personality trait that caused them to be narcissistic, cold, and uncaring. Bettelheim called these women *refrigerator mothers.*

Thankfully, Bettelheim's theory was disproved. In *Infantile Autism: The Syndrome and Its Implications for a Neural Theory of Behavior,* Dr. Bernard Rimland revolutionized the world of ASDs by defining them as biological disorders, not as emotional illnesses.[11] By so doing, he paved the way for the more enlightened perspective we have on ASDs today.

Why do so many more boys than girls have ASDs?

The overall ratio of boys with ASDs to girls with ASDs is 4:1.

Dr. Lorna Wing has found that among people with Asperger's and high-functioning autistic disorder, the ratio of boys to girls is 15:1. But Dr. Wing notes that this number may not be accurate because there is speculation that many girls with Asperger's, especially those with high verbal skills, may not receive a proper diagnosis.

In any case, it is certainly clear that there is a much higher incidence of boys with ASDs than girls with ASDs. Researchers are trying to figure out the reason for the disproportion.

In 1964, Bernard Rimland conducted studies that showed boys tend to be more vulnerable to hereditary diseases and infections than girls, demonstrating that boys are more susceptible to organic damage than girls. In 2000, Dr. David Skuse of the Institute of Child Health in the United Kingdom concluded that the gene or genes for ASDs are located on the X chromosome. Since boys only inherit one X chromosome from their mother and girls inherit two X chromosomes, one from each parent, the hypothesis is that girls carry an imprinted gene from their fathers that may protect them from ASDs and, therefore, make them less likely than boys to have the disorder.[12] A team of geneticists at UCLA have located the probable region of an autism gene on chromosome 17, which they discovered contributes to autism only in boys. This may be the reason why girls have a lower incidence of ASDs than boys.[13] Further research in this area is being conducted.

A more recent theory of gender differences was proposed by Simon Baron-Cohen, who found and labeled essential differences between gender types; he labeled females as "Type E" for empathy and males as "Type S" for systemization. According to Baron-Cohen's research, females are more genetically predisposed to have highly developed people skills that enable them to be more effective communicators—or "little empathizers." Males are more genetically predisposed to have higher visual-spatial abilities that enable them to become "little engineers" who are interested in details and the mechanics of the way things work. Baron-Cohen surmises that ASDs represent the extreme effect of this form of male behavior—that is, males with ASDs have very poor social skills and psychological tunnel vision. This exaggeration of typical gender differences and the male-brain theory could explain why there are so many boys with ASDs, and why some of their major characteristics include a lack of social skills and a propensity toward rigid behavior such as lining up toys, following strict routines and rituals, and focusing on minute details.[14] These behaviors, however, when combined with a higher IQ, can be useful in areas such as engineering and science, which require heightened attention to detail.

Research into why more boys than girls are diagnosed with ASDs continues, but until science identifies beyond a doubt what causes ASDs, the disproportion of diagnoses between the genders is one of the disorder's many mysteries waiting to be solved.

Why are so many more children diagnosed with ASDs today?

If you're reading this book, you are probably the parent or loved one of a child with an ASD or you know someone with an ASD. There are an estimated 48 million people worldwide who have ASDs.

Decades ago, ASDs were considered rare disorders. Hardly anyone even knew what they were. Only 1 in 10,000 children were diagnosed. Now, the statistics are staggering. According to the CDC, ASDs strike 1 out of 166 children, and more than 425,000 children in the United States have an ASD. Today, thanks to extensive research and media exposure, almost everyone has heard of this once hidden disorder.

There have been news reports of an epidemic of autism. Autism is the fastest-growing serious developmental disability in the United States. It is five times more common than Down syndrome, three times more common than juvenile diabetes, and more common than multiple sclerosis, cystic fibrosis, and childhood cancer. ASDs are not only confined to the United States; there are reports of increased rates of diagnoses on a worldwide basis.

According to Autism Speaks, the fund-raising drive of an organization called the Autism Coalition

- there are 1.77 million cases of autism in the United States;

- every twenty minutes, a new case of autism is diagnosed; and

- there are 24,000 new cases of autism in the United States per year.

When did we first notice an increase in cases of ASDs in the United States? In the 1990s, concerned citizens in Brick Township, New Jersey, notified the CDC that there were an extraordinary number of reported cases of autism in their schools. No one knew why. At the same time, epidemiologists at the CDC were receiving calls about an increase of cases in Atlanta. Then, in 1999, the California Department of Developmental Services reported a 273 percent increase in the number of children in California being treated for autism between 1987 and 1998. In 2002, the U.S. Department of Education reported that nationwide autism rates had increased 556 percent in one decade. Researchers found that what was being reported in California appeared to be a "phenomenon throughout the industrialized world."[15]

Marshalyn Yeargin-Allsopp, an epidemiologist at the CDC, recalls training to become a developmental pediatrician in the 1970s and being told that autism was very rare.

So why the sudden increase?

No one knows for sure.

The most widely held theory about the increased number of cases of autism spectrum disorders points to both an improved definition of the disorder and the ability of doctors to make more complete assessments. The ultimate authority on psychiatric conditions, the DSM-IV-TR, has been revised to include ASDs (referred to as PDD in the manual) as disorders that encompass many different diagnoses but eliminate mental retardation and learning disabilities. According to this theory, more children are diagnosed because of a heightened awareness of symptoms and a broader definition of ASDs. But does an increase in diagnoses reflect an actual increase in the number of people who have the disorder? Some experts would argue that there are other factors responsible for the escalating cases of ASDs, such as prenatal or environmental causes or childhood immunizations.

What is the economic impact of the rise in cases of ASDs?

Autism has been called the fastest growing developmental disorder, and its impact is reflected in the amount of money that is spent in the United States on research, treatment, and education. According to the ASA, the annual cost of ASDs is $90 billion. Ninety percent of those costs currently occur in adult services. Through early diagnosis and early intervention, the cost of lifelong care can be reduced by two-thirds. Yet, it is estimated that the annual cost of ASDs in ten years will be $200 to $400 billion.[16]

Is there a cure for ASDs?

There is no cure for ASDs. In fact, even using the word *cure* with regard to ASDs can be tricky simply because *cure* is usually used in reference to diseases, not disorders. Having said that and knowing that *cure* may not be the most politically correct term to use, it is nonetheless the term that most parents and practitioners use. Researchers are working hard to locate the causes of ASDs that will pave the way for a cure to the disorder.

Gary Goldstein, M.D., child neurologist and president of Baltimore's Kennedy Krieger Institute says, "I think you can compare it to the progress that's been made in cancer research and treatment. At one point there was no cure for cancer. Now, there are subtypes of cancer that are curable and some that, so far, are not. We will most likely find subtypes of autism that will respond to treatment, and others that will take longer. The brain is so mysterious, and the [disorder] is so baffling. It will be a slow process. But will we get there? Absolutely."[17]

While there is no single cure for ASDs at the present time, we do know one thing for sure—children with ASDs can benefit greatly from intensive early intervention. As a result of early treatment, a child's symptoms of ASDs may lessen or disappear. Children who aren't responsive may learn to look at you when you call their names. Children who don't like to be touched may learn to give or receive hugs. Children who don't speak may learn to how to have a conversation, ask for cookie, or say one precious word—"Mommy."

The world of ASDs is one that is filled with hope and people just like you— you are not alone on the journey to help your child. You have a major part to play in helping your children get treatment and reach their fullest potential.

PART II:
TREATMENT

It takes a whole village to raise a child.

—AFRICAN PROVERB

Never doubt that a small group of thoughtful citizens can change the world. Indeed, it is the only thing that ever has.

—MARGARET MEAD

The best place to find a helping hand is at the end of your own arm.

—UNKNOWN

Choosing a treatment for our son, Jake, was like going to a restaurant with too many choices on the menu. Instead of choosing from among a reasonable selection of pasta and chicken dishes, we found ourselves having to choose from among an overwhelming number of treatments with unfamiliar names like ABA and Floortime and side dishes like speech therapy and occupational therapy.

When Jake was diagnosed, there were (and still are) so many treatments for ASDs offered by so many specialists, and there wasn't (and still isn't) any consensus on which treatment is best. Authorities touted the virtues of their own therapies while rejecting many others. Treatments for ASDs ranged from traditional, such as speech, physical, and behavioral therapy, to all sorts of alternatives, such as riding horses, hormone therapy, and swimming with dolphins. Which one to choose? We were afraid to make the wrong decision, so we wanted to take the time to make the right one. But all the professionals agreed that we had to decide sooner rather than later. Early intervention was crucial; the younger Jake was when he started, the better the odds were for any kind of success. The clock was ticking, and time spent researching meant precious time lost from treatment. But deciding in favor of one treatment meant deciding against some of the others, ones that might potentially be better for Jake. We had never faced a more pressing deadline.

I spent weeks researching, reading, talking to professionals and other parents of children with ASDs, and agonizing over a final decision. When I felt we had looked absolutely everywhere for answers, we made our decision. We would use ABA as the foundation for Jake's therapy. ABA had been highly recommended by both doctors who had diagnosed Jake, and scientific studies confirmed its effectiveness.

Yet, when I spoke with other parents, their responses were not at all what I expected. . . .

"It's like training a dog," one mother told me.

"A robotic way of teaching," another said.

"Cruel and unusual punishment," a father declared.

"Torture for a two-year-old," a special education teacher said.

In the phone calls that followed, I got mixed feedback. People either swore by ABA or swore at it. It was clearly a treatment method that evoked a great deal of passion either way.

But the research told a different story. ABA was scientifically proven to be a successful treatment method for many children with ASDs. There was more research to support ABA than any other treatment. So why did ABA get such a bad rap? Well, some of those parents were right—ABA was pretty intense. Research showed that you were supposed to do between 25 and 40 hours of one-on-one treatment a week. How would Jake manage that? He was only two years old. But the studies said that all of the intense practice and learning was what made it so effective, especially at such a young age as two when the brain could make new connections.

And why were people comparing ABA with training pets? Because kids were rewarded with treats, toys, or hugs during their sessions when they performed skills, such as waving, clapping, making eye contact, or demonstrated other behaviors. I guess you could say it was similar to rewarding a dog when you're teaching him to sit on command. But it was also similar to what I'd experienced in the corporate world. When employees did a good job, they were rewarded for their accomplishments with a salary increase or promotion. However, while you might punish a dog or fire an employee for bad behavior, during an ABA session, you simply withheld the rewards and continued teaching the child until he learned. So, after doing all of the research, ABA made sense to me intellectually. But emotionally, I still wasn't so sure—until one night when I made one of my many phone calls to parents. . . .

"Mitchell was diagnosed at the same age as your son," one mother said. She had done extensive research on treatments for autism before choosing ABA.

With the phone receiver pressed to my ear, I heard a little voice in the background.

"Mommy, can I go out and play now . . . pleeeeaze?"

"Wait a minute sweetie. I'm almost done," the mother said.

"Now! You promised!"

I smiled. "Who was that? Your older son?" I asked.

"No, that was Mitchell."

I cried. Hearing that little boy's voice erased any doubts about our decision to choose ABA. I wanted more than anything to hear my own son speak—and if ABA was a way to get him there, to get him just to say "Mommy," then we had to try it. This mother went on to refute the negative claims made by other parents. Her son's ABA therapists were gentle and loving, and while the 2-hour sessions were highly structured, they were also filled with hugs and fun play breaks.

With ABA, I learned that we couldn't just get our feet wet. We'd have to take the plunge. "It's a huge commitment," one of the ABA therapists explained to Franklin and me. "It's not just about his therapy sessions. You'll have to adjust your entire lifestyle to accommodate your son."

And so we did. We made a total commitment to ABA. Franklin and I were coached by our ABA team to conduct ABA sessions with our son. Our babysitter was trained as well. We converted the downstairs of our house into Jake's therapy room. We bought all of the supplies, furniture, and special toys, food treats, and other rewards (known as reinforcers) that the therapists told us to buy. I put my management consulting business on hold. Managing my son's therapy became my full-time job. "Autism doesn't take a break," we were told, and neither could we.

When Jake was two years old, an age at which most typical children take naps and play in the park, he was in 40 hours of ABA therapy per week. It was as if our little boy had a full-time job. During his ABA sessions, Jake would sit in a little chair across from his ABA therapist, who had a box of assorted food treats and toys beside her on a table.

"Jake!" his ABA therapist would say encouragingly, holding up an M&M candy a few inches from her face to get his attention.

Jake remained seated in his chair across from her, gazing at his feet.

"Jake!" she'd repeat, drawing an invisible line between her eyes and his.

No response.

"Jake!" she'd say again, this time gently using her hands as blinders around his face to try to shift his gaze to her.

Jake looked up at her.

"Good boy! That's looking at me!" she'd say happily, as she put the M&M in his mouth.

And then it all started again. "Jake!" I'd hear her repeat for a total of thirty times, before taking a play break to do a puzzle or run around the room. Then it was time to learn another skill, such as pointing to objects, matching items, or responding to simple instructions. "Jake!" was repeated in every ABA session of the day, every day of the week, until Jake learned to respond to his name. ABA seemed to be taking the expression "practice makes perfect" to the extreme. But our hope was that the constant repetition would somehow rewire Jake's brain.

While ABA therapy took up the majority of Jake's time, he also had two weekly 30-minute sessions of speech therapy to help him speak and occupational therapy to help his coordination so that he could jump and climb like other kids. In addition, he had biweekly visits to a cranial-sacral osteopath in Manhattan; he'd lie on a table while the doctor subtly manipulated his body to improve his central nervous system functioning. While most children his age ate chicken nuggets and grilled cheese sandwiches, Jake was on a special diet that eliminated gluten, wheat, and dairy. While other kids took their fruit-flavored Flintstone vitamins, Jake took a B_6 magnesium mixture that looked and tasted like stale mustard. Then there were all the homeopathic remedies in little brown bottles with unusual names I couldn't pronounce that we lined up like little soldiers every morning so Jake could gag them down.

I tried to remain optimistic about Jake's future, but his progress in therapy was excruciatingly slow. The ABA therapists remained positive. The speech therapist did not.

"Your son will probably never speak," she told me.

Jake proved her wrong. After thousands of hours of treatment over the course of a year, Jake began to slowly recreate sounds, the same sounds that had come so easily to him as a baby. He was three years old. Isolated sounds became words that *ultimately led to sentences that, although initially somewhat rote-like (having been learned and memorized in ABA sessions), became more naturalistic and gave Jake a way to communicate in the world.*

Then one day near his fourth birthday, as if by magic, Jake developed what the experts called spontaneous language. It was the end of his second year of intensive therapy, and I had taken him to the playground. Using his limited vocabulary, Jake tried to socialize with a group of boys. He chased after them around the swings and the slide, but he couldn't keep up. He could run fast enough, but the boys were talking too fast. The boys ignored Jake and took off, leaving him standing by himself in the middle of the playground. My heart sank. I didn't know what to do, so I resorted to what I thought any typical mother would do in this situation: I took Jake out for ice cream. The man behind the counter at the ice cream parlor waited patiently as I perused the flavors. Then he asked for our order. Just as I was about to answer, a little voice spoke.

"Nilla."

Jake said "Nilla." My son spoke his first word that had not been rehearsed hundreds of times in an ABA session. He had understood the man's question and answered him. All by himself. The ice cream man handed Jake a cup of vanilla ice cream, unaware that this moment marked the day that Jake turned a corner. . . .

HOW TO MAKE THE RIGHT TREATMENT AND INTERVENTION DECISIONS FOR YOUR CHILD

Today, thanks to extensive research and advances in the field of ASDs, there are many effective treatments available. (In the past, there were few effective treatment options, and as a result, many children were institutionalized). Parents now have a full menu of treatment options from which to choose. While this is wonderful news, sometimes it can seem like there are too many options, especially to parents who are trying to find just the right treatments for their newly diagnosed children.

In your search for treatments, you will hear many varying, even conflicting, opinions from parents and professionals. As you already know from reading this book, some people will wholeheartedly endorse certain treatments, while others will reject those very same treatments. There are treatments that are considered to be more conventional, such as speech therapy and occupational therapy, and others that are considered to be alternative or nonestablished, such as homeopathy and accupuncture. The more parents and practitioners you talk to, the more opinions you will get about which treatments to choose. Initially, it can be a confusing process, but it will become less confusing as you become more familiar with the treatments and know what questions to ask.

To avoid overwhelming you with a lot of different jargon in this chapter, I'm using the terms *treatment* and *intervention* interchangeably, to indicate a specific treatment tool, treatment methodology, approach, or intervention designed to help a child with an ASD. Because there is an overload of information on all of the different treatments for ASDs, this chapter will focus on some of the more widely accepted treatments.

HOW EARLY TO BEGIN TREATMENT

There are two key words that you need to know when it comes to getting your child treatment: early intervention.

Early intervention means that you must step in and begin treatment for your child as soon as possible after he or she is diagnosed with an ASD: The earlier the better. Why so early? Studies show that a child's neural plasticity—or the brain's ability to be shaped—is at its maximum when the child is very young. Have you ever wondered how it's possible for some typical children to learn a foreign language at such a young age? It's because their brains are especially receptive to taking in new information and can form new connections. In essence, a brain can be rewired.

The importance of intensive early intervention for children with ASDs cannot be overstated. Studies show that intensive early intervention can improve the overall prognosis for children with ASDs. According to the American Academy of Pediatrics, "early diagnosis resulting in early, appropriate, and consistent intervention has also been shown to be associated with improved long-term outcomes."[1]

How early should you begin an intervention program with your child? Treatment can begin as early as twelve or fourteen months of age, but in most cases, treatment begins later. Dr. Sally Ozonoff, associate professor of psychiatry at the University of California Davis M.I.N.D. Institute states, "It's been shown pretty clearly that starting an intervention at age 3 is better than 5, or starting intervention at 2 or potentially even earlier than that is better."[2] Yet even with the emphasis on the importance of early intervention, many children with ASDs still aren't getting treated until well after their third birthdays. "Diagnosing an infant with autism at 6 months or a year—maybe even one day in the delivery room—could mean the difference between baby steps and giant leaps," writes health correspondent Claudia Kalb in the February 28, 2005 *Newsweek* cover story, "When Does Autism Start?"

Dr. Rebecca Landa, director of the Center for Autism and Related Disorders (CARD) at the Kennedy Krieger Institute in Baltimore, is running an NIH-funded study to determine if early intervention before the age of three can improve the course of a child's social and cognitive development. Dr. Landa's research reveals that there are subtle signs of ASDs before the age of fourteen months. She has identified certain "sensitive periods" of an infant's life when he becomes hyper-focused on understanding parts of his environment. For example, from birth to twelve weeks of age, typically developing babies focus on trying to read faces, and between six and twelve months of age, they focus on trying to understand sounds that lead to language and speech perception. Her theory is that if you provide early intervention to children during these sensitive periods, there is the possibility that brain signals can be rerouted.[3] The study's initial results revealed that children with ASDs at six months of age were similar in development to typically developing children, but by fourteen months, there was a clear discrepancy in three three-fourths of the children—particularly in the area of language. These results may point to the effectiveness of starting treatment as early as (or earlier than) fourteen months of age.[4]

There is other exciting research underway that may help to detect and treat ASDs even before age one. The National Alliance for Autism Research (NAAR) and the NIH have launched a project called the High Risk Baby Sibling Autism Research Project. Known as the Baby Sibs project, researchers at various prestigious universities and medical centers are studying the visual, verbal, and social skills of infant siblings of children with ASDs to see if they can develop early detection of ASDs before age one. Baby siblings of children with ASDs are chosen for this research because they represent a high-risk population—they are more likely to be genetically predisposed to an ASD (there is a 2 to 8 percent chance that a sibling will have an ASD if there is already another child in the family with an ASD). "If we had a way of screening for autism at birth and then could begin very early to retrain the brain, that would really be the ticket," said Dr. Thomas Insel, head of the National Institute of Mental Health, in *Newsweek*.[5]

Intensive early intervention maximizes a child's rate of learning and can help minimize or eliminate problem behaviors such as stimming or self-injurious behaviors. It is crucial to helping children with ASDs gain strength in cognitive and communication, play, and overall developmental skills. Research shows that possibly half of all children with ASDs can recover enough to develop friendships, be mainstreamed in school, have jobs, and lead productive lives if they partake in early intensive intervention. Even those children who don't reach this level of success can do much better than they would without treatment.[6]

WHAT "INTENSIVE" INTERVENTION MEANS

What constitutes an *intensive* early intervention program? Intensive usually means giving a child between 25 to 40 hours of treatment services per week. This may sound like an extraordinary number of hours, especially if you have an infant or a toddler. But in fact, research suggests that it's the intensity (as well as the timing of early intervention) that has a great effect on a child's development. Intensive treatment is much more helpful than a slow and steady approach spread out over time.

According to the NRC, "Services should include a minimum of 25 hours per week, 12 months a year in which the child is engaged in systematically planned, and developmentally appropriate educational activity toward identified objectives. What constitutes these hours, however, will vary according to a child's chronological age, developmental level, specific strengths and weaknesses, and family needs. Each child must receive sufficient individualized attention on a daily basis so that adequate implementation of objectives can be carried out effectively. The priorities of focus include functional spontaneous communication, social instruction delivered throughout the day in various settings, cognitive development and play skills, and proactive approaches to behavior problems. To the extent that it leads to the acquisition of children's educational goals, young children with an autism spectrum disorder should receive specialized instruction in a setting in which ongoing interactions occur with typically developing children."[7]

What does this 25-hour-per-week recommendation mean? The amount of hours per week refers to comprehensive programs that provide a foundation for your child's intervention program, including treatments such as ABA or TEACCH (to be described in the next few pages), which are supplemented with services such as speech therapy and/or occupational therapy. Twenty-five hours of treatment services may be conducted at home, in a school setting, or both, depending on your child's age and needs. But just because a specific treatment is well established doesn't mean that it requires 25 hours per week. For example, speech therapy and occupational therapy are usually incorporated into a comprehensive program or given in addition to a comprehensive program, meaning that a child may receive 5 hours per week of speech therapy as part of a 25-hour-per-week school-based program or may receive 3 hours of occupational therapy per week in addition to 25 hours per week of ABA.

Keep in mind, however, that 25 hours of treatment per week does not mean trying 1 hour of a certain kind of therapy, 1 hour of a different kind of therapy, and continuing on up to 25 different treatments. A hodgepodge of too many different treatments has been shown to be ineffective when treating children with ASDs. Your child's time is precious, especially in the early years. Neurologists refer to this time as the window of opportunity during which your child can make significant changes in learning and behavior. You want to be sure every moment your child spends in treatment is a good investment. The treatment process can be extremely time-consuming and costly—and there's no money back guarantee or any way to turn back the clock and make up for time lost on ineffective treatments. But don't fret. You *can* make the right decisions about treatments for your child by beginning your search in an intelligent and thoughtful manner.

WHAT YOU NEED TO KNOW BEFORE BEGINNING YOUR SEARCH FOR TREATMENTS

Many parents find themselves in highly emotional states as a result of their children's diagnoses (I certainly did), which can make them want to postpone the search for treatments or cloud their abilities to make a decision. If you are having trouble coping emotionally, there are many options available to help you through this often stressful and difficult time. Talk to friends, seek out professional help, or consult with professionals on ASDs or autism organizations for advice (see Appendices D and E for a list of national and international organizations and Appendix F for resources where you can access information about local support groups). You'll also find good coping tips in Part III: Coping.

Speaking with other parents of children with ASDs who've experienced what you're going through can be extremely helpful; they can be both empathetic when sharing their own personal experiences and rational when getting you in the right mindset to find treatments. One mother suggested that instead of thinking of myself as "Jake's Mom" during my research, I should think of myself as a researcher for another child. This helped me become less emotional and more objective in making an intelligent decision for our son. Choose whatever method helps you focus and motivates you. Just don't delay in getting your child treatment.

The best way to begin the process of deciding what treatment is right for your child is to consider the treatment recommendations made by the doctor or professional who diagnosed and evaluated your child. Recommendations usually include more than one treatment based on your child's needs, but because intensive treatment is recommended, usually one treatment is used as the foundation, and others are added on. For example, the foundation of Jake's treatment at age two was 40 hours per week of one-on-one ABA therapy in a home-program. In addition, he had two 30-minute sessions of speech therapy and two 30-minute sessions of occupational therapy per week. Another child with an ASD attended a school for autism that used the TEACCH method (Treatment and Education of Autistic and Related Communication Handicapped Children) as the foundation of his treatment program, which is a highly structured and organized teaching method. This was supplemented with three 30-minute sessions of physical therapy and three 30-minute sessions of occupational therapy per week.

Your child's treatment services should be personalized to meet your child's specific needs. Treatments can take place at home, at a clinic, in a specialized school for ASD or for special needs children, or in a general education school (either in a special needs classroom or in a mainstream classroom). The optimal setting for your child's treatment depends on age, needs, skills, and abilities. Most very young children (under age three) begin treatment at home. In this case, treatment providers come to your home on a regularly scheduled basis to hold treatment sessions with your child and offer you tips on how to help your child. When these children reach preschool age, many of them attend schools, but some continue to have supplemental home programs as well.

KNOWING WHAT TO ASK IN YOUR SEARCH FOR TREATMENTS

The first step in finding the right treatment for your child is to know which questions to ask. Here are some good basic questions that can serve as your guidelines.

What Is This Treatment and What Does It Do?

Ask what the treatment is and what it does and have it explained to you in plain, simple language that you can understand. Don't feel intimidated by complicated scientific jargon; if you don't understand, ask questions. It's crucial that you have a good understanding of the treatment and how it works—after all, it pertains to your child's well-being. Find out the history, philosophy, and goal(s) of the treatment. Who developed this treatment, and what qualifies this person as an expert? Ask yourself, "Does this treatment make sense to me? Is its philosophy in line with my own values? Do the treatment goals relate to the goals I have set for my child?"

Ask the treatment provider if you can observe a treatment session. Be wary if the provider tells you that you can't observe a session because your child needs to "experience it himself." Ask to speak with other parents who have used this treatment. Providers can usually give out contact names. Find out who will be administering the treatment to your child. Will he or she be a trained professional? The provider doesn't have to be an M.D. but must have qualifications that go beyond taking a few weekend courses in the treatment modality.

Ask what the likelihood is that this treatment will actually help your child and how that likelihood is determined. The provider can tell you about the treatment results in other cases similar to your child's. Find out if there are (or have been) any negative side effects to the treatment or any potential negative effects.

Also, find out how many children with ASDs have been through this treatment, and ask about the results. What is the success rate? Look at different measures for success. Did children using this treatment end up being mainstreamed (attending general education schools)? Did this method teach children to accomplish the skills that you seek for your child, such as speaking, interacting, or playing? What are the short- and long-term effects? Be wary if you are told that the treatment has only been used on a few children or is in the pilot study phase, which is often the case with new treatments.

Treatment methods are supposed to be standardized, meaning that no matter which school, clinic, or home-based program you use, you should find the same methodologies interpreted and delivered in the same way. Therefore, standardized treatments should *always* follow the same original training protocols no matter where they are being replicated. But the reality is that there are some variations among the training protocols of different treatment sites, depending on how a school or provider interprets the treatment and on the qualifications of the provider. Slight variations are okay, but beware of providers who say that they are using a reputable methodology such as ABA or TEACCH but interpreting them in a whole new way. For example, an ABA program should include direct observation and measurement of specific target behaviors, which includes data-collecting. Be cautious of schools or providers that don't collect data for their ABA programs. A TEACCH program should be highly structured; beware of a school or classroom teacher who takes a more relaxed approach to TEACCH.

Even though treatments are supposed to be personalized to meet your child's specific needs, there should be standards that are followed when implementing programs. You'll find some good, basic information in this book about most of the treatments for ASDs so you'll be prepared when you pursue them.

Ultimately, when choosing a treatment, in addition to doing the research, make sure to use your common sense and trust your intuition.

What Is the Intensity of the Treatment?

The intensity of the treatment can depend on the philosophy of the treatment itself and/or your child's needs. In the case of ABA, studies show that the treatment's effectiveness depends in large part on its intensity; in most cases, between 25 and 40 hours per week of one-to-one ABA treatment is recommended. Most ABA sessions are 1.5 to 2 hours long; a child may have several ABA sessions in a day that amount to a total of 6 to 8 hours. But this is not the case with other treatments such as speech and occupational therapy. Typical speech and occupational therapy sessions are 30, 45, or 60 minutes long. The frequency and intensity of speech and occupational therapy sessions depend upon the specific needs of the child. For example, some children require five 45-minute sessions of speech therapy per week, while others require only two 45-minute sessions per week. Some children need one-on-one treatment, which means that a teacher or therapist works with your child individually. Other children need group therapy in which the teacher/student ratio is usually 1:3.

There are some alternative treatment programs that are only given for a set number of hours over a set number of weeks, conducted as intensives. This may mean that you have to pull your child out of school or regularly scheduled treatment sessions. Be careful that this kind of commitment won't have an adverse effect on your child's current treatment plan or prove to be counterproductive, either by conflicting philosophically with your child's current program or by causing undue stress on your child who is used to regular routines. Also, keep in mind that, although intensity is most easily quantified as time, a lot of time with a poor provider is not as good as a shorter amount of time with an excellent provider. Other standards of measurement come into play as well, such as the nature of the program, how well it is structured, the amount of exposure to peers, and so on.

Is There Real Science to Support This Treatment?

Real science refers to controlled studies done by scientists on children with ASDs that involve experiments with direct objective observation and rigorous methods by which research is produced. A key component of a study's authenticity is that it is performed by outside, independent investigators. There are treatments that claim to be scientific and look impressive to the layperson, but they are actually considered either pseudoscientific or antiscientific. Such treatments may involve technical jargon that's even endorsed by a doctor when in fact either little or no real objective scientific evidence exists to support them. For example, in some cases, experiments have only been conducted in the promoter's own in-house studies, making them biased and subjective. In other cases, the research sounds scientific when in fact it's only based on testimonials, anecdotes, and/or personal stories from parents or professionals.

This is not to say you should never try a treatment that does not have concrete scientific basis. We ventured outside of the scientific box with Jake and tried some alternative and nonstandard treatments for ASDs, but the foundation of Jake's treatment was ABA, which has its foundation in sound science. Just because a treatment hasn't been proven scientifically doesn't mean that it isn't good, but science can provide that extra dose of confidence when choosing a treatment for your child.

Will This Treatment Complement the Rest of My Child's Treatments?

When choosing different treatments for your child, make sure all of the treatment providers are on the same page. When Franklin and I decided to choose ABA as the foundation for Jake's treatment, we also spoke with potential speech and occupational therapists and told them of our decision. The first occupational therapist we spoke with was completely on board with the principles of ABA—in fact, she abided by many of the behavioral tenets, including rewarding Jake's behaviors with lots of positive reinforcement in her sessions.

But the first three speech therapists we spoke with refused to work with Jake because they did not believe in ABA (the biggest complaints were that the ABA sessions were too long and that ABA taught robotic language—complaints that were unfounded and proved to be no problem for Jake). The speech therapist who was ultimately assigned to us by our early intervention agency (the one who told us he would never speak) told us that she supported ABA, when in reality she didn't. She provided very little positive reinforcement and had a negative attitude in general. The speech therapist who ultimately worked with Jake advocated and incorporated ABA principles in her sessions.

It's important to find out upfront whether or not the providers working with your child follow the same basic philosophies of treating ASDs. If they are conflicting, your child will become confused, and the treatments will be ineffective or counterproductive. In fact, they may even cancel each other out. For example, while one of your treatment providers may be trying to reduce or eliminate your child's hand flapping and other stimming behaviors, another provider may be accepting of these behaviors.

Make sure to discuss treatment philosophies in the beginning of setting up your child's treatment program. This will help you avoid any potential conflicts in the future.

How Am I Involved in Supporting My Child's Treatment?

Make sure the treatment can offer ways for you to help your child. Be cautious of any treatments in which there aren't ways to support your child outside of the session. Find out what you, your child's siblings, other family members, and babysitters can do at home to help reinforce the new skills and behaviors that your child is learning. Often, these suggestions can be great ways to bond with your child and aid in the overall treatment progress. For example, to help Jake develop his upper body strength, his occupational therapist taught us to pick up his legs while his hands were on the floor and run around the house with him as if in a wheelbarrow race. We also had that special plastic brush that we used on his arms and legs to help him overcome his hypersensitivity to touch. Jake liked to be brushed and eventually began to brush us, too. The speech therapist cut out pictures of dinosaur feet and placed them all over the floor, so we could play a game when Jake was having trouble with making the "K" sound; we'd stomp around the room holding Jake's hand making "keh, keh, keh" dinosaur sounds. The ABA therapists worked with us to improve

Jake's imagination skills; for example, we'd zoom Jake around the house, pretending to be airplanes, and we'd make faces, pretending to be scary monsters.

Parents can be instrumental in helping their children generalize skills that are taught in the treatment sessions to other settings—around the house, at school, or in the community. According to "Educating Children with Autism (2001)," the NRC emphasizes the role of families in helping their children with ASDs, and recognizes that families can be involved on multiple levels. "Parents can learn to successfully apply skills to changing their children's behavior. Parents' use of effective teaching methods, support from within the family and the community, and access to balanced information about autism spectrum disorders and the range of appropriate services can contribute to successful child and family functioning. It is crucially important to make information available to parents to ensure their active role in advocacy for their children's education."[8]

How Will My Child's Progress Be Measured?

Ask about the evaluation process. How often will your child be assessed and by whom? You do not have to wait for an official assessment to find out how your child is doing. Often parents call weekly, bimonthly, or monthly team meetings, where all of the treatment providers join together to give feedback, brainstorm, and discuss the child's progress. You should also be able to set up private meetings or phone conferences with your child's treatment providers.

Sometimes, over the course of treatment, your child's progress will be obvious to you: Your child can now form words, no longer throws tantrums, or has stopped engaging in self-injurious head banging. At other times, progress will be more subtle: Your child is just beginning to make sounds or has fewer and shorter outbursts. In all cases, your child's progress should be continually monitored, measured, and updated so that the treatment continues to meet your child's specific needs. For example, ABA therapy maintains comprehensive graphs and charts detailing your child's progress, and team meetings are held to troubleshoot problem areas and keep the programs moving forward. Speech therapy and occupational therapy provide standardized evaluations that target specific components of your child's skills and abilities, including an array of areas such as receptive and expressive language (speech) and fine and gross motor skills (occupational). Beware of treatments that don't offer ways to measure their effectiveness. Even if there is no standardized testing for a particular treatment, the treatment should have measurement criteria. For example, social skills therapists write up reports on a child's skills based on experiential and observational analysis. They include specific goals and objectives as well as games and exercises to promote learning.

Overall, having an independent assessment (carried out by someone who doesn't have a vested interest in the results) with standard measures of areas such as language, cognitive ability, and adaptive skills is the most helpful. This can be conducted by a psychologist, speech pathologist, or another professional in the field of ASDs. The advantage to having this kind of assessment is that you can see if gains reflected at home or in the classroom, such as learning to point and label objects or initiate a conversation, have generalized to other settings.

What Is the Cost of the Treatment?

The financial cost of treatments for ASDs is a hot topic. As you may already know, costs can be exorbitant. Which is why, in your search for treatments, you need to find out which ones are covered by your health insurance company and which are covered by your state agency or school district. In chapter 7, I'll give you tips on how to exercise your legal rights to get treatments at no cost to you through your early intervention program or school district. In chapter 8, you will learn other ways to relieve financial stress, including ways to work effectively with your health insurance company for coverage and reimbursement, steps on how to get Medicaid and other services, and tips from other families on ways to handle finances.

If you do make the choice to pay out-of-pocket for treatments (in the case of most alternative treatments, it's a forced choice), be careful. Many desperate parents who have made initial snap decisions to take on the costs of their children's treatments privately have regretted it later. It's not easy to see in the beginning just how much treatment costs can add up over time. Treatment sessions are usually billed on an hourly basis and range from $40 to $150 per hour. Intensive six- or eight-week programs may require extensive travel, a full- or half-time daily commitment, and cost thousands of dollars. Home programs and special schools for autism can cost between $25,000 and $80,000 per year. In your search for treatments and treatment providers, be aware of large upfront costs or large discrepancies in fees for the same services.

There are other costs that should be considered as well—such as your time and emotional energy. Look for treatments that reasonably suit your lifestyle. If you are just starting the process, it may be difficult to anticipate what will work.

There are certain basic considerations to keep in mind. Home-based programs require a parent or caretaker to be at home. Center-based programs, such as special schools or clinics for ASDs, are possible alternatives to home-based programs. If you have other children, you need to consider the feasibility of transporting your child with an ASD to different treatment offices or clinics for services. How will you deal with the emotional cost of all these changes in your life? Adjusting to driving your child to speech and physical therapy rather than to the things you had imagined, such as toddler music class or a play date in the park, can take an emotional toll. Just know that the beginning is the most difficult part and have faith that daily routines will come more easily to you and your family over time. Ask any parent who's been there. I will discuss the emotional costs of the treatment process in more detail in Part III: Coping.

All the costs—financial, lifestyle, and emotional—will need to be considered when choosing a treatment.

WHAT TO ASK IF YOU'RE CONSIDERING A SPECIAL SCHOOL OR CENTER-BASED PROGRAM

If you are thinking of enrolling your child in a special school or center-based program for ASDs, make sure to evaluate the environment, staff credentials, scheduling, and philosophy or mission of the programs. How long has the school been in existence? What is the school's philosophy? Has it changed over the years? Is it consistent with your values? Has the school or program been consistent in its use and application of certain treatment interventions? Watch out for schools that change their treatments based on the latest trends.

Walk through the school setting and imagine seeing it through your child's eyes. Is it free of distractions that may trigger an outburst from your child? The environment should be positive, highly supportive, and conducive to meeting your child's specific needs. Will your child receive one-on-one treatment, group treatment, or a combination of both? How is progress measured and how often? Be sure there are standard assessments in place to measure your child's progress on a regular basis. What is the class size? You'll want a small class with a teacher/student ratio of no more than 1:3 so that your child can receive as much individual attention as possible. What is the makeup of the class? Is it a general special needs class that's made up of children with various disorders, or is it exclusively a class for children on the autism spectrum? If it is a general special needs class, make sure the teacher has experience and training in working with children with ASDs. If the school is exclusively for children on the autism spectrum, find out (or see for yourself) if the children's profiles seem similar to your child's. Does the setting have peers that could be good role models?

Make sure the staff has real expertise in working with children with ASDs. There are usually certified teachers and teaching assistants on staff. Does the school offer on-site ancillary services such as speech and language therapy, physical therapy, and occupational therapy? The availability of these on-site services can result in great savings of your time and/or transportation expenses.

Look at how the school day is organized. Is there a well-organized structure? How are activities planned? The teaching environment should be highly structured and include generalization strategies previously mentioned so that your child can transfer what he learns inside the classroom to outside of the classroom—generalizing skills (such as imitating or following instructions) at home and out in the community. Ask how many hours of programming your child will receive weekly. Your child should receive a total of 15 to 40 hours per week (parents who receive only 15 hours per week of school or center-based programming usually supplement them with an additional 10 or more hours of home-based programming). The curriculum should emphasize teaching communication and social skills such as language, attending, imitation, play, and social interaction. The overall goal should be to teach your child to develop independence skills.

Is there an opportunity for your child to engage in physical activities at the school, such as gym class or sports? Physical activity has been shown to have positive effects on children with ASDs, in terms of elevating moods and reducing anxiety and stimming behaviors. Participating in sports can provide your child with a great opportunity to develop and practice social skills.

As you walk through the school, look at the other children. Do they seem happy? Are they working productively? Look at the staff. Do they seem happy? If you observe disruptive behavior, how does the staff handle it? Positive programs should be in place to reduce problem behaviors such as stimming and/or self-injurious behaviors. Find out if the school will provide you with recommendations for how to help your child at home and in the outside community. Some schools offer parent and sibling training sessions. Also, ask about extended year programs, since some programs follow the school year calendar and may not offer summer programs. If you are interested in having your child transition to a general education environment, find out if the special school or center has a transition program or a supported inclusion program (where a trained aide accompanies your child to a general education school).

When you have to decide which educational option is best for your child—a special school or center-based program (or general education setting, which will be discussed in chapter 8)—you won't have to make this decision by yourself. If your child has been recently evaluated, you can receive guidance from the professionals who assessed her or from your local early intervention agency or school district committee (more on this to come later in the text). If your child is currently in a home program, your treatment providers can help you choose the right educational setting for your child.

TREATMENTS AND SCHOOLS THAT SOUND TOO GOOD TO BE TRUE

Now that you're armed with all of the questions you need to ask about your child's treatments and schools, there are a few other things to consider. Parents who feel vulnerable after their child is diagnosed with an ASD often become targets for treatments that sound too good to be true. Rule of thumb: If a treatment or school sounds too good to be true, it probably is. When considering a treatment, ask yourself the following questions and pick up on the early warning signs.

WHAT'S IN A NAME? Just as fancy product names lure us to buy certain brands of laundry detergent or celebrities persuade us to try those miracle weight-loss diets, there are promoters who package treatments and schools for ASDs with impressive names and catchy slogans and make false claims of cures. Look out for self-involved promoters who claim to have all the answers and insist that you use their product exclusively. Also, look behind the labels on the products; a company that lists itself as nonprofit may appear to have philanthropic intentions when in fact its primary goal is to turn a profit. Find out where your money is going—into more research or into the promoter's bank account?

JUST BECAUSE IT'S IN WRITING OR ON TV, IS IT NECESSARILY TRUE? Just because information about a treatment or school is published doesn't mean it's reliable. These days, anything can get published, and you may find treatment literature that reads more like a glossy sales brochure for selling a car than a reliable scientific article. In the Internet age, people can write and publish whatever they want, and you'll find that so-called experts, professionals, or parents make definitive statements about treatments for ASDs that simply aren't true or reflect only one person's opinion.

Read with a critical eye. On the Internet, note who sponsors the site. The best sites include those that are sponsored by government agencies, medical schools, and public service agencies. Unless a treatment is reported in a reputable, scientific, peer-reviewed journal, it's not scientifically valid. If you're choosing alternative treatments, look to see if there are references or links to credible autism organizations, scientific books, or research. You must also watch news programs and TV specials with a critical eye, as each one will be written and produced from a specific point of view. Even though most news programs exercise journalistic integrity, they too can get caught up in the excitement of reporting and promoting the latest fad treatment for ASDs.

AM I TOO EAGER TO SIGN MY CHILD UP FOR HIT-OR-MISS AND FLAVOR-OF-THE-MONTH TREATMENTS? New treatments for ASDs turn up all the time, and it can be tempting to try each new treatment just to see if it's the one. When Jake was diagnosed, I remember wishing there were more hours in a day so that I could pile on more and more treatments, hoping for that magic formula that would make him speak and relate. During this time, the hormone secretin was touted in the press as the miracle cure for ASDs, and I attended seminars and read studies to see if it would help our son. In the end, we decided not to use it based on inconclusive studies and parent testimonials—but I must confess that it was still a difficult choice. My heart tried to convince my head that even if secretin worked for only one child, maybe that child would be mine. (The National Institute of Child Health and Human Development (NICHD) has since found no statistically significant improvement in children with ASDs who were given secretin.)

All of us have fantasies about that magic pill that will make our children better, but be careful that your decisions about your child's treatments are based on facts rather than emotions. Establish a foundation for your child's treatment, then add on a few other treatments that will enhance the foundation. But don't make the mistake of trying too many conflicting treatments that may cause undue stress on your child. And remember to be careful about constantly changing treatments because you don't see immediate results or out of a desire to keep up with the latest miracle cure.

6

STANDARD TREATMENTS AND INTERVENTIONS FOR ASDs

From my experience working as a consultant to families of newly diagnosed children on the autism spectrum, I've learned that even those parents who receive specific treatment recommendations from their doctors or other professionals still try to find out about each and every treatment that exists for ASDs. I know that's what I did. Therefore, to save you the trouble of wading through countless books and websites to find out what these treatments are, I've compiled a list of treatments with brief descriptions of each in Appendix C. (Keep in mind that this is a comprehensive list, not a recommended list, of treatments—simply to let you know what's available.)

There are also two newly founded organizations that will be offering treatment recommendations in the near future for parents and professionals: The Autism Treatment Network (ATN) and The Studies to Advance Autism Research and Treatment Network (STAART). ATN is a national nonprofit organization of hospitals and physicians from six leading medical centers that are working collaboratively to evaluate the medical conditions in children with ASDs and determine the best practices for their identification and treatment. STAART was formed as a result of the Autism Coordinating Committee under the NIH. The STAART Centers Program, established in response to the Children's Health Act of 2000, is made up of eight centers across the country, which will contribute by researching the causes, diagnoses, early detection, prevention, and treatment of ASDs.

The following treatments are among the more popular treatments for children with ASDs. I've chosen to list these specific treatments because most of them are more commonly granted by local early intervention agencies and school districts. Remember that I use the terms *treatment* and *intervention* interchangeably to describe the treatment, methodology, therapy, or service. Likewise, I use the terms *treatment provider, therapist,* and *teacher* interchangeably to describe the person conducting the treatment services. I've listed the treatments in alphabetical order.

APPLIED BEHAVIOR ANALYSIS (ABA)

ABA is a treatment methodology that was pioneered by Dr. Ivar Lovaas and is based on theories of operant conditioning by B. F. Skinner. In 1987, Lovaas published a study showing that almost half of the 19 preschoolers who underwent intensive behavioral intervention—40 hours per week of one-on-one therapy—achieved "normal functioning."[1] ABA is supported by more scientific research than any other treatment for ASDs. Hundreds of researchers have documented the effectiveness of ABA for building a wide range of important skills and reducing problem behavior in individuals with ASDs.[2] A report of the Surgeon General states that "thirty years of research demonstrated the efficacy of applied behavioral methods in reducing inappropriate behavior and in increasing communication, learning and appropriate social behavior."[3]

ABA uses different procedures to teach new skills to children. The best-known one, called Discrete Trial Training, breaks down tasks into small teachable steps that children can learn more easily. ABA uses a reward system to motivate and reinforce children while they are learning new skills and behaviors. For example, to teach a child to respond to his name, the therapist will say the child's name and wait a designated amount of time for the child to respond. If the child responds, the therapist rewards him with a special treat, such as a favorite food or toy. No punishment is used. (In the past, Lovaas did use mild aversives—but they haven't been used for years.) If the child does not demonstrate the correct behavior, the reward is simply withheld. The theory is that rewarded behavior will be repeated. When first learning a new behavior, a child is rewarded for just trying. In a Discrete Trial Training session, sets of repeated trials are given to a child. A trial is simply another word for a try or an opportunity—a child is given many opportunities during an ABA session to demonstrate the correct behavior. ABA regards repetition as critical for the brain to process new behaviors and skills.

Good ABA programs incorporate both therapist-directed and child-directed interventions. For example, if a child were learning his colors in a therapist-directed setting, the therapist would hold up a blue card and ask, "What color is this?" prompting the child to answer, "Blue." If a child were learning his colors in a child-directed sequence (also known as *incidental teaching procedure*), the therapist would put an array of M&Ms on the table, prompting the child to reach for one, whereupon the therapist would ask, "What color is it?" ABA strives to make learning fun and enjoyable for the child by offering lots of positive reinforcement and positive interactions.

In addition to teaching children basic skills, ABA also teaches play, social, communication, and relationship-building skills through peer modeling (incorporating other children in the session), activity schedules (visual sequences that teach everyday activities such as brushing teeth to more complex skills such as making friends), and inclusion support (an aide who accompanies the child) in the classroom. ABA can help a child decrease or eliminate stimming, self-injurious behaviors, and disruptive behaviors.

ABA can be taught in formal one-on-one treatment sessions at home or school and in a variety of other community settings, such as the playground or park. Parents are encouraged to be involved in their child's treatment so they can help to generalize their child's skills to the outside world. For example, if your child learns to wave good-bye in a treatment session, the goal of ABA is for your child to be able to transfer this behavior into a real-life setting, such as when you leave the house. This teaching and generalizing technique can be used for simple skills, such as clapping, or more complex skills, such as initiating and holding a two-way conversation.

ABA progress is frequently measured, recorded in written reports, and reviewed so that treatment can be updated and customized to meet a child's specific needs. ABA is the most studied psychosocial intervention for people with ASDs and is available at many locations in the United States and around the world. There are different models for implementing ABA. One well-known approach is the UCLA model developed by Lovaas and his colleagues. Eleven research sites, supported by the NIMH, and a private agency with twelve clinics around the United States (Lovaas Institute for Early Intervention) offer services based on the UCLA model.

FLOORTIME

Also known as the DIR (Developmental, Individual-Difference, Relationship Based) Floortime approach, Floortime was developed by child psychiatrist Dr. Stanley Greenspan. Floortime is an intensive one-on-one intervention that focuses on children's individual strengths and their relationships to others. It is based on the premise that individuals learn best when they are emotionally engaged. Rather than focusing solely on a child's symptoms, Floortime focuses on helping children learn the building blocks of relating, communicating, and thinking. It creates a circle of interaction between the child and parent, professional, or peer. Parents and professionals follow the child's lead to encourage maintaining attention, relatedness, and two-way communication. By capitalizing on children's interests and motivations, Floortime helps children master interpersonal, emotional, and intellectual skills.

In a Floortime session, the parent, therapist, or teacher often gets down on the floor to interact and play with the child. The Floortime experience is a spontaneous, unstructured time. During Floortime sessions, which are typically 20 to 30 minutes long, the parent or therapist strives to create "circles of communication" that engage the child and give him the opportunity to practice back and forth communication. For example, if a child is stacking red blocks, his mother may add a blue block to the tower, prompting the child to engage with her rather than remaining absorbed in a solitary activity. Back and forth play helps the child make the link between cause and effect and provides him with the opportunity to engage in a personal interaction. In this intervention, parents play a particularly active and critical role.

The DIR/Floortime approach recognizes that every child is unique and that no single approach will work for all children. Understanding where the child is developmentally, respecting a child's individual differences, and building relationships are the cornerstones of DIR/Floortime.

MEDICATIONS

While there is no medication to "cure" ASDs, there are a number of medications that can be prescribed to alleviate specific symptoms associated with them. Medication may be used to treat behavioral problems, attention disorders, anxiety, and depression. It can also help improve social and communication skills for individuals with ASDs. Research shows that medication can help reduce hyperactivity, impulsivity, aggression, and obsessive preoccupations. In addition to targeting symptoms that interfere with a child's ability to participate in educational, social, and family settings, medications can also help increase the benefits of other interventions.

Medications most frequently used for children with ASDs include selective serotonin reuptake inhibitors (SSRIs), neuroleptics, stimulants, mood stabilizers, and antipsychotics (particularly the newer atypical forms that have fewer side effects). Sedatives may be used in rare situations for occasional sleep problems. Because children with ASDs do not always respond to medications in the same way that typically developing children do, it is critical that parents consult with a physician who treats children with ASDs. Any treatment plan should be monitored regularly to assess a medication's effectiveness and toxicity.

Children with ASDs often present other medical conditions, and may be treated with multiple medications. As all medications have side effects and interact with other medications, the child's doctor(s) must be well informed about all treatments. Parents should keep written records of all the medications their children are taking, reactions to these medications, and objective data about symptoms (e.g., number of tantrums per day, sleep patterns, ability to focus, and self-injurious behaviors).

OCCUPATIONAL THERAPY (OT)

Occupational Therapy, or OT, does not have to do with job skills as its name may imply. Rather, OT is used to help children with ASDs achieve competence in all areas of their lives, including self-help, play, socialization, and communication.

OT provides support for children with ASDs who have difficulty with sensory, motor, neuromuscular, and/or visual skills. Through OT, children can learn skills such as how to balance their body weight, respond to touch, communicate with others, and accomplish daily tasks. OT can also help children to develop appropriate social, play, and learning skills.

OT sessions are usually held in a clinician's office or in a school setting with the aid of special equipment. Occupational therapists may use swings, trampolines, climbing walls, and slides to help a child with gross motor coordination and sensory issues. OT also addresses fine motor skills, such as writing and drawing. Depending on a child's needs, therapists may use a variety of treatments. Many OT techniques that are used in therapy sessions—such as brushing, wearing a weighted vest, deep pressure, and joint compressions—can be reinforced at home or in other settings. OT may also incorporate sensory integration techniques. Sensory Integration Therapy is described in more detail later in this chapter.

PIVOTAL RESPONSE TRAINING (PRT)

Pivotal Response Training (PRT) is gaining recognition as one of the newer treatments for children with ASDs. Drawing on more than twenty years of research experience, Doctors Robert and Lynn Koegel, cofounders of the Autism Research Center at the University of California, Santa Barbara, have expanded upon the principles of Applied Behavioral Analysis to develop a comprehensive approach to working with children with ASDs. In pivotal response training, specific behaviors, known as *pivotal behaviors,* are seen as central in affecting general areas of functioning. By changing these pivotal behaviors, it is believed that other associated behaviors will change without being specifically targeted.

Pivotal response techniques include positive reinforcement, changing and correcting behaviors, and child choice (where the child expresses a preference). Because children with ASDs have communication and behavioral challenges (they may be self-absorbed or have difficulty forming reciprocal relationships), PRT focuses on teaching children how to engage in effective social interactions. Learning how to ask questions and initiate social contact not only opens the door to relationships, but also can fundamentally change how others perceive children with ASDs.

PRT draws upon the natural motivations and individual interests of each child to make learning engaging and fun. This treatment provides guidelines to improve pivotal behaviors such as motivation and the ability to respond to multiple cues and stimuli. Emphasizing functional communication and skill development, PRT has been successful in helping children with ASDs expand their communication and language skills, reduce interfering and challenging behaviors, and improve their attention spans. In the classroom, PRT is a valuable teaching tool that helps broaden children's interests and improve their academic performance. Most significantly, PRT helps children learn the skills they need to enjoy positive social interactions and make friends.

Unlike more clinical treatments, PRT is designed to fit into a child's everyday life. It is an intervention that uses natural learning opportunities at home, in school, or in any inclusive setting. Because PRT encompasses a child's whole world, parent involvement is critical to its success. As partners in the process, parents learn PRT strategies and train teachers, family members, and others on how to use this approach.

PHYSICAL THERAPY

Physical therapy sessions are prescribed for children with ASDs to enhance their physical abilities. Impairments of movement can interfere with developmentally appropriate functioning. Some children with ASDs can have low muscle tone, as well as poor posture, balance, and coordination. Physical therapy sessions can treat these impairments by providing passive, active, resistive, or aerobic exercise as well as training in functional and developmental skills. Physical therapists implement procedures to increase endurance, motor control, and motor planning. They incorporate therapeutic exercises along with equipment such as weights, exercise balls, and BAPS boards (balance boards) to increase muscle strength and endurance and to facilitate body awareness and coordination. Aquatic, aerobic, and breathing exercises can also be part of your child's treatment. Physical therapy sessions are typically one-on-one and last 45 minutes. They can be administered in the therapist's office or in school by a trained physical therapist.

SENSORY INTEGRATION THERAPY

The goal of Sensory Integration Therapy is to help children better absorb and process sensory information. Sensory integration involves taking in information through the senses and organizing and integrating the information in the brain. Sensory integration therapy focuses on the basic senses: tactile (touch), auditory (hearing), vestibular (sense of movement), and proprioceptive (body position). A child can have a dysfunctional sensory system in which one or more senses is over-responsive or under-responsive to stimulation from the environment. For example, a child may overreact to certain sounds, textures, or visual stimuli or underreact to pain. Sensory dysfunction can affect a child's posture or coordination skills. Therapy for sensory integration dysfunction is usually done by an occupational, physical, or speech therapist who provides sensory and motor activities, often in the forms of games, exercises, and play. One popular form of sensory integration is auditory integration training (AIT), described in Appendix C.

SOCIAL SKILLS TRAINING

Social Skills Training is an umbrella term that can include social skills groups, one-on-one social skills therapy, peer modeling, and video modeling. The goal of Social Skills Training is to help children with ASDs make friends, establish relationships, and have appropriate social interactions. Social Skills Training sessions are usually run by a trained facilitator such as a psychologist, behavior therapist, speech therapist, play therapist, or special education teacher. Parents can even be taught to facilitate sessions with their children by playing fun games that promote social interactions.

Social Skills Training can take place in different venues such as in a treatment session, at school, or at home. In a treatment session, a child can learn and practice social and play skills with the facilitator before transferring these skills to outside social situations. Social Skills Training can also take place in at school during recess in the forms of games and exercises. Social Skills Training can be incorporated in the classroom by a child's classroom aide, who can facilitate social interactions by prompting the child to initiate conversations or join in a game with other children.

The social skills facilitator uses role-playing, discussions, games, and activities to develop social understanding, teamwork, empathy, and improved interpersonal relationships. One technique used to enhance social skills is called "Social Stories," developed by Carol Gray. Social Stories are short narratives that parents use to teach children how to respond appropriately in typical situations. For example, a story teaches children when to say "thank you," when to wash their hands, how to share toys, or how to follow mealtime or classroom routines. Social Stories are usually written in the first person by a therapist, teacher, or parent and can include pictures, photographs, or music. Video modeling works in much the same way as Social Stories to demonstrate appropriate social skills. Another social skills technique called peer modeling places children with ASDs in play situations with typical same-age children who model appropriate play behavior. A therapist facilitates the interaction. A therapist or an aide may also be used in the classroom to assist a child with peer interactions.

SPEECH AND LANGUAGE THERAPY

Speech and language therapy helps a child to communicate more effectively both verbally and nonverbally, using words and/or body language. The speech and language pathologist (SLP) provides appropriate interventions that help children form words or communication systems, process information, and express themselves. The SLP also teaches children the pragmatics of language (how to use language), such as how to initiate and sustain a conversation. Children may be taught to read body language and facial expressions, as well as how to organize their thinking.

In a speech therapy session, children are taught in individual and/or small group sessions, depending on their skill level. Sessions usually last 30 to 45 minutes and are run by an SLP in the office, your home, or your child's school. Sessions may incorporate language-based exercises, games, and activities. For nonverbal children, the therapist may use prompted speech therapy or augmentative treatments such as American Sign Language, communication boards, Voice Output Communication Devices, or PECS (Picture Exchange Communication Systems).

A common misconception is that the application of these augmentative treatments means you have to give up on spoken language for your child. In fact, studies indicate that the opposite is true—augmentative communication techniques can often help speech and language emerge.

TREATMENT AND EDUCATION OF AUTISTIC AND RELATED COMMUNICATION HANDICAPPED CHILDREN (TEACCH)

TEACCH was developed in the 1970s at the University of North Carolina's School of Medicine and was the first statewide program for diagnosis, treatment, and education for people with ASDs. Its philosophy is that the environment should be modified to meet the needs of children with ASDs, not vice versa. For example, if a child is overstimulated in a certain environment, either the environment must be adapted or the child must be removed from the environment and placed somewhere that promotes his learning needs.

TEACCH is a structured teaching approach that does not rely on one specific technique; it is a complete program of services that incorporates several techniques and methodologies. Teaching programs are developed to meet children's specific communication, social, and overall coping needs. Children are assessed through the multidimensional Psychoeducational Profile (PEP). The goal of TEACCH is to help people with ASDs learn functional skills to reach their full potential so they may live more effectively at home, at school, and in the community. Proponents of TEACCH feel that the program encourages an environment that is conducive to their children's specific learning needs and maximizes their children's autonomy through teaching enhanced communication, social, and adaptive skills.

TEACCH has been replicated in different schools and classrooms in the United States and internationally (Denmark, France, Norway, Sweden, and Switzerland). It offers teacher training workshops in North Carolina and at other locations around the country. You can contact your local school district to see if they offer TEACCH.

ALTERNATIVE AND COMPLEMENTARY TREATMENTS FOR ASDs

Parents also use alternative and/or complementary treatments to supplement the more standard treatments. Alternative treatments are considered to be those used in place of conventional treatments, whereas complementary treatments (some of which may in fact be alternative) are used in combination with more conventional treatments. Often these two categories are known as non-established treatments—the implication being that there isn't enough research or science backing them to be considered standard.

Choosing an alternative and/or complementary treatment requires the same amount of research that choosing a more conventional treatment does; but your research will probably involve more parent and practitioner testimonials and less science.

While I am a huge advocate of scientific treatments, I admit that I'm not a purist. I was (and still am) open to alternative and complementary approaches. In Jake's case, when he was two, we used the more conventional treatments (one-on-one sessions of ABA, speech therapy, and OT) as the foundation for his treatment regimen, and added on others that may be considered alternative and complementary (cranial-sacral osteopathy, gluten-free/casein-free diet, vitamin supplements, such as B_6/magnesium, homeopathy, and even energetic therapy). As Jake got older we discontinued some treatments (the GF/CF diet and homeopathy), modified others (fewer one-on-one ABA sessions, more group social skills therapy, and fewer visits to the cranial-sacral osteopath), kept some the same (vitamins, speech therapy, and OT), and added other treatments as well (auditory treatments like Earobics and Fast ForWord, music therapy, and piano lessons, all recommended by Jake's new and optimistic speech therapist to help improve his auditory processing). Why did we modify his overall treatment plan? Did we drop the diet or stop the one-on-one ABA sessions because they weren't working? No. We simply modified Jake's schedule to meet his changing needs. Your child's treatment plan is like a living and breathing organism—it will change and evolve as your child does.

What works for some children may or may not work for your child. So much depends on your child's specific needs and neurological makeup. Some parents I work with have seen great results from alternative and complementary treatments such as AIT, the gluten-free/casein-free diet, and chiropractic, while other parents who've tried these very same treatments saw no changes in their children's skills or behaviors.

There are many alternative and complementary treatments, including but not limited to creative treatments such as art and music therapy, animal treatments such as swimming with dolphins and therapeutic horseback riding, body manipulation therapies such as massage and acupuncture, and many more. In this chapter, I have included two of the more standard alternative and complementary approaches, which are dietary intervention and vitamin/mineral intervention. These treatments are not meant to be used alone; they are used in conjunction with other treatments that form the foundation of your child's treatment program, such as ABA or Floortime. If you decide to choose dietary or vitamin/mineral treatments for your child, make sure to receive nutritional counseling before you begin.

Dietary Intervention

The most useful diet for children with ASDs is the gluten-free/casein-free (GF/CF) diet. This diet was developed based on the observation that children with ASDs are more likely to have food allergies and higher levels of yeast, gastrointestinal problems, and an inability to break down certain proteins. There is evidence that children with ASDs have deficiencies in vitamins and minerals and cannot properly digest gluten and casein. Therefore, the proteins gluten and casein leak into the gut undigested and attach to the opiate receptors of the brain. As a result, children may have behavioral problems such as lack of focus and irritability, as well as digestive problems that may exacerbate their symptoms of ASD. The GF/CF diet strives to eliminate peptides that may cross into the brain and alter typical brain activity so that these symptoms are alleviated. Thus, the GF/CF diet removes all foods containing gluten, including wheat, oats, barley, and rye, and all dairy products—a source of casein.

Other diets for ASDs are listed in Appendix C.

Vitamins and Minerals

The megavitamin approach is based on evidence that some children with ASDs have metabolic errors that may be overcome by larger amounts of certain vitamins. The most popular supplement for children with ASDs is the vitamin B_6 and magnesium mixture, which has been used to decrease behavior problems and increase concentration and eye contact. Other vitamins and minerals that are used include cod liver oil supplements, calcium, and vitamins A, B_1, B_5, B_{12}, and C. Children vary enormously in their need for various nutrients. Parents should seek help from a nutritionist or a nutritionally informed physician.

NOW THAT YOU KNOW ABOUT SOME OF THE TREATMENTS . . .

You will most likely want to do more research on your own and collect further information to make an informed decision about what's best for your child. There is a list of recommended websites in Appendix F and a list of recommended reading in Appendix G that will give you further information. Remember to consider what would work in terms of your lifestyle. A home ABA program is not for everyone; some parents prefer a center-based program. When you research, also keep in mind that most alternative and complementary approaches have little scientific backing, so you'll have to make a judgment call based on your child's specific needs, your level of comfort, and how well the treatment fits your lifestyle. For example, a restrictive gluten-free/casein-free diet works well for some families but can cause stress in others.

It's important to educate yourself when it comes to treatment approaches. Talk to other parents with children with ASDs and professionals in the field—they can be tremendous resources. Make sure the information you read is up-to-date. Even though the clock is ticking and you must make a treatment decision soon for your child, make sure your decision is not impulsive. At the very least, take the time to absorb what you've learned about treatments and think about how they would apply to your child's specific needs.

PARENTS TALK ABOUT TREATMENTS

As you continue your search for treatments, parents will share with you stories about what worked and what didn't for their children. Here are some of their stories, which I collected from my questionnaires.

> Charlie is three years old and has been in intensive ABA and sensory integration therapy for one year. He used to be a child who couldn't talk, had tantrums, and threw himself off the back of the sofa or the bookshelves and crashed into everything in the house. Now he's completely changed. He's a boy who is sweet and attentive and points things out just for the sake of approval. It is amazing and heartening. His language is nearly age-appropriate. He still has some fixation on trains, but is able to engage in pretend play and some peer interaction.

> The day that our son was diagnosed with autism was the day I started making phone calls. I called friends who had worked with autistic children. I called anyone that I knew who had or knew of someone with an autistic child. Everyone said the same thing. "You need to get ABA going for your son." So, this is the first step that we took. He began having approximately 20 to 28 hours of ABA a week. On top of this, he received 1 hour of speech therapy per week, 1 hour of OT per week, 4 hours of a special play group led by occupational and speech therapists, and 1 hour of special therapy integrating speech and OT with what the play group was working on. He still receives all of these services. The most beneficial has been ABA. It has improved his speech and his behaviors. Now when he tantrums for something, we can say, "Use your words." He then tells us what he wants.

> David began treatment at age three and a half. We enrolled him in a program that combined different modes of therapy—ABA, TEACCH, Floortime. The speech therapist used Floortime and the behavioral therapist used ABA. We had success with all of them. It's been approximately sixteen months since we first began therapy. Our son is almost to the point of being conversational; he is more attentive and verbal and has fewer stims, although some days are better than others. He asks many "why" questions and is in general more aware of his surroundings. He's seeking

out friends and adults for feedback and responses. He has developed a sense of humor and is a happy child.

⌣

We tried just about everything. You name it, we tried it—the special diet, ABA, Floortime, speech therapy, AIT, chiropractic. But nothing seemed to work. Our son is now three and a half, and he's still acting out and still not speaking. But we're not giving up. We just put him into a special preschool for autism. They use some of the same techniques as the ones that we tried at home, but I'm hoping that the school will have better results. We have our fingers crossed that something will work for our son.

⌣

We started with ABA home programming for Danny, but it was too hard for me. The time commitment was too much, and because I had another child at home at the same time, I felt guilty that I was spending so much time with Danny and hardly any time with his baby sister. At first I was worried that Danny might not receive services that were as good outside of the home, but I was wrong. We found this wonderful school that we adore. They use TEACCH, and he also gets OT and PT. He still doesn't speak, but he can use PECS to show us pictures of what he wants. He gets lots of individual attention and continues to show progress. The school even potty trained him, which we thought was going to be impossible. Danny also takes a medication called Abilify, which helps him focus.

⌣

We used a home ABA program, the GF/CF diet, and extra B_6 vitamins. Our daughter's progress took off. She was only [twenty-one] months when she started and at first she only did 20 hours a week of ABA, but after a few months she was doing 40 hours a week. She's been doing ABA for just over two years now with amazing miraculous results—she now has emotions, feelings, and language skills and likes to play with her older sister. Her progress has so far exceeded our expectations! Our pediatric neurologist rated her an 8 or 10 severity when he diagnosed her. He is astonished at how close to typical she has become. She still has some issues, like memory retention and low muscle tone, which contribute to an increased difficulty in writing, but she's still doing treatment and showing progress. We're so thankful—she was gone and now she's back!

Why will the same treatment work wonders for one child and be completely ineffective for another? Researchers still aren't sure how to predict which children will improve with a particular treatment. Some suggest that the differences lie in the structural properties of the children's brains. Others blame improper treatment applications—such as a lack of intensity or an inconsistent approach. Researchers continue to look for definitive answers to these treatment questions.

7

YOU HAVE THE POWER: ADVOCATING FOR YOUR CHILD'S LEGAL RIGHTS

THE LAW AND YOUR POWER AS A PARENT

As a parent, you hold more power than you may imagine when it comes to helping your child get services. This is due in large measure to the provisions of the Individuals with Disabilities Education Act (IDEA). Actually, as of 2004, the name was changed to Individuals with Disabilities Education Improvement Act (IDEIA), but most people still refer to it as IDEA. It applies to children with various disabilities, including ASDs. This law provides the states with federal funding for special education programs, but only if the state programs meet criteria specified in the act. All fifty states have opted to comply with the requirements of the IDEA to qualify for the federal funding.

Two of the criteria specified in the act are crucial to you as a parent because they give you the ability to become a powerful advocate for your child within the educational system. First, the IDEA requires that the state provide your child with a free and appropriate public education that meets his or her unique individual needs. Therefore, if it is clear that your child needs a particular service, the state or the school district must provide it. Second, the IDEA establishes an explicit role for you as a parent in planning and monitoring your child's individual education program. You are entitled to be treated as an equal partner in deciding on an educational plan that contains the elements that your child needs. This means that you have the ability to present your ideas regarding the needs of your child and how you believe those needs must be met.

You should understand that the right to advocate for your child is a bit of a double-edged sword. The provisions of the IDEA that give you this right are both empowering and demanding. They don't just put you in a position where you can do a great deal to improve your child's education; they put you in a position where you really must become actively involved to accomplish this goal.

The reason why you must become actively involved with the state in obtaining services for your child lies in the definition of *appropriate* under the IDEA. Obviously, you want the best possible services that you can obtain for your child. However, as we will see later in this chapter, the state is not required to provide the *best* educational services that money can buy. Rather, it is required to provide those services that are determined to be *appropriate* for your child, the very ones that are to meet your child's educational needs. The two educational standards—*best* versus *appropriate*—may differ substantially. Therefore, your role as a participant in the process of planning and implementing your child's educational program is critical. Your job is to demonstrate your child's unique educational needs and to achieve a consensus with the representatives of the local or state agency and the school district regarding how those needs will be met.

This job can be a bit intimidating for parents. It requires that you attend group meetings and become sufficiently well informed regarding educational options so you can make meaningful contributions in these meetings. It requires you to work with a group of professionals who may have a tendency to use technical language that they may or may not explain adequately. It may require you to challenge recommendations made by professionals and suggest alternatives. When confronting this potentially daunting responsibility, always remember that you know your child better than anyone else, including the experts who have evaluated your child and the professionals with whom you will be determining your child's educational program. Don't allow yourself to be intimidated by the process or the people involved in it. If you don't understand something, ask for it to be explained. Getting your child the help that he or she needs is a collaborative process. You as a parent have equal power in working with the professionals to decide upon a treatment plan for your child.

This chapter is designed to help you navigate the system created by the IDEA and exercise your parental rights effectively within this system. The chapter begins with a review of some of the specific elements of the IDEA, giving you a clearer picture of exactly what your child is entitled to and exactly how you are expected to be involved in the educational planning process. Then the chapter presents specific guidelines on what you must do to access and utilize the appropriate state and district systems responsible for choosing and implementing the treatment services and educational programming that your child needs. These guidelines are organized under two headings and correspond to the current age of your child. When your child is under the age of three, you begin by working with the state early intervention office to develop and implement an individualized family service plan (IFSP) that focuses not only on the needs of your child with an ASD, but also on the needs of your entire family. After your child has reached the age of three, you work with your school district's special education personnel, focusing on your child's individual educational needs and program.

YOUR CHILD'S RIGHTS

The first major federal legislation entitling children with disabilities to an appropriate education was passed in 1975 under the title the Education for All Handicapped Children Act. It is this act that establishes the rights to which your child with an ASD is entitled. As a monetary appropriations law, this statute has to be reauthorized by Congress every few years. In 1990, it was renamed the IDEA. In 1997 and 2004, it was amended substantially during the reauthorization. You don't need to read the IDEA word for word, but as a parent who will be advocating for your child, you do need to understand the meaning of certain key phrases contained in it to understand exactly what your child is and is not guaranteed. The concepts embodied in the law that are really important for you to understand are *eligibility, free and appropriate public education* (FAPE), and *least restrictive environment.*

Eligibility

The IDEA specifies that a child is legally entitled to receive early intervention services or special education services if the child meets the state eligibility requirements that define disability. Autism is mentioned specifically in the IDEA as a condition that constitutes a disability. Therefore, if your child has been diagnosed with an ASD, this diagnosis is generally sufficient to determine that your child is entitled to the rights afforded by the IDEA.

If your child has not been formally diagnosed with an ASD, he will fall under the purview of the act if he has experienced significant developmental delays. Early intervention also applies to physical or mental conditions that are likely to result in developmental delays (e.g., Down syndrome). This issue is determined by an assessment that is arranged by the state office of early intervention or by the school district office of special education, depending on your child's age.

Free and Appropriate Public Education (FAPE)

The IDEA specifies that children who are determined to be eligible should be provided, at public expense, *free and appropriate public education* that meets their individual needs. The *free* part of this phrase is pretty clear. All the treatment services and any educational placements that are deemed necessary must be provided by the state or by the school district, free to the parents of the child. This is obviously a tremendous benefit to all but the wealthiest parents, since treatment interventions and special education programming for children with ASDs can be extremely costly. However, the *free* part of the IDEA requirement is meaningful only if agreement can be reached on what is *appropriate* for your child, and the determination of what is *appropriate* to the needs of your child is not always straightforward.

Again, you will naturally want the very best for your child. And you will no doubt be well informed regarding the latest interventions that have been reported to be highly effective. But the state early intervention department or the school district may not have in place the specific treatments or interventions that you would prefer, and they are not required by law to provide your child with any specific treatment or instructional modality. The law does require that the states provide disabled students with services that give them the opportunity to achieve educational success. The state must provide special education services that match children's needs and enable them to progress toward achieving developmental milestones in the near term and economic independence and employment as adults. In fact, determining which services and interventions are appropriate for your child, and therefore which ones will be provided for him, is a collaborative process that may involve considerable negotiation.

You (as your child's advocate) and the official representatives of the state early intervention office or the school district must reach consensus on at least four aspects of your child's educational program: present levels of performance and goals, placement, the related services required to facilitate learning, and any additional educational components that are appropriate to your child's needs.

Present levels of performance and goals refers to your child's current progress at school. Objectives are developed to meet your child's individual needs to help him or her achieve specific goals.

Placement refers to the program or class to which your child will be assigned. Among the options available are an integrated class, a special education class within a regular school, a special education school, a school designed specifically for children with autism, and/or a home-based program.

Related services may include transportation to placements, as well as additional developmental services that may be considered appropriate to help your child benefit from the special education she is receiving. These developmental services may include speech and language therapy, occupational therapy, physical therapy, psychological treatment, and/or social work interventions. Since communication difficulties are a common characteristic of ASDs, speech and language therapy are often included as related services in the educational programs of children with ASDs. You and the representatives of the state early intervention program or the school district must agree upon the related services that your child will receive. This agreement involves more than just deciding whether your child should receive a particular service or services; it involves specifying exactly how many sessions of each supportive service should be provided each week. The provision of a classroom aide would also fall within the category of related services.

Additional educational components include the use of specific curricula or specific instructional modalities that suit your child's learning style; the provision of classroom accommodations, such as distraction-free study environments, and the use of modified testing formats such as tests with extended time limits.

Each and every one of these aspects of your child's free and appropriate public education must be agreed upon, and securing the agreement of the agents of the state early intervention office or the local school district is pretty much a function of demonstrating what your child needs. This is one of the most challenging tasks that you will face in your ongoing relationship with the educational professionals with whom you must collaborate in determining and monitoring your child's educational plan. But fear not: You are more than capable of negotiating effectively with these professionals. Although legal jargon and the technical terms contained in educational and psychological test reports can be confusing, you can request explanations and assert your power as a parent to secure the services your child needs. In these pages, you'll learn exactly how the legal framework and educational system work so that you can make them work for you and your child.

Least Restrictive Environment

Another key concept in the IDEA is *least restrictive environment* defined as the environment in which your child has the greatest possible opportunity to interact with children who do not have a disability and to participate in the general education curriculum. This element of the IDEA is based on the conviction that children with disabilities benefit socially and linguistically from contact with their nondisabled, same-age peers.

In a way, however, this type of mainstreaming is a rebuttal presumption. Thus, the IDEA presumes that a child will be placed in the general education classroom environment unless the presumption is rebutted. This means you must be able to prove that your child can't succeed in a general education setting (even with supports and services) so you can have her moved to a more restrictive setting, such as a special school for children with ASDs. While there is some debate regarding the relative benefits to be gained by children with ASDs from placement in regular classrooms versus separate, special settings, it has become commonplace for children with ASDs to spend most of their instructional time in regular classrooms, aided by special education teachers and/or aides who can adapt the curriculum to their specific needs.

Some children with ASDs spend part of their time in regular classrooms and part in separate special education classrooms. However, under the IDEA, even students who spend most of their time in separate classrooms may still be included in school-wide activities such as assemblies, physical education, sports teams, music, and recess. The manner and extent of your child's inclusion in mainstream activities is another decision that you must make with the professionals at the state office of early intervention or the school district department of special education. In your discussions surrounding this issue, keep in mind that your child's diagnosis of an ASD does not constitute a sufficient justification for a school district to deny your child the opportunity to participate in activities with nondisabled, same-age peers. Current thinking on the issue of mainstreaming emphasizes the value of what your child is likely to learn by interacting with students in the regular school population. Same-age peers provide models of developmentally and socially appropriate behaviors and language that are likely to facilitate the development of your child's own social and language skills.

WORKING THE SYSTEM

Now that you have some idea of what your child is entitled to under the law and what your role is in securing the best possible education for your child, let's turn to the specific steps that you should take to access and utilize the system effectively. These steps depend on the age of your child.

If Your Child Is Younger Than Three Years: Early Intervention and the IFSP

The IDEA provides federal grants to states that provide special education services to children with disabilities, beginning at the age of three. The act also provides federal grants to states that institute programs to provide early intervention services for children with disabilities, including ASDs. Any child younger than three years of age who has a developmental delay or a physical or mental condition likely to result in a developmental delay is eligible to receive early intervention services. If your child is determined to be eligible, these early intervention services must be provided to you at no cost.

Early intervention services may be directed either toward your child or your entire family, and services for your child may include special instruction such as ABA, speech and language instruction, occupational therapy, physical therapy, and psychological evaluation. Early intervention services for families may include training to help the family reinforce or generalize a child's new skills and counseling to help the family adapt to the changed circumstances associated with having a disabled child. Early intervention services are aimed at minimizing the impact of disabilities on the development of your child. The services that are available in early intervention programs vary considerably from state to state, so it is incumbent upon you as a parent to determine which services are available.

It is important that you contact the closest early intervention state office as soon as possible after you come to suspect that your child has a problem or has received a diagnosis of an ASD. Early intervention is available in every state but may be administered by different state agencies. If you're not sure how to get in touch with the early intervention office, you can call your local school district or the National Information Center for Children and Youth with Disabilities for a contact in your state. Other informational contacts include the state or local Department of Human Services, local chapters of autism organizations, the local Department of Health, or local developmental disabilities associations. A list of state resources is included on the website for the Autism Society of America at www.autism-society.org.

Once you have located the nearest early intervention office, there is a series of steps that you must take to secure early intervention services. You must provide a referral for services, provide consent for your child to be evaluated, participate in a meeting to develop an IFSP and participate on an ongoing basis in the evaluation and revision of this plan. In the following sections of this chapter, we will address each of these steps in turn.

Referral

Many parents who contact the early intervention office have been referred by a pediatrician or other medical professional or by child/day care centers, schoolteachers, administrators, or other social service programs. However, a referral from a professional source is not required to contact the early intervention office. As a parent, you may contact the office directly to request that your child be evaluated, based on your suspicion that there may be a developmental problem.

Most parents make initial contact with the early intervention office by phone. However, in addition to the phone call, it is a good idea to send a letter certified/return receipt requested to confirm that you have made the request for an evaluation and to ensure that your request is honored in a timely manner.

Once you've contacted the early intervention office with a request for an evaluation, an early intervention service coordinator will contact you. The coordinator will explain to you how the system works, including how to schedule evaluations and get your child the services he needs.

> **Early Intervention Referral TIP #1**: Be proactive! Make sure to follow up with another phone call and/or letter if you don't hear back from your early intervention service coordinator within a week after your initial call. Even though the early intervention office is legally responsible for responding to your request for an evaluation within a timely manner, the office handles many cases, and it is quite possible for a child to fall between the cracks. Don't let this happen. As you know, time is of the essence in securing necessary services for your child. Don't let bureaucratic delays impede the task of arranging for these services.

Consent for Early Intervention Evaluation

As a parent, you will need to provide consent for your child to be screened and evaluated. An initial screening will determine whether or not your child has developmental delays and what specific evaluations should be conducted.

Evaluations are conducted by at least two professionals. Depending on your child's needs, the evaluators may be a speech and language pathologist, an occupational therapist, a special education evaluator, or other specialists in the field of developmental disabilities. The goal of the evaluations is to verify the presence of developmental delays and assess the nature and extensiveness of these delays. The evaluations provide the basis for professional recommendations for specific early intervention services that are most appropriate for your child.

Evaluations usually include the following five components: a review of your child's health and medical history, a parent interview, a general developmental assessment of your child's strengths and weaknesses, assessments by specialists addressing your child's suspected areas of delays, and an assessment of the potential utility of various forms of assistive technology. In addition, your child's evaluation will include an assessment of transportation needs.

It is important to give consent promptly to all reasonable requests for evaluations. It is to your advantage that the early intervention specialists have as much data as possible with which to formulate an impression of your child—including his developmental difficulties as well as his strengths and resiliencies. Providing consent for requested evaluations in a timely manner conveys to the professionals your support of their efforts to help your child and represents an initial step toward developing a cooperative working relationship. If you unreasonably withhold or delay consent, it may generate a perception that you are less than thoroughly motivated to help your child or that you are difficult or insufficiently cooperative.

> **Early Intervention Evaluation TIP #2**: You have an important role in the evaluation process. You will be asked for information about your child and your perceptions of her abilities and disabilities. Be honest! It's crucial that you tell the truth about your child's symptoms. Many parents try to hide or minimize the symptoms of their children's ASDs. This is a natural tendency, but it's not in your child's best interests. The professionals must understand the full extent of your child's difficulties if they are to recommend appropriate interventions. Therefore, strive to be as cooperative and honest as you can possibly be. This approach to the evaluations will help you get the services that your child needs. On the day of an evaluation, if you notice that your child isn't acting like herself, let the evaluator know your concerns and describe how your child generally behaves. If your child is ill or you believe that another assessment is necessary to evaluate your child accurately, schedule another appointment.

After your child's evaluations have been completed, make sure to request a full copy of all screening and/or evaluation reports (keep them in a special file at home—you'll probably need to access them in the future). You have a right to receive these reports, and it is important that you scrutinize them to satisfy yourself that the evaluators have adequately assessed your child's difficulties and have recommended interventions with which you agree. Familiarizing yourself with the recommendations contained in the evaluation report, in advance of any related discussion, will enable you to identify areas where additional or more intensive services may be necessary. In making this judgment, you may wish to consult with an expert of your own choosing.

If you are not satisfied with the nature of the evaluation or with the results, you can request a second evaluation. To do so, you should send a letter to your early intervention service coordinator that clearly states the specific nature of your reservations regarding the evaluation. Valid reasons for requesting a new evaluation include demonstrable observations that important developmental areas have not been assessed, demonstrable assertions that aspects of the evaluation are inaccurate, and reservations regarding the qualifications of the evaluator(s). Whether or not you liked the evaluator personally is not an appropriate subject for such a letter. The evaluator's personality is most likely irrelevant to the accuracy of the results, and criticizing the evaluator in this manner may alienate your service coordinator or other involved professionals. Make sure to send the letter requesting a second evaluation certified/return receipt requested.

Following the completion of the evaluation, you will attend a meeting to determine your child's eligibility for early intervention services, discuss your child's service needs, and develop and agree upon a formal IFSP.

The Individual Family Service Plan Meeting

In the IFSP meeting, your child's Individual Family Service Plan will be developed. The IFSP is a written document that describes your child's current levels of functioning and anticipated outcomes (goals) and enumerates the specific services that will be provided to meet the skill-based needs of your child and the needs of your family. It is formulated according to your child's diagnosis, as well as his specific challenges and strengths and details your child's and family's service needs, the goals and objectives of the services to be provided, and the source, frequency, and location of services. It also describes how the family can support the child's needs. By law, this meeting must take place at a location and time that is convenient for you, but within forty-five days from the day of your initial referral.

The IFSP meeting is a collaborative effort that involves you and the professionals who have evaluated your child. The early intervention service coordinator who has been assigned to you will typically take a lead role in facilitating the development, implementation, and evaluation of your child's IFSP. You also have the right to invite to the meeting a specialist who has special knowledge of your child and/or special expertise regarding services that you may feel are necessary to meet your child's developmental needs.

In preparing for the IFSP meeting, it is important that you become aware of the services that are available for your child. The services that are most likely to be relevant for children with ASDs include speech therapy, occupational therapy, physical therapy, ABA, sensory integration therapy, parent training, and team meetings. However, not all of these services may be provided routinely in every state early intervention program. It is unlikely that the professionals representing the state early intervention programs will recommend a service that they know is not readily available through existing programs. Therefore, it is up to you as the parent to be aware of services that may benefit your child. Keep in mind, however, that a request for services that are not recommended by the early intervention evaluators are likely to be granted only if you can demonstrate that your child needs these specific services and that the same benefits cannot be derived from available service modalities.

Services specified in the IFSP can also include transportation, such as busing your child to a specific treatment location. The location of your child's therapy will be determined depending on your child's needs. Options include services in the home, at the local day care center, in the preschool, or in center-based or school settings.

As the name implies, the IFSP involves the family's needs as well. Family counseling and parent training are likely to be available. The IFSP may also include suggested ways for your family to help your child perform everyday routines and activities (such as bedtime or mealtime routines or playground activities). The IFSP may specify that services provided by several different agencies be integrated into the overall service plan.

The IFSP can be updated as necessary. The IDEA requires that periodic reviews be conducted (every six months or sooner at your request) and that the IFSP be evaluated and revised annually. This updating process provides ongoing support for both the family and the child. When your child reaches the age of two years and six months, the *transition plan* of the IFSP goes into effect. This transition plan specifies the services to be provided until your child is three years old, at which point the plan recommends preschool educational options for your child and is forwarded to the special education department of your child's school district. The education department must then determine whether your child should be classified as a preschooler with a disability and therefore be entitled to the appropriate preschool educational services.

IFSP Meeting Tip #1: Arrive at your IFSP meeting with a plan in mind about which services you are requesting, and be prepared to demonstrate that these services are necessary for your child to have an appropriate education. Bring documents that will help you make your case, including assessments and recommendations made by outside specialists (such as developmental pediatricians, neurologists or neuropsychologists, special educators, or curriculum specialists). You must understand that the members of the early intervention team may experience some pressure from their administrative superiors to contain costs. They often need to justify to their superiors any recommendation that they make for services above and beyond those which can be provided easily by existing programs that are already funded. Therefore, the supporting documentation that you bring to the IFSP meeting not only may convince the other participants that your requests are reasonable, but also may provide them with ammunition they need to justify a recommendation to provide these services.

IFSP Meeting Tip # 2: When advocating for your child, choose your words carefully. Although your goal is clearly to get the best services for your child that you possibly can, *do not ask for what is best*. This may sound like strange advice, but remember that the law does not require the state to provide your child with the *best* possible services, but only with the services that are deemed *appropriate* to his or her needs. Therefore, in requesting the services that you want, use expressions such as *appropriate* and *necessary*. Make sure the supporting documentation you furnish also speaks in terms of *needed services*. Using the right words may play a crucial role in determining whether or not your requests are granted.

IFSP Meeting Tip # 3: Choose the attitude that you present at the IFSP carefully. It's natural for you to feel scared, anxious, or intimidated either before or during the IFSP meeting. When confronting this new experience, you may feel emotionally charged or overwhelmed. *But whatever you do, try not to act angry or combative*. You want the committee to be on your side. Conduct yourself in a calm, businesslike manner. Adopt an attitude that says you can be taken seriously and you're there to work together with the committee as a team. Be assertive, not aggressive. Using your powers of persuasion and presenting evidence to support your position is much more likely to be productive than raising your voice.

Some parents ask whether they should involve a lawyer in their dealings with the early intervention office or whether they should bring a lawyer to the IFSP meeting. These are judgment calls. Involving a lawyer has both a potential upside and downside. Sometimes lawyers are necessary to help you get the services you want. But the presence of a lawyer may also alienate the early intervention professionals and create a stressful and defensive environment. Whether or not you should involve an attorney depends on your perception of the likelihood that the early intervention professionals will give due attention to your requests or whether they will seek to minimize the services they provide your child in an effort to contain costs. You may be able to get an idea of how the process works in your area by talking to other parents who have already been through early intervention evaluations and IFSP meetings. You may also consider how carefully your wishes were considered in your initial interactions with the early intervention office. If you don't want to hire a lawyer or simply can't afford one, you can get advice from your local advocacy groups. (You may also contact your local ASA office for more information at www.autism-society.org. If you live outside of the United States, see Appendix E for a list of international organizations compiled by the National Autistic Society at www.autism.org.uk.

In our son's case, we consulted a lawyer from the start because we realized very early in the process that our early intervention office was not coming through with services that we needed. Even before our initial IFSP meeting, we sensed an adversarial relationship developing. Hiring a lawyer was the best decision for us because he helped us get services that we needed.

IFSP TIP # 4: Whether or not you bring a lawyer, you need to act like one. Wear business attire if possible. Take notes. Speak up. Represent your client, who in this case is your child. It's often easier for parents to think of themselves as representatives of their children, rather than as Mommy and Daddy. As much as you love and care about your child, the IFSP is a business meeting, and it can be difficult to achieve your goals if you allow your emotions to get in the way of making rational judgments and decisions.

Lastly, keep in mind that you do not have to sign the IFSP document that is presented to you in the meeting. You have the right to take it home and reread it on your own time. Make sure the IFSP contains the services that you think your child requires. If it does not, you must let the early intervention chairperson know the areas of the plan with which you are dissatisfied. In some cases, a simple negotiation over the phone may be sufficient to resolve the disputed areas. In other cases, however, another IFSP meeting must be held. If you cannot come up with a mutually agreeable IFSP for your child, you are entitled to take advantage of the procedural remedies of mediation and a due process hearing, which we'll come back to later in this chapter.

If Your Child Is Age Three to Twenty-one: Special Education and the IEP

The IDEA requires that states provide special education services to children with disabilities beginning at the age of three. Special education services are provided by local school districts. Therefore, if your child has been receiving early intervention services through the state early intervention office, you will stop working with this office, and you will begin to work with the special education department within your local school district. If your child is three years old or older and you have not received early intervention services through the state, your first contact will be with the district's special education department.

If your child is between the ages of three and five, you will work with the district (in some cases regional) Committee for Preschool Special Education (CPSE). If your child is older than five, you will work with the district Committee for Special Education (CSE). These committees may be known by different names in your state. For example, in some states the term MDT is used (an acronym for Multidisciplinary Team) or ARD Committee (an acronym for Admission, Review, and Dismissal Committee). If your child has been receiving early intervention services, her last IFSP will include a transition plan to facilitate the transfer from early intervention services to special education. (Make sure you keep good records. Sometimes transitions can be difficult, but they are much easier if you are organized and plan ahead).

The focus of special education is different from that of early intervention. Whereas early intervention focuses on the entire family and seeks to minimize the overall developmental impact of your child's disability, preschool special education focuses on your child as an individual, and more specifically on preparing your child to succeed in school. In order for your child to qualify for preschool special education, it must be shown that your child has a definitive handicapping condition that impacts her social skills, preschool readiness, academic skills, and/or speech and language skills. To make this determination, the Committee for Preschool Special Education will require, at a minimum, a social history, an educational evaluation, and a psychological evaluation. The

CPSE may also require supplemental evaluations depending on your child's unique needs. These may include an occupational therapy evaluation or a speech and language evaluation.

When these evaluations have been completed, a meeting will be held, attended by the parent, the CPSE chairperson, your child's early intervention service providers (if applicable), and representatives of the evaluating agencies. The purpose of this meeting is to determine your child's eligibility for preschool special education and decide what educational services will be provided. These services will be described in a detailed Individualized Education Program (IEP). If your child is older than five and you work with the district's CSE, the evaluation process and the meeting to determine eligibility and develop an IEP will be similar.

The steps you take when your child is under the age of three (working with the early intervention department to develop and monitor the IFSP) are echoed in the steps that you must take when your child is age three to twenty-one: referral to either the CPSE or the CSE, giving consent for evaluations, facilitating and monitoring the evaluation process, and participating in the meeting conducted to develop your child's IEP.

Referral

Although your child may be referred to the CSE, if he is five years or older (or to the CPSE, if he is from three to five years old) by his school or a professional, the IDEA gives you—the parent—the power to refer your child directly to the CSE for an evaluation. Regardless of whether a school or another professional is involved, you will be calling the CSE to initiate the evaluation process, and you will be responsible for working with the committee to facilitate the evaluation process.

If you are the one who is referring your child for an evaluation, in addition to calling the CSE, you must also formally initiate the referral by writing to the chairperson of the CSE to request an evaluation. Make sure to mail this letter certified/return receipt requested or any other method that will ensure you receive a dated confirmation of delivery and thereby ensure that your child will be evaluated and receive services in a timely manner. State regulations specify time limits from the date of referral until the date that delivery of appropriate services is initiated. New York State regulations, for example, require that an eligible child should begin to receive appropriate services within 65 school days from the date of the referral or 60 school days from the date of the parent's consent for an evaluation.

Recognize that you are dealing with a bureaucracy and that slipups can occur. Once you have made the call to the CSE and mailed the formal request for an evaluation, expect to hear from them within a week or so. If you do not hear from them promptly about getting the evaluation process started, call back. You must take responsibility for ensuring that the process moves along expeditiously.

Consent for Special Education Evaluation

You must consent to your child's evaluation. The CSE typically requires a social history, an educational evaluation, and a psychological evaluation. If deemed appropriate for your child's specific challenges and strengths, additional evaluations may be requested. These additional evaluations may include a speech and/or language evaluation, an assessment of the need for physical and/or occupational therapy, an evaluation of auditory processing, and/or a neurological evaluation.

It is best to consent promptly to all requests for evaluations. The more data that is available to use in determining your child's needs, the better. Also, it is important that you convey a respectful attitude toward the expertise of the members of the CSE, acknowledging that their goal is to determine and provide for your child's educational needs. If these professionals have the sense that you respect their opinions and intentions, they will most likely find it easier to hear and process your input should you eventually determine that your child needs something different from or in addition to the CSE's recommendations. Try to establish a cooperative and collegial working relationship right from the start.

Some parents don't want their children to be evaluated either because they have already been evaluated by professionals or because they don't believe that their children will be given fair assessments. If you don't want an evaluation for your child, you are not required to consent. On the one hand, my advice is to always consent to requests that are reasonable. Failure to consent will likely lead to an adversarial relationship between you and the CSE, which should be avoided if at all possible. On the other hand, there are cases where parents accurately perceive that the district tends to provide only the most minimal special education services and that an evaluation could jeopardize their child's opportunity for an adequate education. In such instances, it may be necessary to raise reasonable objections.

You have the right to ask for the qlualifications of any evaluator proposed by the CSE. If you can show that an evaluator lacks appropriate qualifications or if you can demonstrate that the evaluations proposed by the CSE are inappropriate for your child, you have the right to request an independent evalua-tion that is paid for by the school district. If you make this request, however, you run the risk of alienating the members of the CSE, and the school district may respond by seeking an impartial hearing to prove the appropriateness of its evaluation. If the district can prove this, they will not be required to pay for the independent evaluation. Regardless of who pays for the evaluation, the dis-trict is obligated to consider any evaluations presented by either side. If you choose this course of action, know in advance what you're getting yourself into. Private evaluations are costly (anywhere from $150 to $5,000 per evalua-tion), and while some insurance companies have providers that accept partial or full payment, there are usually long waiting lists.

Even if you have reservations about what to expect from the CSE evaluation, consider your time. Don't wait months and/or spend exorbitant sums of money to have your child evaluated by a private evaluator if you can have your child evaluated free within a reasonable amount of time by your district. Also, choose your battles carefully. Even if your child has already been evaluated by your own private doctors and you are not certain of what is to be gained by further evalu-ation, don't put up a fight by refusing to let the CSE evaluate your child again. They may have good reasons for requesting an evaluation that you're unaware of—and even if they don't, it is probably better to avoid alienating the CSE members by refusing an innocuous request. The people on the committee will ultimately be the key players in deciding your child's services. Don't assume an adversarial position unless it becomes quite clear that they are unwilling to pro-vide something that you consider essential to your child's education.

Your Participation in the CSE Evaluation

As a parent, you fill several important roles in the evaluation process. First of all, you must see that the evaluation is carried out in a timely manner and strive dili-gently to ensure that the members of the CSE obtain an accurate and detailed profile of your child (including her challenges and strengths). If you have not received an evaluation within 30 days of the referral, you should find out why. If the CSE evaluation is not forthcoming in a timely manner, you have the right to request an independent evaluation at the expense of the district. Although it is doubtful that the district would comply immediately with this request and also unlikely that you could then arrange to have an independent evaluation com-pleted in a significantly shorter time span, this right gives you leverage to secure the best efforts of the CSE members and the evaluation personnel.

Your role in managing and expediting the evaluation process also requires you to get your child to scheduled evaluations. You are usually allowed to observe your child's evaluation, which can be helpful in terms of giving feedback to the evaluator about your child's behavior. It's worth noting again that on the day of a scheduled evaluation, if you notice that your child isn't acting the way she normally does, tell the assessor and indicate how your child generally behaves. If you believe that your child is ill or will need another assessment to get a more accurate evaluation, schedule another appointment.

You also have the right to submit additional data to be considered as the committee develops recommendations for your child's Individualized Educational Program. Additional data may include specific evaluations that you had carried out to supplement any evaluations requested by the CSE. If there is a particular service that you feel is essential to your child's education, an evaluation from a professional supporting this assertion may help to persuade the CSE members.

Last but not least, you will play a crucial role in your child's evaluation as a source of data. You will almost certainly be asked for your perceptions of your child and her abilities and disabilities (and if for some reason you are not asked, you should assert yourself and offer your perceptions). It is important that you be candid about your child's symptoms.

> **CSE Evaluation TIP**: When you are asked about your child's symptoms, be as open and honest as you can be, even if you need to describe unpleasant symptoms or behaviors. Focus on your child's disabilities rather than abilities. Don't be surprised or upset when you receive the written evaluations and see that they focus more on the negative than positive attributes of your child's behaviors and skills. This will ultimately help you receive better services for your child.

The Individualized Education Program Meeting

The IEP is a detailed document that describes your child's level of development in various areas (as well as his challenges and strengths), states short-term and annual goals, and indicates in specific terms the educational services that he will receive (for example, if your child is to receive speech therapy, it will indicate the number and duration of weekly sessions). The IEP also indicates your child's placement and the extent to which he will participate in regular education programs, as well as any special services or interventions that will be used to enable him to participate in mainstream classrooms.

The IEP meeting is paramount to your child's education. It is at this meeting that the formal determination is made regarding your child's eligibility for special education services. At this meeting, you can discuss the services that the CSE members recommend for your child, and you can present any ideas that you may have about additional services you feel are necessary. IEP meetings are usually held in a school or school administration building. Most IEP meetings last approximately one hour, but they can last as long as three hours when there are questions regarding the nature and extensiveness of special education services that may be required.

The individuals who typically attend the initial IEP meeting are the parent, the child's current general education teacher, the CSE member responsible for coordinating the child's case, an educational specialist who can interpret the results of the various evaluations, a school psychologist, and a representative of the school district. (Once your child is in the system, future IEP meetings will include your child's general or special education teacher and may include one or more specialists, such as the speech therapist or occupational therapist currently working with your child). You have the right to bring in a specialist of your own choosing to discuss aspects of your child's situation that may require particular services. You may also bring in a person from an outside advocacy group or consult with an advocacy group before the meeting. (In New York State, the IEP meeting may also be attended by a parent-member—a volunteer who lives in the district, has been through the special education process, and helps you by sharing his or her own experience). Your child does not have to be present at the meeting. In fact, most parents do not bring young children to the meetings. However, if your child is fourteen years old or older, the district will probably invite him to participate, which can be valuable in terms of getting your child involved in planning his own future.

Here's what a typical IEP meeting looks like: The chairperson begins the meeting by introducing him or herself. Then all the people at the table introduce themselves and sign in. At some point, generally quite early in the meeting, you will probably be asked to tell the committee how your child is doing. This is a very general question to which many parents respond with little more than a general observation that their children are doing "pretty well" or "not so well." Don't make this mistake. Such a response would indicate to the committee that parents are not prepared to offer much information about what their children need. This kind of response would be a cue to CSE members that they are pretty much in charge and need to do little more than inform parents of their recommendations.

It's important that you avoid giving such an impression. Therefore, when you are asked to tell the committee about your child, identify specific areas in which your child has deficits that may be improved by specific special educational or related services. Refer to relevant documentation whenever possible while making these points. Treat this question as an invitation to give a short presentation making the case for the services you are seeking for your child. Focus primarily on your child's deficits when sharing your description. If you focus on your child's positive behaviors and downplay the deficits, the committee may not think that your child merits receiving the services you are requesting.

> **IEP Meeting Tip # 1**: Be prepared to give an informal yet well-organized and convincing presentation that describes your child and indicates clearly what your child needs. Invite professionals (such as your child's speech therapist or the doctor who diagnosed your child) and/or bring documentation (such as doctor/specialist reports) to the IEP meeting to help support your service requests. Dress in appropriate business attire that shows you expect to be taken seriously.

All the participants at the IEP meeting will review copies of your child's evaluations (which they should have already read prior to the meeting). Either the chairperson or the evaluation specialist reads the test results and highlights significant points from the evaluations. At this juncture, the chairperson may open the discussion to ask for the opinions of others at the table. It's more and more common for the district to draft present levels of performance and goals that are then discussed and added to, omitted, or revised, as deemed appropriate by the entire team.

Your own knowledge of your child can supplement the evaluations and help the committee better understand who your child is. Describe your child and your child's history so that they have a mental picture of who your child is, how your child behaves, and why he needs the services you are requesting.

> **IEP Meeting Tip #2:** If your child is not present at the meeting, bring a picture of him to show the members. This will humanize your child by giving him a face. Connecting a face with the evaluation data will predispose the CSE members to want to help your child as much as they possibly can. Presenting a picture will also give you an opportunity to show the members how proud you are of your child. This will be a completely inoffensive way of demonstrating, without articulating, how determined you are to obtain the services that your child requires.

You may also speak up at any time during the meeting to add to or comment on points that are made by the evaluators. You can also reference documentation that you've brought in from private evaluators to support requests that you are making for specific services. If you do bring such documentation, make sure you provide copies of the evaluations to the committee before the meeting.

> **IEP Meeting Tip # 3**: Be creative in describing your child's educational needs. In one of the IEP meetings we had for Jake, we presented a video that we made documenting Jake's behavior at various stages in his treatment program. We did this to show that he was making progress to support our case for continuing the therapy that he had been receiving.

Of course, you must go into the IEP meeting knowing what special education programs are available and which may be most appropriate for your child. The best way to find out which programs exist is by asking your child's teacher, school evaluator, district special education administrator, or other parents. Many school districts have a Special Education Parent-Teacher Association (SEPTA). SEPTA can be a treasure trove of information. There are four basic placement options: a regular, mainstream classroom (with supplementary support such as an aide or a consultant-teacher); integrated classes (with a general education teacher and a special education teacher); a special classroom for children with special needs (with the possible support of an aide); or a private school or outreach or residential program. Whenever possible, visit schools or programs to see which ones may be most appropriate for your child.

To understand the importance of your participation at the IEP meeting, you need to know that just because a doctor or specialist has made a recommendation for the inclusion of a specific service in your child's IEP, that doesn't mean the IEP committee is required to follow that recommendation. For example, even if a speech and language pathologist states, "Alex needs five 30-minute sessions of speech therapy per week," the IEP committee may elect to provide only three weekly sessions. Although Alex's parents may argue that their son needs more intensive speech therapy services, the committee may argue that providing more services would remove Alex from the classroom too much. The IEP committee is only required to give Alex services that meet the standards of an *appropriate* education. In other words, it is quite likely that the level of services you would like your child to receive will be somewhat greater than the level the CSE is immediately willing to provide. Therefore, in the IEP meeting, the burden is on you to demonstrate that what you are asking for is in fact necessary. This is why simply asking for the best services for your child may get you into trouble. I was advised early on to describe appropriate or necessary services for my child to receive an adequate education. I advise you to do the same thing.

> **IEP Meeting Tip #4**: Always describe your recommendations and requests for services as "needs." Make it clear that these services are required to make sure your child has an opportunity to achieve an adequate level of educational progress. Never argue that the service you are requesting has been shown to be the best.

At the end of the IEP meeting, you will be asked to sign the IEP document. School officials will be asked to sign the document as well. You do not have to sign the document right at that moment unless you're absolutely sure it's what you want (although it's fine to sign the attendance form at the beginning of the meeting, which only documents your presence in the meeting and does not imply your agreement to anything that is discussed during the meeting). It's okay to take the proposed IEP home and read it over carefully by yourself, so you will not feel any pressure from the CSE members. You may also show the proposed IEP to experts of your own choosing, including legal experts, before agreeing to its terms.

If you are not satisfied with one or more particular aspects of the IEP, you should contact the chairperson of the CSE and negotiate these areas. Often an informal discussion over the phone can produce the results you want or at least a reasonable approximation of what you had in mind. If you still cannot accept what is being offered after an informal discussion, you have the right to request mediation or a due process hearing to resolve the disagreements. (These courses of action are considered in the final section of this chapter.)

Once you are satisfied with your child's IEP and have signed the necessary paperwork, you can usually expect services to begin within a reasonable amount of time. For example, in New York State, an IEP must be implemented within 30 days from the date of the IEP meeting. Check with your CSE to see what your state regulations are and when your child is eligible to begin receiving services. Very soon, there will be a national standard for IEP development and implementation. The IDEA has a provision about beginning services immediately unless additional time is required to make necessary arrangements.

Once an IEP is in place, it must be reviewed annually (unless you elect a three-year IEP, as allowed under the latest IDEA statute). After your child begins receiving special education services, you will meet with the CSE each school year to review your child's IEP, evaluate your child's progress, and determine if changes need to be made. This is referred to as an annual review. In terms of evaluations, the law states that the district is required to formally re-evaluate children at least once every three years, which is known as a triennial evaluation.

> **IEP Meeting TIP #5**: If you have a positive experience as a result of your IEP meeting, follow up with a thank-you call or note to the chairperson. This thoughtful gesture can help to build supportive relationships.

When the IFSP or IEP Meeting Doesn't Produce the Results You Want

Unfortunately, there are times when your best efforts as a parent and advocate do not produce a proposed IFSP or IEP that you feel is adequate for your child's needs. If this happens to you and you are unable to secure what your child requires in subsequent informal negotiation with the committee chairperson, you have the legal right to seek mediation and/or a due process hearing.

Mediation

Mediation is a meeting that includes you, a member of the professional group proposing the disputed IFSP or IEP, and an independent mediator. The mediator acts as a referee and facilitator in trying to help you and the committee come to a mutual agreement. The hope is that you will resolve your differences at this stage so that you will not have to go on to the next step, which is a due process hearing.

While it is not necessary to bring a lawyer to a mediation meeting, make sure to consult with a lawyer or legal consultant beforehand. This will give you some idea of what concessions you may reasonably expect to extract from the committee during mediation. If you think that the state has violated procedures under state or federal special education laws and regulations, you can file a complaint to the state education department. This is a complex issue that you should definitely consult an attorney about.

The Due Process Hearing

If you cannot resolve your differences with the early intervention or special education professionals through mediation, you have the right to request a fair hearing before a neutral administrative judge, who will have the power to decide on the services to be included in your child's IFSP or IEP. In the event of a due process hearing, both you and the state (or school district) will present testimony and evidence regarding the disputed areas of your child's IFSP or IEP. Most cases are resolved in a hearing. Yet in the off chance that yours is not, you have the right to appeal to a federal or state court or even take your case to the U.S. Supreme Court. (In some states, like New York, you have the right to appeal to the State Review Officer, followed by a federal or state court. Other states have a one-tiered system where you appeal directly to court.)

If you must go through a due process hearing, contact a lawyer who specializes in representing children with special needs and/or ASDs. As much as you may want to try to save money by representing yourself in a hearing, it's not a good idea. The school district will send their lawyer to represent them, and their lawyer will certainly be an expert in the field. Your lawyer can handle everything from writing a letter requesting a due process hearing to helping you plan your new IEP and representing you in court.

But before you initiate due process procedures, think about why you are going to due process and if it's really necessary. What circumstances necessitate due process? You should use due process only when there is a disagreement regarding a very important issue that is crucial to your child's healing. A dispute concerning your child's placement and related services may qualify. However, a dispute regarding details of your child's evaluation reports probably doesn't. (You do have a right to challenge inaccuracies in evaluation reports using the Family Educational Rights and Privacy Acts (FERPA), also known as the Buckley Amendment.)

Know what you're getting yourself into. Lawyers' fees differ drastically throughout the country. Lawyers can charge between $100 and $300 per hour and may require an upfront retainer fee of around $3,000. Some will negotiate a flat rate. Even if you do hire a lawyer, the lawyer cannot do all of the work; you need to keep strict records of every letter and phone correspondence between you and the district for your lawyer.

Although you can reap significant benefits by engaging in a due process hearing, the entire process can be extremely stressful. I know this because

Franklin and I were involved in two cases concerning Jake. One case lasted more than a year and involved a trial that required me to sit on the witness stand for six hours. I mistakenly thought that my corporate experience had prepared me for this kind of situation, but when it came to advocating for my child, my emotions were in high gear. Ultimately, the financial and emotional toll of the lawsuit was overwhelming. In the end, the case was settled. The second case was settled out of court (much to my relief). Although I may dissuade parents from suing their district for smaller issues, these issues were crucial to getting our son the help he needed, and I must admit that I would do it again if I had to. As a result of our cases, other families in our district now receive a higher level of services without difficulty.

Lessons from Parents Who Learned the Hard Way . . .

Sometimes when things aren't going your way in the IEP or IFSP process, you can try certain tactics to turn things around. Any parent who has experienced this will tell you that you must be ready to stand alone against an entire committee. Here is what one set of parents did.

> After our initial IEP meeting, there were things that we wanted to change on our son's IEP. We had been paying out-of-pocket for extra hours of ABA, and we couldn't afford to do that anymore. We felt the district should pay. We anticipated a fight from the administration, and because we did not want to pay lawyers' fees, we got the phone numbers of several advocacy groups. (Most states have advocacy groups for children with special needs.) They told us exactly what to do and what to say. We were totally prepared when we went into the meeting.
>
> Sure enough, we got the fight we expected. It turned out that the main reason why the district didn't want to give us extra ABA hours was because they'd never done that before with any child and because they didn't know anything about the latest ABA studies. We came in with research studies and doctors' reports.
>
> In the end, we reached a compromise. The school would pay for our son's additional therapy, as long as his extra ABA hours would be done at school, not at our house.

Lesson: It pays to come prepared. Sometimes you will encounter a committee that has expertise in dealing with learning disabilities or conditions other than ASDs. In this case, it may be up to you to educate the committee. For example, at the IFSP meeting of one family I consult with, the committee head kept using incorrect language, referring to the child's condition as "PPD" instead of PDD, and refused to give the child more than 10 hours per week of services. The parents had to fight back with information. They found themselves at the next meeting armed with research studies documenting cases similar to theirs in other states, as well as a lawyer who specialized in such cases. It took a lot of hard work and mediation, but the family ultimately did receive the services they requested.

Here's what another parent said.

We spent most of the IFSP meeting really angry and upset. My husband kept saying, "We want what's best for our son, and we're not leaving until we get it." Maybe he was being heavy-handed, but this is our only child and he's taken this whole thing really hard. Our son is only two years old, and he doesn't speak at all. The committee kept saying that they didn't have to give us what was best because the law said they only had to give us what was appropriate. How was that possible? I thought the law protected us! My husband was so upset. I've never seen him so upset. It wasn't until the end of the meeting that we realized we weren't getting what we wanted. So the meeting ended, and we left and didn't know what to do. We called a lawyer and she said we shouldn't have asked for the *best* services. We should've said the "most appropriate" not "best." But how were we supposed to know that? So we're going back for another meeting. This time we know what to say.

Lesson: Again, remember to use the right language. I can't emphasize enough that you should not ask for the *best* services. That will trigger alarms and may put the committee on the defensive right from the start. Ask for *appropriate* services.

Here's what yet another parent experienced.

I knew which treatments I wanted for my daughter, and I even printed out information about these treatments to hand them out in the IEP meeting.

Even though most of the treatments were alternative, I had evidence showing they worked with other kids who had the same issues as my daughter, who was hyperactive and unfocused. I thought the meeting was going well because everyone was listening and being polite, but at the end of the meeting, the head of the committee said that they would not consider alternative treatments because they made educational decisions and the treatments that I wanted were not considered educational. I showed them the website addresses where I got the information so that they would realize the treatments were legitimate. The next day, I spoke with a woman from an advocacy agency who said I was basically barking up the wrong tree. There was no way that I was going to get my school district or any school district to pay for alternative treatments. If I wanted them so badly, I'd have to pay for them myself. The advocacy person suggested that I take the services the committee offered because she said they were good services (ABA, speech, and OT) and that I should start my daughter's treatment. She said it wasn't worth it to even think about suing or fighting the committee to get alternative treatments because I wouldn't get them.

> Lesson: Choose your battles wisely. Don't try to fight for things you cannot win. While you may firmly believe in alternative treatments or that your child should get 50 hours of treatment a week, these are unrealistic goals. Try to set yourself up for success.

On a final note, if you are in the process of asserting your due process rights, your child has the right to stay put in her present educational placement until a resolution has been achieved. This legal rule is called *pendency*. Your child's placement according to the last agreed IEP cannot be changed prior to an adjudication of the dispute, unless you and the district mutually agree on a new placement.

IEP Success Stories from Parents

At this point, you may be feeling intimidated by the prospect of working with a school district's CSE that may not be predisposed to provide meaningful services for your child and apprehensive regarding the amount of work and level of contentiousness that may be required to secure the help your child needs. But it's really not always like that! Even though we had to fight for Jake's early

intervention services, we ended up having wonderful experiences with his preschool and CSE committees. The committee members were gracious and compassionate and demonstrated how much they cared for our son and his needs.
It was truly a collaborative effort, and as a result, Jake was provided with all the
services that he needed. Let me reassure you that many of the parents I consult
with have had positive experiences in getting services for their children. Here
are a couple of their stories.

One father said the following:
We just moved to New Jersey from another state, and we are now receiving all of our services free for our son. The reason we moved was because
we were paying for everything ourselves, and in a year, we'd already spent
$50,000. Only $2,000 was covered by our health insurance company for
speech therapy. We'd heard good things about the schools and services in
New Jersey. I wasn't sure about moving at first, but I'm so glad we did it.
Our IEP went really smoothly. The committee was so helpful. We got all
of the services we needed for our son.

One mother said the following:
My son, who has autism and a severe seizure disorder, is almost three,
and on his birthday, the local school district will take over where the
state's early intervention program left off. I have been dreading his IEP
meeting(s) for months. We live in New Hampshire, and we do not have a
state sales tax or income tax. As a result, education seems to bear the
brunt of the state's money deficit. So, before our IEP meetings, I was
warned by teacher friends, parents of special needs children, and my family members in Massachusetts that we were probably going to have to
move to a state that had better services.

Although my fears were well founded, they haven't come to fruition.
Our meetings went really well. The school system seems to truly want to
help my son. I feel overwhelming relief, but I keep asking myself why do
things seem to be going so well for us when other parents have nightmare
stories? As a result, I've made a quick checklist of things that were done
before and during our IEP meetings. Just for the record, my son's very
helpful and dedicated group of therapists instituted many of these ideas
and procedures.

First, I developed communication with our school's special needs
coordinator and preschool teacher. I visited the school by myself one day,

and then I brought my son in for an afternoon. Basically, I developed a channel of communication with his future educators.

We had a total of three meetings to organize his IEP. At every meeting, his father and I were both there. Some people do not have a spouse to attend meetings with them, but a grandparent or a close family friend will show a support system for your child.

I brought multiple copies of our son's autism diagnosis and psychological workup. I also had copies of other pertinent medical information. I highlighted his doctor's recommendations. I gave these copies to his future educators. Basically, I was letting them know that I was well aware of what my son's needs were.

I was a part of every meeting. I didn't assume that the professionals were the only ones with input. Nobody knows more about the needs of my child than my husband and I. Also, I took specific notes. This way, if something gets changed, I'll have the day and time that an original comment was made.

Before his final meeting, my son's occupational therapist, speech therapists, and ABA coordinator met to finalize our goals. Once they knew what my goals were, and once I got their input, we had an organized proposal.

We live in a rural area, and things are pretty casual here. Nonetheless, I wore a nice outfit to every meeting. As the saying goes, "dress to impress." It has always worked for me at job interviews, sales meetings, and so on. So looking professional when discussing my child's future seemed appropriate.

Now, here's the most important thing that we did for our son. We brought an advocate who was 100 percent in line with our goals—my son's ABA coordinator. She is not a lawyer, but she's sat in on enough IEP meetings with attorneys to know what to say and how to say it. In other words, you can get along with your child's educators, you can have an organized set of goals, you can be the best dressed in the room, but if you bring an advocate, it will get you further than anything else on my checklist. Our school system was well aware that we had an advocate who knew exactly what she was doing. We got what we wanted.

The final step in our IEP process was waiting to sign my son's IEP. We brought it home and read it in a quiet, unrushed setting. Then, we signed it.

FREQUENTLY ASKED QUESTIONS ABOUT THE IFSP AND IEP

Will my child be entitled to treatment services through early intervention or the school district over the summer?

The treatment services granted through your child's IEP are provided during your school district's public school calendar year. In some cases, parents can negotiate in an IEP meeting for what is called an extended school year (ESY). The only way children are entitled to an ESY is if it can be proven that they will experience *substantial regression* without services between the end of the school year and the beginning of the next. While every child with an ASD may experience some level of regression over the summer, parents must prove that their child will regress to the point that it would take him until the following November to catch up to where he left off in June. This is often difficult to prove because, in essence, you are trying to predict your child's future—but it can be done. Make sure you keep good records of your child's progress, including written progress reports, results of standardized tests, and doctors' recommendations. Be prepared for a battle, but go into the IEP meeting with an open mind. Many parents who do not receive services during the summer through their district choose to continue services on their own and pay out-of-pocket for the same providers who worked with their children during the school year.

We have an IEP in place where we live now, but we are moving. Do we use the same IEP in our new school district?

Services not only vary from state to state but also from district to district. This means that even if you move a few miles away from your current address and enter a new school district, your current IEP or IFSP may not be honored in that district.

If you do move, you will need to contact your county or district as soon as possible to request an IEP meeting. Make sure to send in advance or bring with you a copy of your current IEP, as well as all the documentation necessary to support your child's current service needs, such as referrals from doctors and specialists. Also bring in the results of all evaluations, including those conducted prior to the initial IEP meeting and current teacher and/or therapist evaluations.

At the new IEP meeting, make a case for why your child should continue to keep these services or express your concerns about why you think your child's current IEP should be changed. Often, your new county or district will be amenable to honoring your child's current IEP. In some cases, you may hear, "We don't offer that service in this district." If this occurs and you feel that this particular service is crucial for your child, you may request that it be provided by outside agencies at the expense of the school district. In this case, it will be incumbent on you to demonstrate that the service in question is essential to your child's educational progress.

Our district has offered to give us everything we want in terms of services. In fact, they've even offered us more than we asked! They offered 25 hours of ABA when we only requested 20. They offered speech therapy three times a week when we only requested once a week. Is it okay to turn down some of the services?

Parents who are offered a lot of services are in an incredibly fortunate position. Most parents have to fight for them!

My advice is to never turn down services. Although it is within your right to reject services, you almost certainly do not want to do so. First of all, take a step back and evaluate the entire situation. If the committee is recommending these services and hours, there's probably a very good reason. Perhaps they see more than you do that your child really needs the intensity of services. Secondly, if you do decide to turn down services or hours, know the consequences. Rejecting services or hours this year may prevent them from being offered again next year when you may really need them. Thirdly, all of the research studies recommend intensive early intervention. Some parents mistakenly think that by turning down services, they are providing a kinder and gentler alternative to intensive intervention.

Some parents of older children with ASDs now regret that they did not give their children more hours of treatment when their children were younger. Parents who did 10 hours of ABA with their children wish they had done 30 or 40. Parents who never tried other treatments such as OT, PT, or sensory integration wish they had. It's not too late to intensify your child's treatment plan if he is older, but it helps to make it as intense as possible during those early intervention years.

8

ON YOUR MARK, GET SET . . . START TREATMENT

We started treatment and while most of our child's services are covered, some are not. How can we get our health insurance company to help cover at least some of our child's expenses?

Whether or not you will be able to obtain insurance benefits to cover the cost of treatment for ASDs is largely a function of the laws of the state in which you reside. Be sure to check with your health insurance company about what treatments may be covered.

There are currently several states in the United States that have state mandates where coverage for ASDs is required by law, among them California, Texas, New Jersey, Connecticut, Colorado, and Indiana. These mandates are rooted in state laws that require mental health coverage comparable to benefits received for physical ailments. The insurance mandate for ASDs under Indiana State law now defines ASDs as "neurological disorders" and covers certain services such as ABA therapy. In Colorado, several health insurance carriers agreed to cover autism as a "congenital (birth) defect" and pay for 20 visits each of "medically necessary" treatments for speech, occupational, and physical therapy.

In states where the law does not explicitly require insurance companies to cover treatment for ASDs, these insurance companies typically will not cover such treatment. For example, Blue Cross officials in Maryland and Indiana have indicated that they do cover therapy for ASDs in those states where they are required to do so. However, the same officials have indicated that Blue Cross does not cover treatment for ASDs in states where they are not specifically mandated to do so. Cigna has a similar policy of covering treatment for ASDs only in states where such coverage is mandated.

However, even if you live in a state where insurance companies are required to cover treatment for ASDs and even if your insurance company has a stated policy of covering treatment for ASDs when required to do so, actually collecting these benefits may require some diligent effort on your part. In a December 21, 2004 *New York Times* article titled "Battling Insurers over Autism Treatment," Milt Freudenheim reported on Mrs. Beverley Chase's experience collecting insurance benefits for her four-year-old son's autism treatments in Indiana. The family was insured by Cigna, which has a stated policy of covering autism treatments when required by state law—which is the case in Indiana. Nevertheless, according to Mrs. Chase, Cigna was unresponsive to her claim for months, and the company's first response was a rejection of the claim on the basis that the therapist providing treatment was not properly accredited. Due largely to Mrs. Chase's persistence in pursuing the claim, the company eventually agreed to cover the treatment. However, they still required a monthly copayment of $500. Mrs. Chase summarized her experience by noting that in her state the law was on her side and that "if you have the tenacity, the mental health, and the stability," you can prevail. Yet, she also acknowledged that "it is not an easy road."

Of course, parents who live in states where the law does not require insurance coverage for treatment for ASDs will likely have a much more difficult time collecting from their health insurance carriers. We worked hard at trying to get our health insurance company to pay for some of Jake's doctors' visits and treatments, but a lot of effort yielded us very little coverage. (The only insurance coverage we received was a lifetime maximum deductible of 30 visits to a speech therapist of which only 50 percent was covered.) But don't give up. With laws changing in our favor, insurance companies may now offer you more coverage than you imagine. One point of leverage for parents is that a diagnosis for Autism Spectrum Disorders is included in the *Diagnostic and Statistical Manual of Mental Disorders,* published by the American Psychiatric Association (APA 2000) under the heading *PDD*. This is significant because most health plans offer coverage of some kind for most of the mental disorders that are recognized in the manual. According to TACA (Talk About Curing

Autism), there are other reimbursement tips that can be used as well. Because children with ASDs may have physiological issues, such as food allergies, yeast overgrowth, chronic diarrhea, constipation, or other medical conditions, a doctor can code the diagnosis and treatment issues so that they reflect these concerns as well, rather than just using one of the diagnoses of Autism Spectrum Disorders.[1]

In the absence of a specific legal requirement for health insurance to cover treatment for ASDs, a parent may have to be creative and persistent. Sometimes, this may require considerable negotiation and possibly the threat of litigation to obtain any meaningful reimbursement.

Our child's service plan is in place. Is there some sort of guarantee that these treatments will work? What can we expect?

As much as all of us wish that the treatments came with a guarantee, they don't. Time will tell whether or not a treatment is right for your child. There are no hard and fast rules about what your child will accomplish at the beginning of therapy. Each child is different and has a different rate of learning. Most children make wonderful progress with early intensive intervention, but some children are not as fortunate. Researchers don't know why some children respond better than others, and more research will have to be conducted before we're able to predict which children will or will not respond to specific treatments.

It's important as a parent that you set realistic expectations for your child's treatment. A few weeks of speech therapy will not necessarily make your child speak. A few weeks of occupational therapy will not necessarily ensure that your child will gain the proper motor coordination to climb and jump. Sometimes it's helpful to think of your child's therapy in terms of sports training. Would you expect someone to be an ace tennis player after a few lessons on the court or a first-class swimmer after a few classes in the pool? Yet many parents of children with ASDs are quick to judge a treatment if they don't see immediate results. It's important to give the treatments a chance to work.

You'll see results sooner with some treatments than others. Do not expect any one treatment to demonstrate results right away. Parents who do this often end up using a hit-or-miss approach to treatments, which we already know is ineffective. Constantly trying new treatments without giving them a chance to work is disruptive and stressful for your child.

Assess your child's treatments in a thoughtful and objective way. Notice your child's behavior and skills set. Have they improved? What feedback are you getting from the therapists or teachers? Sit in on therapy sessions. Attend meetings at your child's school. Offer therapists or teachers suggestions of ways to work with your child that may help their efforts.

One of the biggest challenges of accurately assessing one particular treatment is that it rarely occurs alone. Since most parents choose a combination of treatments, it is often difficult to isolate the variables to determine exactly which treatment is having a positive or negative effect. Consider which skills and behaviors each treatment is supposed to impact and see if your child is progressing toward those goals. If not, find out why. Some treatments need to be tweaked to have the maximum effect; tweaking may involve a change in frequency or intensity or a modification of the approach. For example, once a child has established a foundation of speech and language skills, the therapist may recommend fewer one-on-one sessions and more group sessions to give the child more opportunities for social interaction. The parents of this same child may want to increase the number of hours in social skills therapy and decrease hours in another treatment.

Again, give the treatments time; give them a chance to work. Only stop a program if you notice an immediate, detrimental effect that you can pinpoint to one specific treatment. Allow at least two months to pass before you decide to change a treatment. Remember, it's a process, and you must allow it to progress over time.

Results vary for each child, and in most cases parents must be patient. In our situation, Jake barely responded to ABA during the first few weeks. A little girl named Sarah, who started her treatment at the same time as Jake, cruised through her ABA programs; the therapists added new programs for her on a daily basis. Sometimes your child will show progress in one area sooner than in another. When Jake began speech therapy, he sat and stared at his speech therapist for the first month while she did all the talking, whereas in occupational therapy, he began showing progress right away—climbing up a ladder, sliding down a ramp, and demonstrating other gross motor skills. Sarah, in contrast, excelled at speech therapy but was lacking in motor coordination skills.

Your child's therapists and/or teachers should tell you how your child is progressing in terms of his or her specific needs. Jake's initial progress was demonstrated in his ability to respond to simple instructions such as "sit down" and "stand up." For one rambunctious little boy named Robby, initial progress meant being able to sit quietly in a chair and focus on putting puzzle pieces on a board. Sarah, who excelled at speaking but would never look at the person to whom she was speaking, began to establish eye contact with her therapist when she talked. Children on the autism spectrum have different needs and experience different rates of progress.

Little victories are among the things that parents learn to use as measures of their children's successes. In the beginning, the fact that Jake could sit through an entire therapy session without crying was a little victory. When he learned to wave and clap, that was a little victory. When Robby was able to tolerate a hug, that was a little victory. When Sarah looked up when her name was called, that was a little victory. Celebrate your child's little victories.

How do I measure the effectiveness of the treatments?

There are many ways to measure the effectiveness of treatments—direct observation, standardized tests, written progress reports, and verbal feedback from therapists. You should be receiving objective feedback, sometimes in the forms of progress reports from schools or updated evaluations and standardized testing from speech and language therapists and occupational therapists. ABA therapists keep daily data collection and give progress reports. Programs that rely exclusively on verbal feedback as measures of progress may not be providing a truly objective evaluation of your child's progress.

Another way to measure the effectiveness of your child's treatment programs is to sit in on your child's treatment sessions and observe. How is your child responding in the session? Is he responding at all? Is there a rapport between your child and the therapist? If you're not sure if a treatment is right for your child, let a fresh set of eyes be your guide. Ask your spouse or even another treatment provider to sit in on a session. Tell them beforehand what the objectives of this treatment are. Is your child achieving the goals set out for him? Is this treatment supposed to be teaching your child functional skills that he needs for everyday life or is it supposed to target one specific area of development? For example, if one of the goals of the treatment is to teach your child to imitate, is your child imitating? If the therapist says your child can imitate in his treatment sessions, is he also able to imitate you or only the therapist? You want to be sure your child's skills are being generalized to other people, to your home environment, and to other activities.

Note your child's reactions during a treatment session. A child's discomfort during a session isn't necessarily an indicator that a treatment is not right. Discomfort can simply be an indicator that the child is being asked to do things that may be challenging or that he may not understand yet. Similarly, your child's complacence during a session does not necessarily indicate that the treatment is working.

Also, take note of which behavioral changes you see in your child outside of the therapy sessions. If there is no change in the behaviors that have been targeted by this treatment, the treatment may not be right for your child or it may need to be modified. One mother complained that her child was still having tantrums at home and asked why the treatment wasn't working to stop his tantrums. As it turned out, the treatment provider had no idea that tantrums were a problem for this child because he never had them during sessions. As a parent, you must openly communicate with your treatment providers and help them set goals for your child.

Because you are so close to your child and see him on a daily basis, you may not notice all of the effects of treatment. While you are focused on other goals, you may not notice subtler changes, such as the fact that your child is stimming less frequently or has replaced an idiosyncratic behavior with an appropriate one. Ask friends or relatives if they notice changes in your child's skills set or behaviors. I also recommend that you videotape treatment sessions. We videotaped most of Jake's ABA sessions, and it was incredible to see the positive changes in his behavior over time. Because we were living with him and constantly raising the bar by working on new behaviors, the video helped us to see just how far he had come.

It can also be helpful to keep records of changes in your child's behaviors and skills, much in the same way that you would keep a baby book. Record your child's initial symptoms and dates. Then, on a weekly or monthly basis, note which treatments are taking place and what changes you notice. While it may not be possible to pinpoint exactly which treatment is responsible for your child's progress, especially when your child is receiving several treatments in the same time period, it's helpful to simply note your child's behavioral changes. Sometimes, it's the combination of treatments that is responsible for your child's progress. Other times, you may see more immediate progress when a new treatment is introduced. But is this a result of the new treatment or because the existing treatments have suddenly kicked in? Without doing controlled scientific experiments, it's just too difficult to tell. In any case, if you are observing positive changes in your child, you most likely have the right treatment programs in place.

If you do decide to drop a treatment, make sure it is because the treatment itself isn't working—not because the treatment provider isn't delivering it properly. I consulted with a family who was not happy with a particular treatment. When I went to observe a session, I discovered that the therapist was not delivering the treatment properly. It turned out that she had not been trained effectively. When the family tried a different, better-qualified therapist, they saw immediate positive changes in their child's behavior.

In addition to observing changes in your child's behavior outside of the therapy sessions, there are other ways to measure a treatment's effectiveness. You should be receiving regular feedback from your treatment providers about how your child is doing. Some feedback will be more concrete than other feedback. ABA therapists will chart your child's progress on graphs and provide written reports; speech and occupational therapists will provide written evaluations. You will receive less formal feedback from alternative treatments like therapeutic horseback riding or homeopathic providers, who usually won't give you written evaluations, but should provide you with verbal feedback about your child. Make sure with any treatment that you receive feedback on a continuous basis.

One bit of warning: Don't become so enamored with a treatment or treatment provider that you lose sight of what the treatment is supposed to be doing. Some treatment techniques are more attractive than others. You may find yourself swayed by fancy equipment or the fact that a certain celebrity is using the very same treatment for his or her child. Being enamored with a treatment (or even the idea of a treatment) can cause you to lose your objectivity, especially when you are feeling desperate to help your child.

Don't stick with a treatment if you think it is abusive, if you notice immediate adverse effects in your child's behavior, or if the provider claims that it's your fault that it's not working. For example, Holding Therapy was a popular treatment in the 1980s that was touted on TV and in the news as a treatment that helped parents bond with their children—and it still exists today. Holding Therapy involves parents forcibly holding their child until the child stops resisting or until a fixed time period has elapsed. This treatment is based on the false premise that the mother has failed to bond properly with her child. Holding Therapy has not only been discovered to be ineffective, but also many now consider it to be abusive; children are often restrained against their wills and become distressed. Proponents of the treatment claim that distress is part of what makes the treatment work, and if parents are not seeing positive results, they must be doing the treatment incorrectly. Be wary of such assertions.

While written reports and data are important in measuring the effectiveness of treatments, so are your instincts. Trust your judgment.

Will my child like the treatment sessions?

In the beginning, treatment can be difficult on both children and parents. For the first few weeks of ABA therapy, Jake cried during every session. He had tantrums through his OT sessions, whined through his speech therapy sessions, and shrieked during visits to the cranial-sacral osteopath. When the therapists showed up for home therapy visits, he clung to my leg and sobbed. I felt as if we were sending our two-year-old to the torture chamber by putting him through this intensive therapy regimen. My husband took a more rational approach. He said, "Jake isn't crying because he's hurt or in danger. He's crying because this is all new to him. He's just uncomfortable—he'll get over it."

Sure enough, Franklin was right. After the first few weeks, Jake's crying stopped, and he actually began to look forward to his therapy sessions. He smiled when the therapy team showed up at the front door and easily allowed them to take him downstairs by the hand. He had all these "firsts" that were little victories: His eyes widened when he squished Play-Doh through his fingers for the first time; he giggled when he understood how to touch his nose when asked; and he was so proud when those first sounds started to come out of his mouth.

Many parents report this same trend—the beginning is rough and then it gets better. One child actually bit one of her therapists when she first started treatment. Another lay down on the floor and refused to get up. One boy sat in a corner and rocked back and forth. But in all of these cases, the children adjusted and went on to look forward to their sessions and show progress.

As a parent, it can be difficult to watch your child go through the initial stages of treatment. My advice? Hang in there. Remind yourself that the beginning is difficult for every child, and that it's going to be okay. Your child will adjust to his or her new treatment schedule—and so will you.

Once my child's treatment/school program begins, how involved should I be?

Some parents think that their direct involvement is over once their child is in a treatment program or at school. This is not the case. You play an important role in your child's treatment. Sit in on treatment sessions as an observer. Ask questions after sessions. Whenever possible, videotape sessions to track your child's progress. If you're running a home program, make sure to have at least one team meeting a month, at which the entire team of therapists meets to discuss your child's progress, brainstorm new ideas, and chart future treatment goals and ob-jectives. If your child is in school, be proactive about communicating with teach-ers to find out about your child's progress. Find out if you can sit in on treatment sessions at school and if you can receive parent training on how to help your child at home.

It's important that you remain informed and aware so that you understand your child's treatment and can help support the therapists' or teachers' efforts outside of the treatment or educational session. Decide with your service provider how often you will sit in on your child's sessions. In the beginning, when children are very young, some parents choose to attend sessions more reg-ularly to support their children and better understand what the treatment is. Ul-timately, you want to do what's most beneficial for your child. In some cases, a parent's presence can provide a sense of comfort and security that the child needs to facilitate the session. In other cases, a parent's presence can be a detriment.

Initially, I sat in on every one of Jake's home ABA sessions. In the begin-ning, my presence was supportive, but after the first few weeks, the therapists felt that Jake might have been crying more in my presence. Sure enough, his crying did dissipate after I sat out. I was still able to view his sessions; I actually hooked up a video camera and monitor and watched his sessions from afar so that I could keep up-to-date with what Jake was learning in his ABA sessions and learn how to teach him on my own. Then, after a few weeks, the ABA team incorporated my presense back into the sessions—in addition to rewarding Jake with food treats and toys, they rewarded him with hugs and play breaks with Mom (rewards that were good for both of us!). In addition to watching Jake's ABA sessions, it was helpful for me to watch Jake's speech and OT ses-sions so that I could reinforce his new skills and behaviors at home and in the community. For example, when Jake was learning to climb and swing in his OT sessions, we'd practice these skills at the playground.

If your child is in school, speak with the teacher about observing class-room or treatment sessions. When Jake was in preschool, it was a distraction for him when I sat in the classroom, but I was able to observe through a win-dow in the door. By watching his aide (an ABA therapist assigned to help Jake at school) demonstrate ways to prompt him in social interactions, I learned how to use these skills in his play dates at home. When Jake was in kinder-garten, I was able to sit in on his small group speech-therapy sessions once every two weeks. This didn't prove to be a distraction at all; in fact, Jake liked it when I joined in the games and exercises, and I learned new ways to help him initiate and maintain conversations.

What does a typical treatment schedule look like?

Your child's schedule will vary depending on his particular needs, the year, and the day of the week. It will adapt and change with his needs. You may end up changing your child's hours of treatment and/or adding or removing another treatment. The schedule will also change when your child first attends school. The following is an example of Jake's typical daily schedule when he was two years old:

Jake's Monday Schedule
9:00 A.M.–11:00 A.M. ABA
11:30 A.M.–12:00 P.M. Speech therapy
12:00 P.M.–12:30 P.M. Lunch
12:30 P.M.–2:30 P.M. ABA
2:30 P.M.–3:00 P.M. Snack/nap
3:00 P.M.–5:00 P.M. ABA
5:30 P.M.–6:00 P.M. Occupational therapy
6:30 P.M.–7:00 P.M. Dinner
7:30 P.M. Bedtime

Here are examples of weekly treatment schedules.

Jake, age two
Diagnosis: PDD-NOS
Description: nonverbal, low receptive language, low-to-intermittent eye contact, no social or relatedness skills, and delayed motor skills

ABA	40 hours/week (home)
Speech therapy	1 hour/week (home)
Occupational therapy (OT)	1 hour/week (OT office)
Cranial-sacral osteopathy	1 hour/month
Dietary intervention	DAN protocol (GF/CF diet; vitamin therapy)
Energetic healing	45 mins/week (weekend)
Naturopath	Homeopathic regimen (daily doses/ appointments every 3 months)
Toddler gym class	45 mins/week (weekend)

Nathan, age four
Diagnosis: Autistic Disorder
Description: low functioning and nonverbal

| Center-based program | 5 full days TEACCH-based program with 1:1 aide/week |

Michael, age five
Diagnosis: Asperger's
Description: highly verbal, limited social skills, and hyper and hyposensitive to sensory stimuli

Kindergarten	Half day inclusion program with 1:1 aide
Speech therapy group 1:3	Two 30-minute sessions (in school with speech therapist)
OT/Sensory integration therapy	Two 45-minute sessions/week (in school with occupational therapist)
Medication	Ritalin, Conserta, Metadate

Will my child's treatment schedule change over time?

Treatments may need to be adapted over time depending on your child's needs. Sometimes you will need to add on more hours of a treatment and sometimes you'll need to subtract. You should prioritize which treatments are the most important for your child at a specific point in time. For example, Jake had 40 hours of intensive one-to-one ABA in private sessions for one year, which were adjusted to 25 hours when he attended preschool. His ABA continued, but in a different way. The ABA team worked as aides to support him at school—prompting him in social interactions and helping him to pick up cues from his peers. The therapists' roles simply shifted to accommodate his progress. We also added other treatments, which you can see from his schedule.

Jake, age four

ABA 1:1	25 hours/week (home)
Preschool	9 hours/week with ABA aide
Peer modeling	1 hour/week with ABA aide (home)

Speech therapy 1:1	Two 45-minute sessions/week (therapist's office)
Occupational therapy 1:1	Two 30-minute sessions/week (OT office)
Social skills therapy 3:1	1 hour/week (home)
Music therapy 1:1	45 mins/week (therapist's office)
Piano lessons 1:1	1 hour/week (home)
Gym class 15:1	1 hour/week (8 sessions/weekend with parent aide)
Cranial-sacral osteopathy	1 hour/month
Energetic healing	45 mins/month
Naturopath	Homeopathic regimen (daily doses/appointments every 3 months)

Again, children's schedules change as their needs change. For example, one girl's tactile hyposensitivity was an overwhelming issue that needed to be addressed immediately at the beginning of her treatment. She had a habit of stabbing pencils into the palms of her hands. She had problems taking her feet off the ground because it was disorienting for her, so she would hold onto the walls of her house to keep her balance while walking. After a year of intensive sensory integration therapy, she no longer engaged in self-injurious behavior and could walk with ease. At this stage, her lack of social skills became a higher priority, and her peer modeling and social skills therapy hours were increased, while her sensory integration hours were decreased. Changes in children's schedules also occur once children attend a school or center-based program. If you have been running a home program, you'll find that many of the treatments you had at home are now covered at the school or center. Parents may also supplement school programs with after-school treatments.

Do not overload your child's schedule. If you do decide to add on more hours of treatment to your child's current schedule, you may want to reduce hours from another treatment. Try to maintain a balance.

Naps are essential for every two-year-old. How can I accommodate this basic need in a treatment program that is all-consuming?

Even though it is not unusual for toddlers to take naps, it's crucial that you use your time wisely. In most cases, you must make a judgment call. Some parents report that their children were able to adjust to more therapy hours and the absence of a nap; other parents report that they tried cutting out naps but had to phase them in again because their children became too tired during their therapy sessions.

In most of the cases I work with, parents decide that therapy is a priority over naptime. In the beginning, it can be difficult because your child may get irritable and may even fall asleep during a treatment session (this happened to Jake initially). But parents often find that by changing their children's schedules so that bedtime is earlier and the morning routine more disciplined, their children are able to adjust to new, more demanding schedules with few problems.

The most important thing is to maintain your child's treatment schedule, whether or not it includes naps. If your child is taking naps, make sure to allow ample wake-up time before a session begins. If your child is not taking naps, make sure to keep a strict bedtime schedule. A well-rested child will be able to learn and retain information better than a tired one.

How do I measure the effectiveness of my child's therapists and treatment providers?

One measure of a therapist's effectiveness is your child's progress. Is your child experiencing success with this therapist? If not, why? Watch the way your child reacts to the therapist during a treatment session and vice versa. Is your child happy to be with the therapist? Is the therapist happy to be with your child? We had a team of ABA therapists, and Jake seemed to be happy and showing progress with everyone except one. She had fabulous credentials; she just wasn't fabulous when working with our son. Therapists have their own personalities, and sometimes their personalities don't match your child's. For example, an outspoken therapist may not relate well to your quiet child, or a timid therapist may not relate well to your rambunctious child. Bonding is an important part of the treatment process. Your child will usually do better with a therapist who connects with him.

Be careful how you judge your child's therapists. For example, some therapists are fantastic at relating to children, but not so great at relating to adults. Be clear about why your child's therapist is there. The therapist's priority should be to help your child. Conversely, do not be seduced by a therapist who is paying more attention to you and not enough to your child. Sometimes the treatment provider becomes *your* savior rather than your child's; the therapist is so compassionate and attentive to you that half of your child's treatment session involves you and your needs. It's okay if your child's therapist does become a friend, as long as the friendship does not impact his or her professional relationship with you and your child. Treatment therapists should always be professional when it comes to working with your child; they should be respectful of your time (sessions should run on time as scheduled) and they should be respectful and open to your opinions and feedback. The treatment provider should also offer consistent verbal feedback on how your child is doing, as well as provide you with written evaluations.

How can I work effectively with my therapy team?

First of all, treat your therapy team with respect. Be kind. Keep in mind that these are the key people responsible for helping your child. In some ways, your team becomes part of your family.

Keep communication open. Make sure your therapists feel comfortable coming to you with both positive and negative feedback. Provide feedback to your therapists about your child's behavior outside of the therapy sessions.

Listen openly to suggestions that your therapists give you. If they ask you to practice certain skills with your child, do it. Anything that you can do to reinforce your child's skills outside of the therapy environment is extremely helpful.

In a way, it's like you're running a business. Make sure your employees are happy and motivated. In return, they'll do their best for you and your child. Show your therapy team that you care about them. These individuals work incredibly hard and are not always recognized for all of their work. Tell them what a good job they are doing. Send a birthday card. Offer a snack at a team meeting. Little things count.

What if one of my child's therapists doesn't agree with the other treatments we're using for our child?

As you know, there are many differing opinions about treatments for ASDs. As I mentioned, in Jake's case, we were told by three different speech therapists that they flat out refused to work with our son if we chose to use ABA. If you're getting that kind of feedback up front, don't try to persuade those providers to work with your child. In fact, if there's someone currently on your therapy team who is vehemently opposed to another treatment technique you are using to the point where it is affecting his or her work and relationship with you and your child, you should seriously consider removing this person from your team.

You'll find that some traditional treatment specialists criticize what are considered to be alternative treatments, and alternative therapists criticize traditional treatments.

If one of your therapists disagrees with your current treatment plan, first of all, hear this person out. It's possible that he or she has had experience with other families who have tried the treatment, only to see negative results. Be open to hearing about different treatment experiences. In the end, however, you need to decide what's best for your child. Sometimes another person's opinion is just an opinion. In our case, even though one of our ABA therapists did not support our choice of using cranial-sacral osteopathy with Jake, this did not interfere with her working relationship with us or with Jake. In fact, it turned out that she didn't know exactly what it was and had chalked it up to another alternative therapy. Once we explained it to her, she was more open to accepting it. Sometimes, even though you are working with so-called experts, you don't realize your own expertise as a parent. As much as you will be learning much from your team of therapists, there's much that they will be able to learn from you.

Can I replace a therapist on my treatment team?

Sometimes things just don't work out with a therapist on your team. The therapist may not bond effectively with your child, not carry out the treatment properly, or have a high rate of absenteeism. In any or all of these cases, it's important that you confront the therapist with your concerns. If the concerns are not resolved, contact your service agency, school district, or the supervising therapist. List your concerns in an objective and businesslike manner. Give specific information regarding why this person is not an effective member of your team.

Make sure to weigh the consequences of losing this person from your treatment team. How many hours are they providing? Is it more beneficial for the person to remain on the team until you find a replacement? Keep in mind that you may have to wait a while before receiving a new service provider.

Will I have to buy new equipment or rearrange my home when I start my child's treatment?

Your therapists will usually tell you what is necessary to help support your child's therapy. Nathan's occupational therapist suggested that his parents purchase a big plastic physio-ball and a trampoline and make use of the swing set in their backyard so Nathan could practice swinging and climbing to help him with his balance and coordination skills. Our basement was converted into an ABA therapy room for Jake. We had to purchase a little table and chairs, notebooks for graphing data, learning tools such as exercises and games recommended by the ABA therapists, a plastic bin that we filled with edible reinforcers (rewards) such as peanuts and raisins, and a big basket of wind-up toys, whistles, and puppets that were also used as reinforcers. In some cases, if the child is doing a computer-based program, parents will be required to have a computer and buy necessary software.

My child was progressing in his therapy but now seems to be regressing. What's happening?

Children may experience progressions and regressions during treatment, and it's unclear why this happens. For example, your child may be able to properly label an apple or teddy bear one day, then be unable to label those same objects the next. Sometimes, parents find that their children experience success in one treatment area and regression in another. For example, your child may demonstrate incredible success in speech therapy while experiencing a regression in motor skills. Some parents report that their children regress when they are sick with a fever; others report just the opposite—that their children seem more focused and on-task when they are ill. Your child may also experience a plateau, during which you see no gains and no losses for a period of time.

Some parents I work with see what I refer to as a regression/surge cycle in their children's progress. They report that after a period of successes, their children show periods of regression. For example, one mother reported that her daughter Sam's echolalia sometimes reappeared in full force after she experienced a period of progress in her treatment programs. We noticed this trend with Jake. After months of progress, Jake would revert back to his self-stimulatory behavior, constantly spinning around or tracking the wheels of his truck with his eyes. This would happen for an entire week, during which he'd regress in his therapy sessions—not remembering skills that he'd already mastered, such as clapping or labeling his colors. Then, after a week of full-on stimming, it was as if his brain rewired, and he'd begin to experience success at full speed.

As with most parents, I initially panicked when Jake showed regression, my greatest fear being that he would remain in his regressed state. But he didn't, and after a few rounds of regression/surge cycles, I became more at ease. Try not to panic if your child shows some regression or has a series of bad days. Don't throw the baby out with the bathwater, so to speak, by immediately stopping a treatment program when this happens. Speak to your therapy team and find out if there were changes in your child's programs. Discuss ideas about ways to adapt a current treatment so that your child will experience success. Sometimes the stress of a new program can cause an initial regression, and you'll just need to wait it out. Other times, a quick fix like changing a child's reward system can resolve the problem.

Will early treatment cause such great improvements in my child that he is able to attend our local public school with typical children?

Your treatment team can help you assess your child's individual needs and determine if your child is ready to attend a general education school. When you are considering schools for your child, you will hear the term *mainstream* used. Mainstream refers to the practice of including and integrating a child with special needs into an educational setting with typical children. Mainstreaming is often used synonymously with *inclusion*. You will hear the term *integrated setting* used as well.

There are different ways that your child can be in an integrated setting, including a self-contained special education classroom, full inclusion, partial inclusion, and a collaborative classroom. A *self-contained classroom* is exclusively for children with special needs (not necessarily all with ASDs) and is taught by a special education teacher. *Full inclusion* means that your child is placed in a typical classroom with children who do not have special needs and is taught by a general education teacher. *Partial inclusion* means that your child is placed in a self-contained special education classroom but is given the opportunity to be included in integrated classes for particular subjects or areas of specialty (such as music and art). A *collaborative classroom* is made up of one-third special needs students and two-thirds typical students and is taught by a special education teacher and a regular education teacher. This teaching arrangement is known as collaborative team teaching (CTT).

Whichever of these four types of classrooms your child is in he may be entitled to receive special services, such as speech or occupational therapy, in a general education setting. The type and frequency of special services is determined during your IEP meeting.

Children with ASDs in integrated settings often have full- or part-time professional aides who help them play, learn, understand directions, communicate, and socialize during the school day. Depending on where you live, this aide may be referred to as a *shadow,* special education itinerant teacher (SEIT), or teacher's aide. An aide can be provided free by your state agency or school district if he or she is included in your child's IFSP or IEP.

Currently, there is a strong educational movement to integrate children with ASDs and other disabilities with their peers in a general education setting. Studies have shown that inclusion can greatly benefit a child with an ASD. By observing and imitating the behaviors of typically developing children, children with ASDs can improve their communication, play, and social skills. Inclusion can also benefit typically developing children as well. Teachers report that children in the classroom develop a heightened awareness of the needs of children with disabilities and learn to be more accepting and sensitive to individual differences in general.

Is inclusion right for your child? It depends on your child's needs and whether she has the prerequisite skills to learn in an integrated setting. Usually a professional who is working with your child, such as your case supervisor, team leader, or treatment provider, will give you advice. If you are just starting out, you can seek out recommendations from the professionals who diagnosed and evaluated your child.

When deciding if inclusion is right for your child, according to Sheila Wagner in *Inclusive Programming for Elementary Students with Autism,* you and the professionals who work with your child will want to take into account the following considerations:

- Academic skills: Is your child [at] grade level? Will he need a modified curriculum? Can your child follow directions and work independently? Does your child pick up on verbal cues, such as two- and three-step directions? ("Go get your pencil, and sit down.")

- Social skills: Does your child demonstrate appropriate play skills? How does he or she respond to other children? Does your child share? Request help? Initiate conversations with other children?

– Behavioral skills: Does your child take part in disruptive behavior? Can he or she sit for extended periods of time? Can your child stay on task?[1]

These are only some of the criteria that you will use to determine whether or not inclusion is right for your elementary school-age child. If you are considering inclusion for your preschool child, these criteria would be modified. For example, your child may need to respond to one-step directions ("sit down") or if she doesn't yet speak, have high imitation skills that may enable her to pick up on peers' verbal or social skills.

You'll also want to visit the school and sit in on the classroom that your child will be attending to see if it is right for her. If your child has sensory issues, see if the classroom setting may be too noisy or bright or if the combination may induce sensory overstimulation that may impede your child's learning. Look at the size of the classroom and the makeup of the children. Find out the length of the school day.

Ask the teacher and/or principal these questions: How accepting is your school of children with ASDs? Are there other children with ASDs in inclusion programs here? What experience do the teachers have with children with ASDs? What will be done to support my child's needs in the classroom? It's important to find out how your child's IEP goals will be supported in the classroom. Since in most cases children will have a classroom aide with them (at least initially), you'll want to find out how the aide can work with the teacher to further your child's success (e.g., through daily communication notebooks). Also, ask about what other services are offered for your child at the school, such as speech and occupational therapy, and how they are incorporated into the school day. If your child is in a contained special needs classroom, ask if he will have the opportunity to interact with other typically developing children. In some schools, children from general education classrooms will visit the special needs classrooms to read to the children or do special art projects with them. It's important to ask questions to make sure the inclusion setting is right for your child. Research has shown that inclusion can be beneficial as long as the programming is well-defined and implemented.

In Jake's case, it was recommended by his ABA team that he enter a general education preschool for an initial few hours a week with one of his ABA therapists as a shadow. Even though Jake had very little speech and language skills when he entered preschool, his other imitation skills were high as a result of his intensive ABA teachings. Initially, Jake needed lots of prompting from his shadow to follow group directions, participate in group activities, and learn group routines. For example, when Jake first started school, I'd walk him to the door of his classroom, and he'd just stand there. The other children would race in behind him saying "Hi, Jake!" They would then put their backpacks in their cubbies, hang up their coats, and sit down and play. When you think about it, this is a rather complex sequence that most typical four-year-olds barely think twice about, and yet, we had to break it down into components so that Jake could learn what to do. Jake's shadow would meet us at the door and guide him through this basic routine until he learned how to do it himself. His shadow would sit behind him during circle time and use gestural and verbal prompts to help him throughout the school day—she'd gently nudge his arm and whisper to him when it was time to raise his hand or get in line for snack time.

After a while, Jake was able to pick up cues from his peers. He'd watch the other children and follow their lead when it came to getting out crayons, drawing pictures, or building blocks. The ABA therapists taught him skills in his individual sessions that enhanced his experience at school. For example, the teacher informed us that Jake was rather passive at school when it came to hanging on to his toys. If he was playing with blocks, another child could easily take them from him without protest. So the ABA team taught him to say "That's mine! Give it back!"—expressions that most four-year-olds know and use naturally. They also taught him to say "Look at me! Watch me!" when he was on the slide or the swing at the playground—common expressions that you'll hear from most typical children at any school or playground. These expressions helped Jake to get a response from his peers, which in turn helped his social interactions. Jake was happy when a child watched him push his train around the track after he'd said, "Look at me!" The social reinforcement was key in helping Jake make friends.

Another mother reported that her son benefited from inclusion because he was hyperlexic, meaning he had a precocious ability to read words (he'd been reading since he was two years old). Even though he had limited verbal skills, his mother felt that the contained special education classroom did not meet her son's academic needs, so he began in an inclusion classroom in first grade. He had a full-time shadow and was taken out of the classroom for speech and occupational therapy. When asked how the other first graders reacted to her son, she said, "The other kids in the class knew it was cool not to pick on him and so they didn't." She reports that they still don't. Her son is now in high school and is happily learning geography and history along with his peers. This mother is extremely satisfied with her son's progress in an integrated setting, but she cautions other parents that inclusion is not always the easiest option: "It requires an intense commitment from parents. You really have to be an advocate for your child, and sometimes that means fighting for your child's services and also teaching the teachers how to help your child."

While inclusion may work well for some children with ASDs, it is not right for every child. One father reported that his daughter started out in a full-inclusion setting, but was then transferred to a special education classroom at the same school. "It was too much for her. She was in sensory overload. There were too many kids in the classroom, and it was too loud for her. She started stimming again. Her aide recommended that we move her into a special education class that was smaller. She's doing much better now." Another parent reported that she never even considered inclusion. "Our son was too low-functioning. It was never an option. We knew he had to attend a special school for autism."

Inclusion options may change as a child grows and develops; while it may not be right for a child initially, it may be right for a child once her foundation skills are established through intensive treatment. As a parent, know that you have options for your child's education and work to place your child in the setting that will most benefit her.

What if we don't use any treatment at all? Will my child grow out of his ASD?

Years ago, children with ASDs were considered to be hopeless, and parents were told to either leave them alone or put them into institutions. No treatments were offered. As far as we know, there were no stories of spontaneous recovery. This is because children with ASDs generally do not learn things naturally from their environments the way that typically developing children do. Typical children pick up imitation, speech and language, social, and play skills just by being exposed to other people in a natural environment. Children with ASDs do not. However, now we know that with intensive early intervention in which conditions are optimized for learning the same skills that typical children learn naturally, children with ASDs are able to learn and grow.

Intensive early intervention can have a profound effect on children with ASDs, so if your child has been diagnosed, don't take a wait-and-see approach. Be proactive. Get your child the help he needs as quickly as possible.

Will all of this treatment change my child's unique personality?

There is one school of thought that contends that individuals with ASDs, especially those with high-functioning autism and Asperger's, should not be rid of their ASDs. These individuals believe that their ASDs are what makes them special and resent the thought that treatment may remove their quirkiness and idiosyncratic behaviors. This was the focus of the December 20, 2004 *New York Times* article titled "How About Not 'Curing' Us, Some Autistics Are Pleading" by Amy Harmon. In response to this article, I wrote a letter to the editor, which appeared in the *New York Times* on December 22, 2004.

> To the Editor:
>
> Re: "How About Not 'Curing' Us, Some Autistics Are Pleading" (front page, Dec. 20): As the mother of a child who recovered from autism through intensive behavioral treatment, I respect that individual differences and the need for treatment are not mutually exclusive. The article highlighted the school of thought that people with autism should not be treated because their autism is what makes them special.
>
> Everyone should be respected and appreciated for his or her uniqueness. Parents of children with autism want most of the same things as parents of typical children. They want the best for them: to help their children get along in the world, to communicate, interact and to make friends.
>
> Treatment is not the enemy. Treatment for autism can be seen as the equivalent of schooling for the typical child. Both can help children achieve their full potential by identifying and nurturing core strengths and individual differences.
>
> Why shouldn't children with autism have the same opportunities to learn and grow as typical children?

Parents of children with ASDs have all kinds of hopes and dreams. Some dream of college and marriage for their children, while others hope simply to receive a hug or hear the words "I love you." With treatment, perhaps these children will achieve these goals, but perhaps not. At the very least, I believe that treatment will offer them the opportunity to fulfill their truest potential.

Can treatments "cure" children with ASDs?

Some children with ASDs do experience what is referred to as *recovery*. Children who achieve recovery from ASDs no longer meet the criteria outlined in the DSM-IV-TR. They are considered to be "no longer on the autism spectrum." Some recovered children still exhibit quirky or idiosyncratic behavior (such as minor finger flicking or tapping) or have other developmental issues (such as slower motor coordination or speech and language impairments). There is also a small percentage of children who experience full recovery and look and act like any other typical child. Jake is one of these children. But when Jake was first pronounced recovered, he still had some catching up to do. While he no longer met any of the criteria for PDD-NOS and had no residual stimming or idiosyncratic behaviors, his skills still lagged behind those of other children his own age. Jake did not speak as fluently as his peers, had slower auditory processing, and needed a therapist to support him on play dates. We continued his full treatment program of speech therapy, social skills therapy, and ABA-supported inclusion at his school.

Dr. Deborah Fein and colleagues at the University of Connecticut are currently researching children who experience recovery from ASDs. Dr. Fein recognizes that children who move from "autism to a behavioral picture of nonautism" are in the minority (the actual numbers are unknown), but there are documented cases. In one study, Fein found that eleven children in her practice who initially presented with classic autism or PDD-NOS as young children no longer met the criteria for ASDs after receiving intensive ABA therapy. These children did show some minor residual behaviors and had some attention deficits and social problems, but the children were more similar to the typical ADHD child (who is social and wants friends but is somewhat impulsive and immature). In a second study, Fein and colleagues described fourteen children who moved from autism to nonautism. These children were all mainstreamed with no significant educational support and were receiving only minimal outside therapy, such as 1 hour of speech therapy per week. This study focused on their language at ages six to nine. The researchers found that while this group did show rather subtle residual language impairments, most aspects of their language were well within typical range. As with the first group, these children had also been through intensive ABA therapy at young ages. Because her studies thus far have primarily involved children who have been through ABA therapy, Fein acknowledges that her sample is not a random one; it can't be concluded from her papers that ABA is necessarily the only treatment that can lead to this outcome, nor that ABA guarantees this kind of success with every child.[2]

Children on the autism spectrum experience different levels of success. Just as there is a spectrum for autism disorders, there is a spectrum of success. Some previously nonverbal children learn to speak. Some children remain nonverbal but learn how to communicate through gestures or pictures. Others learn to play, interact, tie their shoes, brush their teeth, establish eye contact, sit quietly in a chair, respond to their name, and hug their parents.

How much can you expect for your child? Time will tell. But if you're in the process of choosing your child's treatment or if your child is already receiving treatment, you're already on the right road.

PART III:
COPING

When you get to the end of your rope, tie a knot and hang on.

—FRANKLIN D. ROOSEVELT

Never, never, never give up.

—WINSTON CHURCHILL

Like Alice of Alice in Wonderland, I was sliding down the rabbit hole. I was so focused on trying to help Jake that I lost sight of everything else around me. I put my work on hold, stopped talking to my friends, and pretty much shut myself away in our house—the house of autism. If it wasn't about autism, I didn't want to know.

When I finally did leave the house, I discovered a side of me that I didn't know existed. I pretty much hated everyone. I hated bank tellers, gas station attendants, grocery store clerks, the dry cleaner with the toupee that was always slightly askew, the deli owner's wife who wore too much perfume and not enough deodorant, and little dogs in sweaters. Basically, I hated anyone or anything that seemed to be leading a typical life.

But most of all, I hated the mothers—especially the mothers who appeared at the playground with their "healthy" children. What had I done wrong? We had all probably read the same pregnancy books, taken the same prenatal vitamins, and attended the same kinds of Lamaze classes. I had even bought a Walkman with an extra headset to pipe Mozart into my belly. And I had tried to keep up that healthy pregnancy diet, only I ended up cheating and substituting the home-made organic zucchini bread with Twinkies.

All of the other children at the playground turned out just fine. They talked, played, and had loads of fun.

Maybe their mothers ate the zucchini bread.

I hated them all. The mothers.

And I desperately wished I could be one of them.

Then there was my marriage. I don't think I even noticed that it was going down the toilet. It happened gradually.

Franklin and I dealt with Jake's autism differently. I spent my days research-ing autism and my nights crying. Franklin left for work earlier and came home later.

"Jake will be just fine," he kept insisting.

Franklin's denial became my bedrock of security.

It was also the force that was driving us apart.

Franklin went through the motions of supporting Jake's therapy, but it took him months before he could finally "see" Jake's autism. When he did, he was dev-astated. His dreams of sharing baseball games and hiking trips with his son were shattered. I thought that on some level his wrenching revelation might actually bring us closer as a couple. It didn't. Instead, every ounce of our combined energy was directed toward healing our son, with none left over to nurture our own rela-tionship. At first we fought, then gave it up. We were too drained to argue. Weeks passed that seemed like years. When Franklin and I finally sat down to talk for the first time in months, the discussion was focused not on Jake, but on whether or not our marriage would survive.

Then there was the money issue. The financial burden of Jake's therapy was almost as intense as the emotional one. We weren't given any early intervention services at first even though we were legally entitled to them, so we had to pay out-of-pocket for all of Jake's treatment. We thought our health insurance would cover it, but it didn't. In the midst of trying to manage all of Jake's treatments, I ended up having to prepare for a court battle with our state agency to get reimbursement for Jake's services, a trial that dragged on for months. Being a witness in a case that involved my son was one of the most difficult things I ever had to do. In the end, we won what we should have been given in the first place. Then, just when I thought our legal battles were finally over, a year later, we were in another lawsuit and our case was settled out of court.

But there was a silver lining to all this: It just took a while to emerge. As a result of our court case, we were told, families in our community now receive treatment services more easily. The other good news is that our marriage did survive—in fact, Franklin and I became even closer, establishing a special and lasting bond as a result of everything that we have gone through together surrounding Jake's diagnosis. Franklin began to work less so that he could spend more time with Jake. I also stopped hating everyone—including all of the mothers—as I became more accepting of Jake's diagnosis and our new life. I began to reclaim a life outside of the house and work again, only instead of returning to my work as a management consultant coaching executives in the business world, I began to consult with families of newly diagnosed children with ASDs.

No one seems to talk about how the diagnosis of ASDs affects every part of your life. After Jake was diagnosed, the focus was on getting him help. All the experts were there to offer opinions on which treatments to choose and how to get services—all of the necessary first steps that are crucial in helping your child with an ASD. But what the experts don't talk about are the effects of the diagnosis on your marriage, family, friendships, other children, work, and everyday life.

"Life as usual" no longer exists and is replaced with another life filled with new rules and expectations. Many of us parents feel like we've landed on another planet: Planet ASDs. It is a place filled with children who exhibit idiosyncratic behaviors and doctors who speak a different language. For a while we don't unpack our bags, hoping that we won't be staying very long, but then it hits us that we're going to be here for a while. So we unpack and figure out a way to make our new lives work. We come to the realization that while we can't control our child's diagnosis, we can control how we choose to respond to it. We can decide how we're going to spend our time and manage our relationships. The more we realize what we can *do, for ourselves and for our children, the more we can move forward on our journeys.*

One of the most poignant examples of this new life is described in an essay by Emily Perl Kingsley, titled "Welcome to Holland."

Welcome to Holland

I am often asked to describe the experience of raising a child with a disability—to try to help people who have not shared that unique experience to understand it, to imagine how it would feel. It's like this. . . .

When you're going to have a baby, it's like planning a fabulous vacation trip—to Italy. You buy a bunch of guide books and make your wonderful plans. The Coliseum. The Michelangelo David. The gondolas in Venice. You may learn some handy phrases in Italian. It's all very exciting.

After months of eager anticipation, the day finally arrives. You pack your bags and off you go. Several hours later, the plane lands. The stewardess comes in and says, "Welcome to Holland."

"*Holland*?!?" you say. "What do you mean Holland?? I signed up for Italy! I'm supposed to be in Italy. All my life I've dreamed of going to Italy."

But there's been a change in the flight plan. They've landed in Holland, and there you must stay.

The important thing is that they haven't taken you to a horrible, disgusting, filthy place, full of pestilence, famine, and disease. It's just a different place.

So you must go out and buy new guide books. And you must learn a whole new language. And you will meet a whole new group of people you would never have met.

It's just a *different* place. It's slower-paced than Italy, less flashy than Italy. But after you've been there for a while and you catch your breath, you look around . . . and you begin to notice that Holland has windmills . . . and Holland has tulips. Holland even has Rembrandts.

But everyone you know is busy coming and going from Italy . . . and they're all bragging about what a wonderful time they had there. And for the rest of your life, you will say "Yes, that's where I was supposed to go. That's what I had planned."

And the pain of that will never, ever, ever, *ever* go away . . . because the loss of that dream is a very, very significant loss.

But . . . if you spend your life mourning the fact that you didn't get to Italy, you may never be free to enjoy the very special, the very lovely things . . . about Holland.

Your trip to Holland may not have been what you planned for or expected, but at some point it will feel like home. You won't be alone in unpacking and settling in—you'll be surrounded by people like you who were just as surprised as you were to find themselves there. The beginning is the most difficult part. Unpacking means that you'll have to accept your child's diagnosis, which can be a big hurdle that exists right at the beginning of the road to your new life. This section will help take you over that hurdle and beyond. You will learn tips on how to cope with issues surrounding diagnosis, treatment, therapists, family, friends, and relationships in the community. You will hear true stories from other parents about how they handled situations in their lives. My hope is that by the end of this section, you will feel less alone on your journey and more comfortable and confident in your new world.

IN THE BEGINNING: COMING TO TERMS WITH THE DIAGNOSIS AND ISSUES SURROUNDING THE DIAGNOSIS

How do I cope with all of the emotions I'm feeling about my child's diagnosis?

You may experience a range of emotions after learning that your child is diagnosed with an ASD. Many parents experience a sense of loss, which may pertain to a loss of one's old life (the way it used to be) or a loss of one's future life (the way it may have been). You may mourn the loss of certain dreams and hopes that you had for your child with an ASD. You may have feelings of fear, worry, confusion, guilt, embarrassment, resentment, and a sense of existential loneliness—as if no one in the entire universe could remotely understand what you are going through. You may find yourself plagued with questions such as *Why me? Why did this have to happen to my child? What have I done to deserve this?* Fantasies about future ballet classes and baseball games are instantly wiped out when we hear the words, "Your child has autism."

Many parents go through something similar to the stages of grief as described by psychiatrist Elizabeth Kübler-Ross.

Denial: *No, not me—this can't be happening to me. My child's diagnosis cannot be true.*

Anger: *Why is this happening to me?*

Bargaining: *I promise I'll be a better person if . . . you make my child's autism go away.*

Depression: *I'm feeling miserable. My life has no meaning.*

Acceptance: *It's okay. I'm ready for whatever life has in store for me.*[1]

Parents pass through these stages in their own time, and sometimes it can be a long road to acceptance. Parents can get stuck in one of the stages and need time to process their feelings before moving on.

As a mother, I had first-hand experience riding this emotional rollercoaster. I thought that on some level I'd feel relieved once Jake was diagnosed and we finally had a name for what was wrong with our son. Instead, I felt numb—in shock. On top of this, I felt as if I'd set myself up for the fall. I was the one who decided to take our son to the doctor. I was the one who insisted on finding answers. It was as if I'd just stood in the middle of the road and allowed myself to get hit by a Mack truck. So after I received my son's diagnosis, I cried, told a few family members and close friends, and untold them a week later.

After conducting my own research, I came to the conclusion that my son did not have PDD-NOS or any diagnosis related to autism. I'd been overreacting to his symptoms, I rationalized. And so I stopped crying. My denial became my shield. That is, until a few days later when I went back to the playground and watched the other children play and laugh while Jake lay silently in the sandbox, repeatedly pushing a plastic truck back and forth in front of his face. Within the confines of our own home, Jake was just fine; I'd grown used to his spinning and silence. But outside, it was as though a spotlight shined on him, magnifying all the things that were wrong with him. My denial faded away, and I passed through all of the other stages of grief.

Isolation came next. We had recently moved to a new city, and the last thing I felt like doing was sharing my grief with new neighbors. Besides, I was having enough trouble dealing with the diagnosis myself. So I stayed in my house, shutting myself off from the rest of the world. I didn't even call my old friends. I felt as if no one could understand what I was going through.

Anger followed. When it hit, I wasn't prepared for the extent of my pent-up rage. I was furious and distressed about the diagnosis, and my anger seemed to extend to every aspect of my life. I was angry at myself, my husband, even at our poor defenseless son. I was angry that I'd have to give up my work. I resented all the mothers (many of whom were my friends) for having children who talked and played, while my own son was silent and passive: *Why me and not them?*

I quickly passed through the bargaining stage where I'd make daily pacts with myself—such as, *I'll be a better person if Jake's autism will go away.*

Then I plunged into depression. Although I understood and recognized that Jake had autism, I remained depressed for months. Some psychologists say that depression is really anger turned inward. That was probably the case with me. After a while, my anger became buried under so much guilt and pain that I began to retreat and draw inward. True acceptance, the last phase of the grief cycle—where I felt comfortable in my own skin and with our new life—would not come for more than a year.

As isolated as I was, I had no idea that most parents of children with ASDs experience similar roller-coaster rides of emotional turmoil. I didn't know that it was okay for me to express my feelings or that I could do so in a constructive manner. I learned the hard way, and it almost cost me my marriage. Most of my pent-up rage was directed at my husband, who still couldn't see that anything was really wrong with our son. My feelings just poured out of me—and onto Franklin. He bore the brunt of my rage. In my eyes, he could do nothing right. In addition to not taking our son's diagnosis seriously, he was not taking out the garbage fast enough or was chewing too loudly. I'd use any excuse to yell at him. If we hadn't found a therapist, I don't think our marriage would have survived. I'm not sure how well *I* would have survived.

Most of us experience intense feelings when our children are diagnosed. One father, Jonathan Shestack, describes what he went through when his son was diagnosed.

> You want your child to get better so much that you literally become that desire. It is the prayer you utter on going to bed, the first thought upon waking, the mantra that floats into consciousness, bidden or unbidden, every ten minutes of every day of every year of your life. Make him whole, make him well, bring him back to us.

Psychologists recommend that you allow yourself to experience your feelings. Holding in feelings can be detrimental to your psychological, emotional, and physical health. Anger turned inward can lead to depression. Bottled-up grief can lead to illness. Even if you feel like isolating yourself, even if you doubt that anyone else can truly understand what you're going through, try to figure out a way to express your feelings constructively. Keep a journal. Speak to a therapist. Confide in a close friend or family member. Join a support group for parents of children with ASDs.

One mother shared the following:

> The autism support group totally saved me. I finally felt like I could talk to people who knew what I was going through. I felt so alone before and then I found out I wasn't the only one.

During this time, the most important thing to remember is to not become isolated. Therapy can be extremely helpful when you're trying to sort out your feelings about the diagnosis. There is individual therapy, couples therapy, and group therapy. Sessions may be run by a psychologist, psychiatrist, psychoanalyst, psychotherapist, or social worker. There are also wonderful support groups in the community of ASDs, both live and online. Contact your local autism organizations to find out about the ones in your community (see Appendices D and E). The following is some advice from parents:

> Find some alone time, even if it means you just sit down and cry. Don't keep your feelings bottled up. Sometimes I just needed a good cry and then I felt better. The beginning is the toughest part. It does get better—I swear. Just hang in there.

> I was feeling so overwhelmed all the time. It felt like I was under so much pressure. So I decided that every day I was going to do just one thing to make myself feel better. One thing. Even if it was only for fifteen minutes. I'd take a walk, read *People* magazine, eat a cupcake, or call my best friend. Doing that one thing for myself every day had a major effect on me. It helped me turn my depression and despair into hope and action.

> I have two kids on the spectrum, so I'm pretty much an expert on coping now. That first month or two or three requires a lot of strength, but it also requires a lot of sorrow. When my first child was diagnosed, I defined a 'good day' as one where I didn't cry before 10:00 A.M. I think that initial stage is essential. You have to let yourself feel it and then use that energy to motivate yourself. Feel it and then get to work. You have to take care of

your own mind before you can help shape your child's. You have to find a balance where you have enough strength and creativity to meet the challenges. As a parent you know your child, and you will be their biggest support, advocate, and healer. But first you have to heal.

The old adage "time heals all wounds" does apply here. How much time you will need to process your emotions is an individual thing. If your child has just been diagnosed with an ASD, you may find it hard to believe that you'll ever feel better. But you will. Be patient. Accept yourself for where you are now. Trust that, eventually, the anger and hurt will subside, and you will reach a place of overall acceptance.

No matter what anyone says, I still feel like I caused my child to have an ASD. How do I deal with the guilt?

Feelings of guilt are natural when you're trying to accept your child's diagnosis. Even though Bettelheim's theory of the refrigerator mother has long been disproved, many parents—especially mothers—still experience feelings of guilt. Studies show that mothers respond with more guilt to a child's diagnosis than fathers (Gray 2002).[2] Through the process of interviews and the parent questionnaire that I distributed to both mothers and fathers of children with ASDs, I discovered this as well. Mothers also harbor many of the same doubts: *Were my genes to blame? Was it my diet during the pregnancy? Was I too old when I was pregnant?* Mothers (more than fathers) also have a tendency to direct "should" scenarios at themselves—such as, *I should have opted for natural childbirth instead of having had the labor-inducing drug pitocin. I should have noticed my child's symptoms earlier. I shouldn't have immunized my child. I should have been more attentive, more loving, less stressed out. . . .*

Sometimes guilt can also lead to blame. Instead of keeping that finger pointed at ourselves, we turn it around and point it at others. We blame our spouses, parents, grandparents, aunts, uncles, in-laws, and any other family members who could have potentially contributed to our child's diagnosis.

Feelings of guilt and blame are common reactions to a child's diagnosis of an ASD. It's important to have your feelings, but don't let them consume or incapacitate you. Find a healthy and constructive way to deal with your feelings. All the energy you spend blaming yourself and/or others could be better spent on treating your child and maintaining familial relationships.

How do I cope with the A-word? I can't even bring myself to say the word *autism* when I'm describing my child.

Some parents don't want to hear or use the A-word in connection with their children. Even though the current term for autism is ASDs, most doctors and professionals still use the word *autism*. This can be devastating because, for many people, autism carries a stigma.

I was one of those parents who was initially uncomfortable with using the A-word. For me, it was less about admitting it to the world and more about admitting it to myself. I could not stand to hear myself say that my son had autism, so I continued to say that Jake had been diagnosed with PDD-NOS. When someone asked me what I meant, I offered an explanation that included the term *developmental disorder,* carefully avoiding the A-word.

During this time, I was on the phone with the father of a child with an ASD. He kept referring to Jake as having autism. When I finally corrected him, he responded by saying, "PDD-NOS, PDD, call it what you will—it's all autism." Besides, he joked, autism is easier to say. I listened to him use the word over and over during the rest of the conversation and, by the end, I had to admit that I was becoming more comfortable with it.

The more I used the word autism, the easier it became to say. As I grew more involved in the world of ASDs, I learned that many parents use the word to describe their children's diagnoses no matter where their children fall on the spectrum. At the very least, they used the word interchangeably with the official diagnosis.

As more and more children have been diagnosed with ASDs, the mainstream media have zeroed in on the subject. Consequently, the disorder has lost a lot of its stigma and become much more acceptable to the public and to parents of kids with the disorder. And yet, not all parents are comfortable with the diagnosis. I consulted with one family who could not accept their son's diagnosis of autism despite the fact that he displayed classic symptoms such as hand flapping, spinning, and no language. They did acknowledge that there was something wrong with him, but refused to accept the A-word. So they took their three-year-old to five different doctors, including a developmental pediatrician, speech pathologist, and three pediatric neurologists in three different states. The first four doctors gave the boy a diagnosis of autism. These parents would have continued their quest if that fifth doctor hadn't offered a diagnosis called Landau Kleffner, which is not on the autism spectrum. That was the diagnosis they accepted. The entire diagnostic process took them more than six months—months that could have been spent treating their son. Ironically, the treatment that the doctor recommended for Landau Kleffner was one that is also recommended for autism.

Call your child's diagnosis whatever makes you feel comfortable, but don't get so hung up on the A-word that you end up losing precious time that could be devoted to getting your child the help he needs. And consider this: If those of us in the community of ASDs can't use the word autism, aren't we just perpetuating the stigma? Perhaps the more we use the word, the more the general public will come to accept it.

My spouse can't even mention our son's name and autism in the same breath. In fact, he's in denial that there's anything wrong with our son at all. What can I do?

It's not uncommon to hear stories about one spouse being in denial about his or her child's diagnosis. As we already know, an ASD is a weighty diagnosis that can elicit a lot of deep emotions. Denial, on the one hand, can often act as a protective coating, allowing us to insulate ourselves from feelings that may seem too difficult to process. Acceptance, on the other hand, allows us to embrace a child who is not perfect and embrace a life that is not at all as we had planned, hoped, or dreamed.

There are also cases where both parents are in denial. I've received calls from concerned grandparents, aunts, and uncles who suspect ASDs in their grandchildren, nieces, or nephews. After hinting around or even directly confronting the parents, these family members are distressed by the parents' inability to accept the fact that anything is wrong with their children. Parents of children with ASDs are not the only ones who go into denial. Other family members and friends may experience it as well. Grandparents often have as much difficulty as parents in accepting the diagnosis. In one case where the parents were struggling to accept the diagnosis, the grandparents insisted that there was nothing wrong with their grandson. They said the parents worried too much and suggested that the parents just leave him alone.

Denial can lead to many kinds of issues—especially relationship issues. When one spouse is in denial, all the work related to a child's diagnosis falls to the other spouse. This spouse often performs a solo act in terms of researching and getting the child help, which can create a buildup of resentment in the relationship. When grandparents, relatives, or friends are in denial, relationships can become strained. The parents of the affected child, who are dealing with their own emotions, are often faced with the additional burden of feeling responsible for the emotions of others. They may expend an inordinate amount of energy trying to convince their relatives and friends that the diagnosis is real. Sometimes, a parent will fall victim to the unresolved feelings of the person in denial and perhaps hear such statements as, "There's nothing wrong with our grandson. You always tend to overreact," or "It's nothing serious. You just didn't read to your daughter enough." Many parents hear that they just don't know how to discipline their child correctly or that the reason for their child's behavior is because they spoil him.

When Franklin was in denial, my instinct was to yell, "Snap out of it!" Initially, I did yell. I tried my hardest to point out what was wrong with our son. But Franklin came up with reasons why Jake was okay. Jake was just a late talker, like Franklin. . . . Jake's shyness prevented him from interacting with other children. His strained eye movements were a result of a nervous habit. And his outbursts were typical of boys his age—remember what the pediatrician had said about the terrible two's? But my instincts and two doctors' diagnoses had already confirmed what he did not want to see—his son had autism.

Franklin did emerge from his denial after three long months, but it was only after I stopped trying so hard to convince him that something was wrong. When I stopped fighting and just let go, he was able to really see his son's condition.

So what do you do if someone close to you is in denial about your child's diagnosis? As difficult as this may sound, the first thing you must try to do is respect them and accept where they are emotionally. Acceptance does not mean agreement; it involves listening and respecting the person's hurt feelings, which are usually deep-seated in someone who is experiencing denial. Your ability to listen openly to those feelings and show empathy will help that person be less defensive and more open to your point of view. All of us have a tendency to react from our own point of view, and in a highly emotional situation, we're often quick to react with disagreement or advice, with little regard for the other person's point of view. Even when we think we are listening, we may be interrupting or formulating new arguments instead. As much as we may want to yell "Snap out of it!" and force the other person to see our reality, it won't help—in fact, it may drive him or her more deeply into a place of denial.

For example, if your spouse says, "There's really nothing wrong with our son—you're just overreacting," instead of responding with, "You don't know what you're talking about," try to see his or her point of view. Why would your spouse think that? What are the unexpressed feelings? Most people don't express their feelings explicitly. Often you must read between the lines—observe their tone of voice and body language. Do they sound angry? Do they look sad? Try to respond on an emotional level. Acknowledge their feelings. Say, "I know you're upset, and I understand that our child's diagnosis is difficult for you."

Reflecting feelings shows that you are listening openly and in good faith. Reflecting feelings is a simple yet incredibly powerful strategy for showing empathy and removing defensiveness. Try it. The next time your child or spouse is upset, instead of becoming defensive or argumentative, say, "You seem upset" or "You seem sad," and watch what happens. The heated emotions will dissipate. Noted psychologist Carl Rogers emphasized the importance of empathetic listening. According to Rogers, "people only listen when they feel listened to." It is only when a person's feelings are acknowledged and respected that he or she can get to the point of feeling deeply understood—of feeling "heard." Feeling heard without judgment can allow a person to go on to express more feelings.[3]

Part of denial can also be a result of not fully understanding the disorder. Many people have preconceived notions about autism spectrum disorders. Provide them with the facts about what your child's diagnosis really is. Share articles, books, or case studies that describe your child. Often, while one parent is shouldering much of the responsibility, the other is left in the dark about the details of the diagnosis and treatment plan. Sharing information can be an extremely useful way to help a loved one "see" and accept a child's diagnosis.

Who do I tell about my child's diagnosis?

Choosing whom to share your child's diagnosis with is a personal decision, but the most important thing is that you do share it with someone. Isolating yourself and withdrawing into a world of grief can be unhealthy for both you and your child.

Some parents choose to share the diagnosis with many people—family, friends, other parents at the playground, and people in the community—as a way to explain why their child's behavior is different. It takes pressure off them by offering the diagnosis as an explanation for their child's horrific tantrum in the supermarket or inappropriate behavior at the neighborhood playground. Parents of children with ASDs can feel unduly judged or blamed if their children are acting out in public, and sharing the diagnosis can often elicit tolerance and compassion.

If you're still feeling raw and vulnerable after your child's diagnosis, however, it's best just to tell the people closest to you. This will help ease your burden and set up a support system. I initially felt the need to be more private. At the playground, surrounded by parents of typical children, it was easier for me to offer excuses for Jake's behavior rather than a full-blown explanation of his condition. "Boys talk later than girls," I'd say if someone commented on his silent behavior. "He's just tired—he missed his nap today," I'd say when someone observed that Jake was lying on his belly in the sandbox. However, I felt comfortable telling complete strangers who had no contact with me or my son about Jake's diagnosis; the customer service representatives at the phone company and credit card companies knew all about Jake's diagnosis because, in my efforts to explain why all of our bills were being paid late, I just let it out. (It felt surprisingly good to vent to complete strangers.)

Even after I came to terms with our son's diagnosis, it still took me a year to begin sharing his diagnosis with the world at large. While I was still struggling with Jake's diagnosis on a personal level, I had been cautioned by other parents of newly diagnosed children that my son may be stigmatized and ostracized in the community if I shared the diagnosis with too many people. Since we had just moved to our new city, I was afraid. But when I started coming out and sharing Jake's diagnosis, I found the opposite reaction to be true. Neighbors and people in the community were extremely generous and understanding. They wanted to know more about the disorder and what they could do to help.

Make sure you share your child's diagnosis with your immediate family. If you have other children at home, it's also important to share the diagnosis with them. Chapter 13 will offer tips on how to explain the disorder to your other children.

How do I handle and respond to some of the well-meaning but frustrating things people are saying to me as a result of my child's diagnosis?

"Everything happens for a reason."

"It could be worse. I know someone whose child was in a car accident. . . ."

"It'll all be okay; you just mark my words."

"This whole experience will make you a stronger person."

"I had a feeling there was something wrong with your child, but I didn't want to say anything to upset you. It's good you finally found out."

"I know exactly how you feel. It's so much worse when it's your own child. My son was sick last year with the flu for two weeks, and it was so difficult."

At some point, you will hear one or more of these types of statements from someone who cares about you, and it will take all of your restraint to not tell them to shut up. Even though you recognize that they are trying to help you, it's still hard to hear these comments. The bottom line is that if they haven't had a child diagnosed with an ASD, they don't know how you feel—which is why they may say all the wrong things in an attempt to make you feel better. For the moment, you may not even want to feel better; you may need to feel angry, depressed, and resentful. And yes, it probably could be worse, but at that moment it's not helpful to hear this because at that moment it feels like the worst thing that could ever happen to you.

Loved ones generally mean well, but in a desperate attempt to help you, they may end up offering unsound advice or clichés. As the parent of a newly diagnosed child, don't be afraid to take control and tell people directly what you need to hear or what you find difficult to hear. In my case, I initially found myself holding in a lot of anger and resentment toward friends and family members because of what they said. But after a while, I learned to ask them to stop telling me that "everything was going to be okay" and that "things happen for a reason" because it caused me too much anxiety. How did they know what was going to happen? And for what reason did we deserve this? I also learned to ask for what I wanted: "I want you to listen to me and be there for me, but please don't offer me condolences, clichés, or advice." Many friends and family reported that it was a relief to hear what I wanted so that they didn't have to guess.

It's okay for you to ask for help. Many of us feel like we must do everything ourselves and that it's a sign of weakness to ask for help. But now is the time to recognize that asking for help is not a sign of weakness. In fact, it takes strength and courage to share with others what you want and need. Remember, you are ultimately asking for help that will benefit your child.

Believe it or not, asking for help will also benefit the person you are asking. All the relatives and friends who feel helpless will be empowered. Be specific about what you want. Ask for help with grocery shopping, running errands, or taking care of your child or children for an hour or an afternoon. Even ask for financial help if necessary. Recognize that friends and family members probably want to help you out during this time. Help them to help you.

10

BEYOND SOCCER GAMES AND BALLET CLASSES: COPING WITH ISSUES SURROUNDING TREATMENTS, SERVICES, AND SCHOOLS

I'm still feeling emotionally drained. Can I wait until I'm feeling stronger to get treatment services for my child?

Don't deny your feelings, but don't allow them to hold you back from getting treatment for your child. Your child needs treatment as soon as possible, and it's up to you to make this happen.

One cognitive technique that psychologists recommend to relieve emotional stress is called *compartmentalizing*. This involves putting your thoughts or feelings into a separate compartment in your mind so that you can focus on what needs to be done in the present moment. For example, if you're feeling emotionally overwhelmed about your child with an ASD, visualize placing your feelings into a box and putting it on a shelf. This can help you focus on making those phone calls for services or taking care of other business without feeling distracted by your emotional state. By removing the emotional component for even an hour, you will feel stronger and more able to make rational decisions.

Another coping tip for when you're feeling emotionally overwhelmed is to do what actors do: Play a role. This was a tip I used to give professionals in the corporate world to help them assume their roles as managers. You already play the role of parent, but now you need to jump into a few other roles—those of researcher, businessperson, advocate, and spokesperson. In a way, you're like an agent who is representing a client, and the client just happens to be your child. How do you do this? Shift your mindset. Even though you are feeling one way, act another way. Get your head into business mode. If you've been moping around the house in your pajamas, get dressed. Go to work, even if it's in your own home. Allow yourself a temporary detachment from your feelings and pretend that you are a researcher. Speak to other parents and professionals in the world of ASDs. Seek out positive mentors who can offer you support and advice. Ask questions. Take notes. Be proactive in getting your child the services he needs. Become your child's advocate.

This acting exercise is much easier than you may think. In fact, many parents report that this intellectual exercise gives them a break from feeling consumed by their emotional reactions to their children's diagnoses.

While my friends are driving their kids to soccer practice and dance classes, I'm driving my child to speech therapy and OT. How do I adjust to my new life?

Adjusting to your new life will take some time, especially since it was completely unplanned. In the meantime, many of your friends are doing with their children the very things that you had planned to do with yours. One way to deal with this situation is to use what's referred to as *cognitive restructuring*. Don't dwell on your friends' lives. Instead of telling yourself how much you wish you were driving your child to soccer practice, try telling yourself that you're doing what's best for your child right now.

You may be surprised at how quickly your life will return to normal—normal, at least, in the sense that driving your child to speech therapy becomes a regular part of your daily or weekly routine. While you may not be a soccer mom or dad right now, you're a speech therapy mom or dad, and you'll soon realize that you're not the only one out there. You'll be able to bond with other parents in the same situation.

We have a home program for our child. There are therapists coming in and out of our house all day long. How do we handle this?

Home programming can be a mixed blessing. On the one hand, you don't have to constantly drive your child from one treatment specialist to another. On the other hand, you do have to deal with various people coming into your private home almost every day.

To make this situation more comfortable and less intrusive, try setting up a separate room or area of the house or apartment that becomes the child's treatment space. Organize it in such a way that is conducive to running a therapy session. Try to keep distractions at a minimum—no phone, TV, or background noise whenever possible—at least in the beginning. After a while, as your child adjusts to sessions, background noises may be added into your child's treatment session as a way to teach him to stay focused even if there are distractions. Your therapists will tell you how to set up the space and what supplies you may need to purchase, such as games, toys, or therapeutic tools.

Be considerate of the therapists' time and your child's needs. If your child's first session begins at 9:00 A.M., make sure your child is dressed and fed before the session begins. If your child has taken a nap before an afternoon session, make sure he has ample waking time before the session begins. Feeling rushed or exhausted when entering a therapy session can cause your child to feel anxious and unfocused.

Be aware of boundaries. Since the therapists are in your home on a daily basis and have formed a special relationship with you and your child, they can begin to feel like part of the family. While they may seem like relatives or close friends, they are there for your child first and foremost. This means that it's not appropriate for you to engage in idle chat with the therapist during your child's session time.

Treat your therapists with respect. After all, they are the ones who are helping you help your child. They are guests in your home. Offer them coffee or a glass of water. Show them that you care by saying thank you and telling them how much you appreciate their help. All of these kindnesses will be returned to you tenfold.

(Note to therapists and treatment providers: Please extend the same aforementioned courtesies to parents. Be respectful, on time, aware of boundaries, and kind. Parents also need to hear that they're doing a good job.)

I have all these therapists who are working to help my son. In some ways, I feel like I'm running a business, but I never went to business school. Any suggestions?

Managing your child's treatment program can be similar to running a business. You are the CEO, your therapy team makes up your employees, and your company's mission is to help your child. Like any business manager, you will need to manage your time effectively, setting priorities and goals, motivating your employees, making sure employees are compensated on a timely basis, and handling day-to-day concerns such as sick days, vacation days, and holidays.

Here are some tips I used to offer in my corporate seminars that can be extremely helpful in running a home therapy program and/or managing your child's treatment schedule.

- *Organize.* Business executives use palm pilots or organizers to plan their schedules. You can do the same. In addition, posting a schedule on the refrigerator or any other central place in your home can help you keep track of your child's time. Since most schedules stay the same on a weekly basis, you can draw up a simple schedule that begins like this.

Day	Treatment/Activity	Time	Provider
Monday	ABA session	9:00 A.M.–11:00 A.M.	Laura
	Speech therapy	11:30 A.M.–12:15 P.M.	Sandy
	Lunch	12:15 P.M.–12:45 P.M.	
	Occupational therapy	1:00 P.M.–1:45 P.M.	Debby

And so on.

- *"Put first things first."* That's what leadership expert Stephen R. Covey suggests. In other words, set your priorities. Your priorities change when your child is diagnosed; therefore, you need to manage your time differently. Learn to delegate. If you're in the habit of doing everything yourself around the house or staying late at work, you need to start assigning responsibilities to others or ask for help. Also, learn to say no; if you're used to saying yes to being on every committee or helping out every friend, accept the fact that you have other priorities right now. Be flexible and learn to roll with the punches. Sometimes unexpected things will come up: Your child is sick and misses therapy sessions, or your therapist has to cancel. Don't let these situations unnerve you. Let go of the feeling that the world will end if your child misses a treatment session. (I know this from personal experience. I used to get extremely upset if a therapist called in sick and would frantically call other therapists to fill in. I felt that Jake would experience some major regression if he missed even one session. Eventually, I realized that my stress level was adversely affecting my son more than his missed session.)

– *Set goals and objectives.* Meet with your child's therapy team to establish goals and ways to achieve those goals. In the corporate world, goals and objectives are revisited on a regular basis. You need to do the same thing when it comes to your child. Your therapy team should serve as a guide to establishing specific goals and objectives. Make sure they are realistic. A goal such as "My child will speak over the next few months" is not appropriate. A goal such as "my child will practice vocal imitations for X amount of time" is more appropriate.

– *Work as a team.* Some parents feel entitled to boss around their therapy team, while others relinquish their power and defer completely to the professionals. Neither of these strategies is effective. Work together with your team on a continual basis. Ask questions. Offer input.

– *Motivate your employees.* Your therapy team sees a lot of different children, and deals with a lot of stressful issues that come up on a daily basis. They are often exhausted and feel unappreciated. Show them respect. Let them know you care. Remember, the best way to reinforce a behavior is to reward it! A sincere "thank you," a holiday gift, or even a tin of cookies can go a long way toward keeping your treatment providers motivated to help your child.

– *Make sure your employees are compensated on a timely basis.* Your team will most likely be paid by your state agency or school district. Sometimes you'll need to follow up with the agency or district if payment is delayed. If you are paying out-of-pocket, make sure to pay as soon as possible after you receive your invoice. Delays in payment may affect your team's motivation.

– *Discuss vacations, sick days, and holidays in advance.* Different therapists will have different policies regarding compensation. Since agencies and districts abide by the local public school calendar, therapists are not paid for times when the schools are closed for holidays or vacations. If you want your therapists to work with your child during these times (and many parents do), you will have to pay them out-of-pocket. Some therapists will charge you for unused hours if you cancel for any reason but will not charge you if they are the ones who have to cancel. Discuss these issues in advance so that there are no surprises.

What can I do to help out my child's treatment?

As I mentioned earlier you need to stay actively involved in your child's treatment. Sit in on some of your child's therapy sessions. Ask questions. Listen to your therapists' feedback. Learn how to reinforce some of the skills that your child is being taught. Offer your own feedback. Let the therapists know how your child is behaving at home.

There are some parents who don't get involved in their children's treatment and just assume that by sending their children to an expert, the expert is somehow fixing them within the confines of the therapy session and therefore needs no parental help. But treatment does not happen in a vacuum. Parents are an integral part of the treatment process. Reinforcing and building on a child's skills can benefit both the child and parent. Your child will be able to practice skills that can lead to success, and as a parent, you will feel more connected with your child.

Sometimes, even though we understand the importance of reinforcing our child's new skills, it's just not that easy to do. For example, when our ABA therapy team was first teaching Jake how to point with his finger to indicate what he wanted, Jake had difficulty because he was used to grunting to get what he wanted. In the sessions, the therapists would hold up an item, such as a toy truck or a cup of juice, and say, "What do you want?" Jake had to point to one of them to get rewarded. In the beginning, the therapists would help him by putting their hand over his and shaping his hands and fingers into a pointing position, and he'd get reinforced for trying. After a while, Jake learned how to point in his therapy sessions, but we still had to reinforce this skill around the house for him to be able to generalize it. So, if Jake came into the kitchen after an ABA session and wanted a cookie, instead of grunting in the direction of the food cabinet, he had to point. Then, I was instructed to say, "What do you want?" and give him the cookie only after he pointed to it. We were told that if we just gave into Jake's grunting and handed him the cookie, he'd become confused and have trouble learning the correct behavior.

It all made perfect sense: Reward the behavior you want repeated. We did our best to reinforce all of Jake's newly taught behaviors and create new opportunities for learning. We invented fun games so that Jake could practice imitating our movements; we repeatedly placed him on the bottom rung of the ladder at the playground and said "Good climbing the ladder," as we guided his little body upward; we purposely dropped pencils and other objects on the floor repeatedly when he was learning to say "Uh oh." Honestly, a life of reinforcing Jake's therapy 24/7 was hard work and could be frustrating at times, both for us and for Jake. There were tears shed (on both Jake's and our part), but there were also humorous moments, like when I started saying to my husband, "Good washing the dishes" and "Good taking out the trash."

In the end, most parents find that the more they stay involved with their children's treatment and the more they reinforce the new skills and behaviors that are being taught, the better for both them and their children.

At first it seemed like every minute was filled with treatment sessions, but now I've become aware that I have pockets of downtime between treatment sessions. What am I supposed to do with my child during this time?

Downtime in the world of ASDs is considered to be the time between treatment sessions or before or after dinner, during which there are no scheduled activities for your child. For instance, there may be a 30-minute break in between home ABA sessions, a total of 40 minutes in the car driving to and from the speech therapist's office, or an hour before dinnertime. Even though your day may seem chock-full of treatment sessions, if you add up all the in-between time, there's actually a lot of downtime. While typical children will use downtime to play games or talk about their days, children with ASDs will often use downtime to engage in stimming or misbehaviors. Jake would stand in line with me at the grocery store and repeatedly open and close his fists or sit in his car seat and mechanically shift his eyes right and left. If I continued to let him stim without interrupting or redirecting his attention, his stimming would grow more intense. So at the grocery store, I'd give Jake something else to do with his hands, like helping me unload the grocery cart. And when he was stimming in the backseat, I'd call his name so he would look at me, and then reward him with a cracker. It was up to me to find ways to use this downtime productively.

The most productive way to use this time is to find or create teachable moments that will allow your child to practice new skills. This is especially important because most children with ASDs do not learn from their environments the way typical children do. For example, a typical child can observe someone waving good-bye and repeat the behavior. But this does not happen with the majority of children with ASDs. Jake had a lot of trouble learning to wave good-bye. This was a skill that he practiced in his ABA sessions, but he still couldn't get it. So Franklin and I made a game of it. Jake and I would stand in the kitchen, and Franklin would walk into the living room. "Bye!" Franklin would say as he rounded the corner to leave. "Wave bye-bye!" I'd prompt Jake, lifting up his hand and showing him how to wave. We'd walk from room to room in the house. We'd also use real opportunities to practice waving good-bye, such as when Franklin left for work in the morning and when therapists left after their sessions.

There were times outside of the house when Jake and I would practice some of the other skills he'd either recently acquired or was just learning in therapy to help him generalize. Of course, sometimes I'd have to create these "real" situations. Waiting in line at the bank, I'd drop a penny on purpose and say, "Jake, pick it up." When he did, I'd say, "Good boy! Good picking up the penny. Give me five!" He'd slap my hand and smile, proud of his accomplishment. I never really thought about how odd we must have looked until one day at the playground, when I was sitting in the sandbox with Jake, and I threw a yellow plastic shovel in the corner. "Go get!" I said. He stood up and ran over to the corner, picked up the shovel, and ran back to me, proudly displaying it. "Good getting the shovel." Then I repeated this exercise with a pail, a truck, and anything else I could dig out of the sand. After about ten minutes of this, we switched to the slide, located right next to the sandbox. Jake had been practicing climbing skills in his OT sessions, and I watched as he put one foot on the ladder, then the other, making his way up the rungs until he reached the top. Then he wriggled onto his bottom, and slid down the slide. "Good sliding down the slide!" After a few rounds of this, a mother who had been sitting on the edge of the sandbox looked at me and said, "Excuse me, I can't help but ask. . . . Is English your son's second language?" I began to laugh. It was the first time that I saw what others saw. This mom who repeated short phrases over and over to her son. In a way, yes, English was Jake's second language. It was replacing grunting and stimming, which seemed to be his first.

Here are some tips on what you can do with your child during downtime.

– *Bring along a bag of toys, games, and learning tools.* When you're in the car or out in the community, carry flashcards and books. This will encourage appropriate play rather than stimming behavior. Make sure to rotate the selection so that your child stays interested and to avoid fixation on a single object.

– *Talk. Sing. Find fun ways to communicate.* Even if your child hasn't learned to speak yet, your child can still learn by listening to you. When you're driving, you can describe the sights and sounds, such as saying, "Look at the red stop sign!" Or put on a fun CD and say, "Listen to the music!" If you're at home, find fun ways to engage your child using pots and pans as musical instruments, or practice what your child is learning in a treatment session, such as "Touch your nose!" or "Clap your hands!"

– *Encourage social awareness.* If you're at the playground, say, "Look at the girl with the ball!" Take your child by the hand and lead her to another child, prompting her to say, "Hi!" If your child cannot speak, sit her down in the sandbox next to another child and show her how to make a sand castle or dig a hole. Encourage your child to imitate what the other child is doing (provided that it's appropriate behavior. You don't want your child to imitate throwing or eating sand). You can also invite the other child to join in helping you build a sand castle.

In an ideal world, you would fill every moment of your child's downtime with learning opportunities. But there are going to be those days when you just need a break, and it's okay to take one. There were stressful days when Jake would be stimming in his car seat, and I just couldn't bring myself to stop the car one more time to interrupt and redirect his behavior. So I just turned up the volume on the radio and pretended that it just wasn't happening. I felt some guilt, but I got over it. You will, too. As parents, it's okay to admit that in the midst of trying our best to fill in our children's downtime productively, sometimes we just need some real downtime for ourselves.

I can't help comparing my child with other kids. At the playground, I compare him with typical kids. Even at his special school for autism, I compare him with other kids with ASDs. Sometimes, I feel hurt that he just isn't doing as well as other kids. What can I do?

It's fairly common for parents to observe their children's peers and note how their own children measure up in terms of behaviors, skills, and abilities—whether or not they have ASDs. But the competitiveness that many parents of children with ASDs experience is often mixed with feelings of hurt or anger, and these emotions can be detrimental to developing a positive attitude toward a child's healing.

It is generally our comparisons that lead our children to be diagnosed in the first place. We compare our children with their siblings, other kids at the playground, or the developmental chart that tells us at what age our children should be sitting up, walking, or talking. Jake's pediatrician accused me of being a "competitive New York mom" because my concerns about Jake's behaviors were based on my comparisons with other children his age. The doctor argued that, as a first-time mother, I didn't know that all children developed at different rates. Yet, in retrospect, I realize that as a first-time mother, had I not compared him with other children at the playground, I wouldn't have realized just how serious his condition was as early as I did.

Some comparisons with other children can be fair and practical, such as using them to identify your child's symptoms of an ASD. But comparing your child with typical peers can set you up for unrealistic expectations and eventual heartache. I'm not suggesting that you prevent yourself from looking at other kids—that's unrealistic. But I am suggesting that you think twice about *how* you're looking. I learned to be an anthropologist of sorts; I observed typical kids playing and interacting so that I knew what appropriate behaviors actually looked like in kids Jake's age. That helped me clarify goals for Jake's treatment and understand some of the things that didn't immediately make sense to me in his therapy.

For example, I wondered why Jake had ABA programs that taught him to slap the therapist's hand in response to "Give me five!" or why he had to learn to say, "Look at me!" when he slid down the slide or climbed up a ladder on the swing set. Sure enough, by observing typical kids at play, I realized that Jake was practicing classic behaviors and skills exhibited by most kids his age. It seemed that every kid at the playground knew how to respond to "Give me five!" and that it was a very common greeting. Also, almost every kid shouted "Watch me!" or "Look at me!" from the top of the slide, while swinging on the swings, or just while running around. It seemed as if there was this whole code of social behaviors that every typical child seemed to be born with but that remained a secret code to kids with ASDs who needed it to be decoded, broken down, and taught in simple steps.

In addition to comparing their children with typical children, parents also tend to compare their children with other children with ASDs. Again, this is not a fair comparison because no two children are the same, even if both are on the autism spectrum. Children with ASDs have different rates of development. One mother of a child in a special school for autism kept parallel tabs on her son's progress and that of another child who started school at the same time as hers. At the end of the school year, she was dismayed to learn that her son was still not speaking, yet the other child was. She began to feel hopeless. But the director of the school reminded her of the many advances her son had accomplished. He no longer had tantrums before every meal. In fact, he could actually sit still at a meal—something that seemed nearly impossible for him when he started the program. Instead of stimming constantly as he once did, this boy now played games with other children. The more the director talked, the more the mother realized that her son had made incredible strides. She had been so focused on the other child that she had neglected to notice just how well her own son had been doing.

You may encounter competitive parents in the world of ASDs. If nothing else, this should make you feel like one of the parents of a typical child, who experience this all the time—in encounters with other parents who want to see how many music, dance, and gym classes their child is enrolled in just so they can brag about their own child's busy schedule. There are parents in the world of ASDs who may drop the name of an obscure treatment to see if you know it or ask how many treatments you've tried, how much language your child has acquired, or whether your child is mainstreamed. My advice to you is to avoid this game. Don't get sucked into the comparisons and competitiveness game. It won't help you at all.

Make a choice. Choose to focus on your own child and her accomplishments, no matter how big or small. Studies show that whatever we choose to focus on in our lives becomes a dominant force. Focusing on the negatives will make us more pessimistic; focusing on the positives will make us more optimistic. If you focus on your child's deficits, those deficits become magnified and overshadow any positives. Comparing your child with another child, typical or with an ASD, is a waste of energy because, at the end of the day, it doesn't change the reality of where your child is developmentally. Focus your energy on your own child—on her personal goals, what makes your child happy, the little victories along the way, and all the positive things in her life. These are the things that are important to your child in the real world, not the relative world. Celebrate your child for who she is and where she is right now.

When my daughter started treatment services, I met another mom whose son had just started his services at the same time. His mom and I have become friends, and we often ask how each other's kids are doing. The problem is that my daughter is doing much better than her son. I know this sounds crazy, but I feel guilty about this. Can you help me?

Just as it can be difficult if your child is not doing as well as other children, it can also be difficult if your child is succeeding. It's not uncommon for parents to feel jealous when their children are not achieving milestones that similar children have reached and guilty when their children reach ones that other children haven't. I experienced both sides of this scenario. In the beginning, I was extremely jealous that another child who had started treatment at the same time as Jake was already talking, while Jake was nonverbal and could barely clap his hands. Jake's progress was extremely slow in the first six months of treatment. On the flip side, when Jake's skills finally did emerge and he began to do well in his treatments, I felt pangs of guilt when he surpassed this other child. If you find yourself in one of these situations, my advice is to have your feelings without acting on them. You can have your feelings of guilt about your child's successes without needing to apologize profusely or make excuses to another parent whose child is not progressing at the same rate as yours. However, don't brag. I know of one mother who is so proud of her son's accomplishments that she unintentionally hurts other moms with her boasting. Be sensitive to others' feelings and connected to your own.

My child has been receiving treatments at home and at facilities near our home. I'm always with him, so I'm on top of everything he's doing. But soon he will be attending a school, and I'm feeling vulnerable. I won't have the same kind of control as I did before. What can I do to stay on top of my child's progress?

Most parents experience anxiety when their children go to school for the first time, and when their children have ASDs, the anxiety may be even greater. You want to make sure your child is okay on his own, that he is safe, and that his individual needs are being met.

If your child is in a special school for autism, you can stay on top of your child's progress by attending and being an active participant at school clinics. Share your observations and thoughts with the teachers, therapists, aides, and service providers who work with your child. Many schools for autism offer weekly or monthly clinics or team meetings, to which parents are invited to meet with the treatment team to discuss their children's current progress and future goals. Make sure you take advantage of this opportunity! Your child is usually present so that you can actually observe how the treatment is delivered and learn what you can do to reinforce the teachings at home. This is a great time for you to ask questions and inform the team about how your child is doing at home. Your input is a crucial component of these meetings. At the team meetings, in addition to discussing your child's current progress, goals, and objectives, you can also discuss your feelings about the treatment process. The treatment process can be confusing and overwhelming to parents, engendering feelings of frustration; you may feel frustrated that the process is taking so long—that your child isn't speaking yet or continues to tantrum. Often the team can offer you explanations, practical advice, and suggestions on how to cope.

In addition to holding team meetings, most schools for autism will also send home written progress reports throughout the school year to let you know how your child is doing. These reports can also be used in your child's IEP meetings.

If your child is in an inclusion program at a general education school, you will not have regularly scheduled team meetings and meetings with your child's speech, occupational, or physical therapists, or any other professional who works with your child. However, you can request parent-teacher meetings. In the classroom, your child will probably have a shadow (also referred to as an aide or a SEIT), who is there specifically to help your child cope and achieve success throughout the school day. Your child's shadow should provide you with daily feedback on your child's progress. Following are some ways to feel more in control and stay on top of how your child is doing:

1. *Be honest about your child's diagnosis and needs. Empower school personnel—the teacher(s), principal, lunchroom supervisor, and anyone else with whom your child may come in contact—with ways to help your child.* Some parents want to keep their child's diagnosis under wraps in an inclusion environment because they feel that an ASD carries a stigma. I'm not suggesting that you make an announcement to the entire classroom of students, but you do need to tell the relevant personnel. Otherwise, your child may be misunderstood and judged unfairly.

   One mother learned the hard way. In her parent-teacher conference, the teacher complained that her son was a troublemaker, always interrupting and blurting out inappropriate comments in the middle of class. She threw up her hands and said to the child's parents, "I'm planning on flunking your son. You should have done a better job of disciplining him." The mother started crying. Both she and her husband and the child's therapists had worked so hard to prepare their child for school. Feeling backed into a corner, the mother broke down and told the teacher about her son's diagnosis. Much to the mother's surprise, the teacher softened. The teacher could now view the child through a different set of eyes. His outbursts were not intentional; they were a manifestation of his disorder. His anxious reactions, which she had found overly dramatic, were real. This was a child who needed order. If the teacher could spend a few minutes at the beginning of the day making sure his schoolbooks were in order, he would feel less anxious throughout the day.

2. *Set up a daily communication system with the teacher and shadow.* Create a chart of approximately ten to twenty skills you want to track for your child, and track approximately five skills at a time. You can organize the chart by time and subject so that you can track whether or not problem behaviors occur at certain times of the day or during certain lessons. By identifying what triggers your child's problems, you can step in and remediate. Make sure to keep the chart simple. Teachers are busy, and it's unrealistic to expect them to fill out a complicated daily journal. The simpler you make it, the easier it will be for a teacher and/or shadow to

keep you updated on a daily basis. A checklist is best. For example, your checklist could include the following:

☐ Follows directions

☐ Stays calm

☐ Completes assigned work

☐ Transitions smoothly from one class to another

☐ Raises hand to answer questions

Simply ask the teacher to check off each skill or behavior that your child accomplishes throughout the day. Next to any items that your child doesn't accomplish, the teacher can write a brief comment about what happened. If your child has more than one teacher, make sure copies are distributed to each one. Have your child bring home the reports in his backpack.

3. *Communicate with and train your child's shadow.* Because many shadows are not professionals in the field of ASDs (they may have a degree in general special education), you can request that the school district send them to a training program to teach them skills specific to shadowing a child with an ASD. You can also ask the district to hire a professional consultant who specializes in teaching social skills. In the meantime, you can train the shadow on what behaviors you are targeting. In fact, the shadow can also fill out the teacher checklist with additional details, such as notes about why your child is not accomplishing a certain skill. To avoid making your child feel singled out in the classroom, especially as he gets older, the shadow can say that she is there to assist the entire class, rather than there only for your child.

4. *Don't blame the teachers—teach the teachers!* This includes the shadows as well. Some parents believe that once children leave the house, it is the teachers' responsibility to fix them, and if parents don't notice progress or a situation isn't handled to their liking, they blame the teachers. Instead of blaming, be proactive in teaching the teachers and shadows how to work with your child. Identify your child's specific

needs. Target problem behaviors and offer solutions. Be specific. General suggestions such as "You've got to handle my son's outbursts better when you see one coming" are not effective. Inform teachers about warning signs. One mother told the teacher that before her son had an outburst, he would stand up and start finger flicking. This was usually a sign that he was feeling overwhelmed. All he needed was to find someplace quiet to collect himself. The teacher worked it out so that when she noticed the boy's early warning signs, she'd gently suggest that he take a walk to the library.

Offer other valuable teaching tips. Teachers can identify your child's strengths and put your child in charge of a particular project that relates to those strengths. For example, if your child is a good artist, the teacher can ask her to do a sketch and ask the other children to color it in. This can boost self-esteem and promote social interaction. Or if your child is good at math, the teacher can partner her up with a child who needs help in math, so that your child can play the role of tutor. This benefits both children and can help your child gain the respect of her peers.

5. *As your child gets older, teach your child how to self-manage.* For example, a child can learn to recognize her own warning signs of mounting frustration or stress, such as finger flicking, foot tapping, or another stimming behavior, and initiate deep breathing or other relaxation techniques. Your child can also learn coping strategies, such as how to ask for a break or for help. You can teach your child good comebacks to teasing. Give your child a logbook where, over the course of the school day, she can write down what bothers, disappoints, or confuses her. Set a specific time for her to review the logbook with you or her teacher. You can also set specific times throughout the day when the child has to "check in" with her teacher.

Whether your child attends a special school for ASDs or a general education school, keep the lines of communication open among you, the teachers, your child's shadow, and school personnel. You play an integral part in helping your child to succeed in school.

I'd always dreamed of my child attending our local public school, and he reached that goal. But now he's in fifth grade, and I'm not so sure it's the right environment for him. What can I do?

It's always valuable for you to reassess your child's school and treatment plan to make sure it's right for him at that point in time. An inclusion kindergarten environment may be the perfect fit for your child, but higher grade levels (especially middle school) may present social challenges that have a negative impact on his self-esteem.

This was the case with one child who was extremely bright and motivated but had difficulty making friends or even sustaining two-way conversations with peers. His lack of social skills was tolerable when he was younger (there are fewer social pressures in lower grades), but his idiosyncratic behaviors and awkward social interactions became more of an issue when he was a preadolescent at age eleven in middle school. Middle school can present a difficult transition for typical children as well. Hormones change and so do peer pressures. Even though this boy had an aide with him in the classroom to help prompt him in challenging social situations, it seemed that now most of his social interactions were with the aide. When he was younger, he didn't think twice about having an aide with him in the classroom, but as he became older, he became self-conscious about having an aide. He also became aware that he had no friends even though he desperately wanted to make friends. He became depressed. Luckily, his parents were aware of his feelings and made a change. Instead of sending him to a large public general education school, they sent him to a small, private school that other children with special needs attended. The boy received intensive social skills training after school to help him make friends. Now, at twelve years old, he's in a classroom with ten other students, where he has a best friend and a renewed sense of confidence.

In another case, parents found that rather than moving their child out of their local public school, they would change the current situation. They hired a social skills therapist who not only helped their son but also taught all the other children lessons on tolerance and compassion and ways to communicate more effectively with children with ASDs. Another set of parents found that by moving their child out of a general education school to a school that taught high-functioning children with ASDs, their child received more individualized attention from special education teachers who understood their son's disorder better than regular education teachers. Yet another set of parents sent their child to a public school, pulled him out for a few years to place him in a smaller private school, and sent him back to a general education public school when he was more socially prepared. As you can see, there are many options when it comes to providing a suitable school environment for your child.

When deciding whether or not your child's school situation is appropriate, be sure to keep your child's needs in mind and not your own. The competitive world that exists among parents of typical children also exists among parents of children with ASDs. Unfortunately, to protect their own egos, some parents will place their children in a general education environment before they are ready or keep them in a general education environment when it is no longer appropriate for them.

I want my child to make friends. I've heard that social skills are important to teach to kids with ASDs, but I don't know how to do it.

The majority of children with ASDs have difficulty employing social interation skills, as previously mentioned. Teaching appropriate peer interactions at a young age is an important part of a comprehensive behavioral treatment program (Taylor 2001).[1] Setting the stage for social interactions when your child is two or three years old can help your child make friends and relate to peers when he is older.

Typical children are wired for socialization from infancy. They naturally engage in joint attention, which we know from chapter three is an early social skill whereby a child and parent (or other adult) share the experience of looking at an object or watching an event together. Most children with ASDs are not intrinsically motivated to socialize, preferring instead to retreat into themselves and focus on certain objects, facts, or routines that they find comforting. Even though socialization may not come naturally to children with ASDs, they can and should be taught to socialize. Research shows that involving typically developing peers in social skills interventions provides children with ASDs the opportunities to observe, imitate, and learn from the social skills and behaviors of their peers (Kamps et al 2002).[2]

Social skills training can be incorporated into existing treatment programs, such as ABA, or into the school day during recess or at lunchtime. Social skills can be taught by parents and caregivers at home as well. Social skills behavior therapist Terese Dana recommends the following at-home tips to promote social skills in your child:[3]

– *Make the games simple and interactive.* Play "Follow the Leader" or a game that involves rolling a ball back and forth between you and your child. Use simple language and imitation to teach new skills. Practice the games repeatedly until your child feels comfortable and confident enough to generalize the play skills in group situations. After your child has mastered simple games, you can introduce more complex games such as playing tag or board games, which are made up of many skills that need to be broken down and taught. If your child is in school, find out what games are being played in physical education class or at recess so that you can teach them to your child in advance.

– *Create or adapt games around topics that will motivate your child to participate.* For example, if your child loves dinosaurs, you can create a game where you pretend that a small ball is a dinosaur egg. The children can pass the ball to one another to keep it away from the T. rex who is chasing them to eat the egg. By creating games around your child's interests, your child will be happier and more motivated to engage socially.

– *Choose or create games that target your child's specific needs.* For instance, Jake had trouble playing catch because he couldn't stand having anything thrown at him. At his preschool, a "snowball fight" was held with his entire class, using snowballs made out of wads of yarn. The kids loved it—and so did Jake. After that, he was able to catch a ball. For Jake's tactile sensitivities (as you'll recall, he didn't like being hugged) and to promote cooperation, a game was created for Jake and his friends that involved a dragon who captured children and put them in a dungeon. The only way they could escape was if another child went in to save them. At first, Jake was wary about being touched, but after repeating the game many times (using different variations) and seeing how all the other kids handled it, he got into the spirit of the game and allowed himself to be captured.

– *Use peer modeling.* Choose a same age/gender typical peer who can serve as a role model for your child. It can be a neighborhood child, classmate, cousin, or friend's child. Try to pick a child who is highly verbal and outgoing, and use only one child per session in the beginning. Including too many children can be overwhelming for your child initially. As your child becomes more attuned socially, you can involve more children, thereby introducing a more advanced social dynamic where the noise and activity level are higher.

If you're not sure of what to say the first time that you invite a child over for a peer-modeling session (since the phrase can sound rather daunting), just explain to the other parent that the session will look like a play date with an adult who leads the children in fun activities. The child's parents can simply tell their child that she is going on a play date; they don't have to explain the child's role. In fact, according to Dana, it's preferable if they don't: "Often it changes the way the children interact. The peer acts like a teacher instead of a friend, which can alter the nature of the social interaction." Sessions should be fun and interactive so that the children enjoy participating and look forward to coming back again.

One of Jake's first peer models was a boy who was energetic and loved to take charge. He was able to interact with Jake on a whole different level than any adults could. He would switch from one activity to the next (common for typical children, whereas children with ASDs tend to stay with one activity), and if Jake didn't join him right away, he would take Jake by the hand and lead him to the activity. He also talked a lot and changed topics frequently, sometimes even in mid-sentence (again, common for typical children). Jake worked to keep up with him, and you could tell that he really wanted to connect with him by the way Jake smiled and followed his lead. The peer felt special and loved the attention.

A peer-modeling session can be led by you at home or by your child's therapist during a treatment session. Plan the activities you will be introducing in the session ahead of time. Switch the leader/follower roles. For example, if the children are involved in an imitation game, let your child lead part of the game while the other child imitates, then switch roles. If the peer has a good idea for a game, do it! It's great motivation for the peer. If the children don't want to play a certain game, don't force it. Move on to another one. Games require cooperation and sharing, not winning or losing. Overall, keep peer-modeling sessions fun and interactive. At first, they should be short—no longer than 30 minutes. Set up situations that motivate your child to interact with the peer. For example, let the peer hold the crayons, snack, toy, and so on. Eventually, the therapist or caregiver should fade out his or her role and observe from afar so that the children play on their own. Specific issues that arise can either be addressed by the therapist through an unobtrusive prompt (such as a quick whispered reminder to look at the boy while he's talking) or can be addressed in a private session at a later date.

- *Practice and reinforce social and play skills.* If your child is in school, coach the shadow or aide, teachers, speech therapists, guidance counselors, and/or school psychologists on how to make your child's social and play experience a success. Have a social skills therapist coach your child's shadow on how to encourage your child to generalize the social and play skills. Lunch and recess are important times during the school day for your child to generalize these skills. The shadow should not do or say things for your child, but should prompt him to interact. He can lead games at recess that have been taught in advance at home, by assuming the role of teacher's assistant and talking up the activity to encourage (not force) other classmates to participate. The shadow should not enable the child by playing the game for him. The shadow can offer some prompting but is there primarily to increase the child's independence.

  The shadow can also prepare the child with appropriate topics of conversation that he can discuss with peers at lunch, or if the child is having trouble initiating or joining in a conversation, the shadow can bring up topics that she knows will help the child participate. For example, if a child has a dog, the shadow can go over to the table and tell a quick story about a dog, which prompts the children to start a conversation about dogs so that the child can join in. (At first, the child may need a direct prompt from the shadow—such as "What's your dog like?")

- *Plan lunch dates.* When your child's schedule is filled with treatment sessions, a lunch play date can be a good time for social skills practice. (Jake used to have a weekly lunch date at our home with a child from his preschool.) Again, if your child eats lunch at school, his shadow can suggest good topics to talk about during lunch.

- *Keep an open door policy for neighborhood children.* Let children of all ages come over to be with your child. The more exposure to social situations your child has, the more comfortable he may feel.

- *Enroll your child in music classes, gym classes, and/or art classes.* If there's no room in your child's treatment schedule for a weekly class commitment, you can always take your child for a visit to a children's museum, a library, or a toy store or to see a puppet show or play. These are all good ways to expose your child to social interactions.

- *Play sports with your child or sign your child up for a sports team.* There are special needs sports teams as well, which you can find out about through your local chamber of commerce or local autism organization. Sports can teach coordination, cooperation, and turn taking. Sports can also greatly benefit your child socially at school. Being on a sports team provides your child with opportunities to make friendships. Many children talk about sports and play them during recess.

- *Teach empathy skills.* Empathy is an important part of friendship. You can teach your child how to become more empathetic by creating games. For example, Jake was taught the "rude/polite" game. He and his peers had to listen to the leader (the teacher, therapist, or me) and determine whether or not what she said was rude or polite. If the leader said something polite (such as, "You are so nice!"), the children would stand still in their places. If the leader said something rude (such as, "You smell terrible!"), the children got to run across to a designated play area and then run back to their places. After a few rounds, the leader would discuss how words can make people feel happy or sad.

   Other ways to help create empathy include taking your child to the playground and having him guess how people are feeling by looking at their body language. What are their facial expressions saying about how they feel? If they are jumping up and down and waving their arms in the air with smiles on their faces, how do they feel? You can use pictures of people in magazines and books to teach children how to clue into facial expressions and body postures. To encourage your child to see things through someone else's eyes, have your child participate in picking out birthday presents for friends. Ask your child, "What do you think Jennifer would like?"

- *Create teamwork games.* This can help with empathy skills and making friends. Make up games during which participants must work together toward a common goal by saving one another or work, rather than pitting them against one another in a competitive match. These types of games can also help children learn empathy skills. In these games, be sure to include everyone at all times. No one should have to sit on the sidelines because they "got out." Praise children after each round for saving their friends.

Teaching children with ASDs the prerequisite skills for social awareness and social interactions is considered to be a key component to successful early childhood treatment and educational programming. Children with ASDs may be more open and willing to interact with others if given the opportunity to practice their newly acquired social skills with typically developing peers in a social skills training program (Koegel, L. K., et al 2001).[4] Overall, social skills training should be fun and engaging and can be a part of your child's treatment sessions, school recess, or even take place in your own backyard.

11

INSIDE AND OUTSIDE THE HOUSE: COPING WITH EVERYDAY LIFE

I need help with some of the basics at home, especially with getting my son to sleep, getting him dressed, and toilet training. Any tips?

– **Sleep**: Many children with ASDs have problems sleeping. It's important that you address them right away to avoid establishing bad habits. Make sure you have a bedtime routine at the same time every night and stick to it. Make going to sleep enjoyable by singing a favorite bedtime song, reading a favorite bedtime story, or giving your child a favorite stuffed animal. Be aware of your child's sensitivities and arrange the bedroom accordingly. For a child with visual sensitivities who needs complete darkness, install window shades. Use plug-in nightlights for a child who needs some light. For a child with auditory sensitivities, keep the noise levels low. Install a white noise machine if necessary. For a child with kinesthetic sensitivities, make sure sheets and blankets are made of fabrics that are tolerable for him. Sometimes a sleeping bag can make a child feel more comforted and secure. Pushing a bed against a wall can also make children feel safer. After you say goodnight, make sure you leave the bedroom. Try not to return, even if your child is crying. If you do return, make it a short visit and instruct your child to go to sleep; do not bring in a snack, lie in bed with him, or tell him a story—these are all ways of rewarding him for *not* going to sleep. While this can be extremely difficult for both you and your child, it is necessary. Your child needs sleep—and so do you! Here is a list of how much sleep your child needs per night, depending on his age.

Infants (birth to 1 year old): 14 to 15 hours
Toddlers (1 to 2 years old): 12 to 14 hours
Preschoolers and kindergartners (3 to 6 years old): 11 to 13 hours
School-aged children (6 to 11 years old): 10 to 11 hours

Children with ASDs often have significant sleep problems, and doctors are finding that many parents underreport them. If you have tried everything and your child is still experiencing sleep disturbances, consider other things that may be adversely affecting your child. Is he drinking sodas with caffeine or consuming foods high in sugar content? Are there distractions in the bedroom such as a TV or computer? Most sleep disturbances can be solved by using behavioral interventions and making the bedroom environment comfortable and conducive to sleep. If your child continues to have difficulties, ask your pediatrician about medications. Prescription and over-the-counter antihistamines have been used to help children sleep. However, these same medications may also produce the opposite effect and increase excitement. Ask your doctor about exogenous melatonin, chloral hydrate, trazodone, clonidine, and benzodiazepines.

 – **Getting Dressed**: Make sure your child's clothes are comfortable, especially if your child is hypersensitive to certain fabrics or textures. For example, wool can be irritating, so check labels to make sure clothes are made of cotton or nylon. Other tips for hypersensitive children include washing clothes using fabric softener before first wearing them, buying socks without seams, cutting out labels from shirts and pants, using unscented laundry detergents, and adapting clothing to meet your child's specific needs (e.g., cutting off tips of gloves, or stretching out the necklines of tight shirts).

If your child has a fixation with a certain item of clothing—such as a favorite shirt with a basketball design on it—and insists on wearing it every day, substitute different shirts with similar designs or set up a visual calendar indicating which days he can wear that particular shirt. You can also use Power

Cards, which are intrinsically motivating learning tools that incorporate a child's special interests, such as an activity or favorite cartoon character into a story that helps him learn or understand appropriate skills and behaviors. The Power Card stories are easy and fun to create—you write short, motivational step-by-step instructions combined with an illustration of your child's special interests, such as a person, place, or activity.[1] For example, a child who is learning how to get dressed could follow Mickey Mouse's or another favorite character's instructions. The child can then use the cards again to help remind him of what to do. In the case of the boy who constantly wore the basketball shirt, you could use his interest in the New York Knicks to help create a story where a player wears different clothing.

Overall, getting dressed should be an organized and structured routine. Lay out your child's clothes the night before to avoid anxiety in the morning. Let your child be part of the process. Again, you can create a visual schedule that includes pictures and words to show your child what will occur in what sequence. For example, you can use the first-then strategy: First you put on your underwear, then you put on your pants. Start out slowly—one step at a time—and only go on to the next step when your child has mastered the one before it. Help the child along. For example, to teach your child how to put on his socks, put a sock on his foot halfway, then take his hands and show him how to pull the sock on the rest of the way. Make sure to give lots of praise while your child is trying to master a step. You can also use humor when helping your child to get dressed. Put your sock on your hand or try to put your child's arms through his pant legs to help teach him what's correct and incorrect.

Children can also learn by imitation. You can demonstrate putting on each item of clothing, one by one, and have your child follow you.

These same tips for getting dressed can be applied to brushing teeth, face washing, hair brushing, and other grooming rituals.

– **Toilet training**: Many children with ASDs have problems with toilet training. Toilet-training skills can be incorporated in treatment sessions by using behavioral models found in TEACCH or ABA programs. These methods break down the activity into smaller, teachable steps. For example, a child can be taught 1. enter the bathroom; 2. pull pants and underpants down or allow adult to help; 3. sit on toilet; 4. get toilet tissue; 5. wipe with tissue; 6. stand up; 7. throw tissue in toilet; 8. pull clothes on; 9. flush toilet; and 10. wash hands. Often a visual support system is set up with a series of pictures and/or instructional words to help prompt the child. It's important to provide positive reinforcement in the form of verbal praise and/or a treat when the child is successful (you can start by rewarding each step and build to the point where you're offering one reward if the child successfully completes the entire sequence). If your child is having trouble with a certain step, such as sitting on the toilet, you can come up with creative ways to help him get over that fear, such as allowing him to sit on the toilet with his clothes on, sit on the toilet with the seat down, or use a potty seat on the floor. You can also use yourself or a doll as a model. If your child becomes overly interested in flushing or playing with the toilet paper, you can give him something else to hold or encourage him to go on to the next step. Other things to consider when toilet training your child include making sure the child is ready to be toilet trained, teaching the child to recognize his own body signals, and making the bathroom environment comfortable, not over-stimulating.[2]

Family meals are becoming a challenge. While the rest of the family is sitting down, I'm rummaging through the cabinets trying to find something for my son to eat. He is the pickiest eater! Please help.

Many parents of toddlers report that their children are picky eaters, but children with ASDs seem to have even more difficulties. This may relate to sensory issues. Some children cannot bear to eat foods that are too soft, too crunchy, too hot, or too cold, while others experience the opposite extreme and will insist on eating only soft, crunchy, hot, or cold foods. As you saw earlier, one boy had to have all of his food heated up—even cereal and peanut butter and jelly sandwiches—and another had to have all of his foods served on different plates—peas on one, corn on another, and so on. Some children prefer to eat all of their foods at room temperature, which means they cannot eat cold foods such as ice cream, and hot foods must be cooled until they are tepid. Some children may only eat mashed potatoes that were the same consistency every time. Other children may eat specific foods in specific ways, the way Jake had to have his Cheerios in the same yellow bowl or his evenly sliced hotdogs on his Winnie-the-Pooh plate. Children with ASDs will sometimes even eat foods that fit into one of four categories: sweet, sour, bitter, or salty. For example, one child may eat only potato chips, crackers, and bacon.

One of the largest challenges for parents is to meet the nutritional needs of their children with ASDs. This can often be difficult, especially for parents who have their children on special diets, such as the GF/CF diet. When we started Jake on the GF/CF diet, which we followed for almost one year, I was worried about finding foods he would eat. All of his favorite foods were now excluded from his diet. No more macaroni and cheese, Oreo cookies, Cheerios, peanut butter and jelly on white bread, or Goldfish crackers. But sure enough, I discovered a whole world of gluten-free/casein-free food in my local health food store. There were cookies, crackers, pasta, and bread that were gluten- and casein-free. Jake liked his new waffles and cookies, but it was still a challenge to find other kid-friendly food that he would eat. To get Jake to eat a balanced diet, we had to use some creative strategies coupled with a big dose of behavioral intervention.

Here's what we learned. To help your child maintain a healthy diet and overcome food fixations, introduce new foods gradually and make sure they are healthy and nutritious. If your child has a favorite food, you can withhold this food until the end of the meal and give it to your child as a reward for eating other foods. With Jake, we modified this strategy in the beginning. After each bite of turkey, we gave him a tiny piece of a gluten/wheat/dairy/ sugar free chocolate chip cookie. After a while, we gave him a cookie piece after three bites of turkey, then five, until he could finish his meal and get a whole cookie at the end. This strategy can also help to replace food fixations.

Another strategy is to gradually introduce foods that are the best sensory fit for your child, such as introducing other soft foods to a child who only likes to eat pudding. Then, you can gradually try to desensitize your child by adding foods with some texture. New foods can be introduced through behavior modeling—you or a sibling could demonstrate eating and enjoying a new food. New foods can also be incorporated in a social story. Some parents suggest hiding healthy foods in other foods, such as mixing finely grated vegetables into a pasta sauce. One mother whose son ate only mashed potatoes was able to hide tiny pieces of meat and tofu in his potatoes. Some parents will use protein drinks to supplement their children's diets. This is okay, provided that it's not for every meal and that you're not inadvertently reinforcing a child's dislike of chewing. There are many helpful and creative ways to get your child to eat; just keep your goal in mind. Ultimately, you want to get your child to eat a balanced and healthy diet. Go slowly at first, but follow through. Small and consistent changes are key to your child's success. You can also ask your ABA therapists or other treatment specialists for behavioral techniques or consult with your occupational therapist, who may offer feeding therapy services.

Sometimes my son has a tantrum right in the middle of family dinner. His tantrums are like no other child's I've ever seen. He shrieks and throws himself on the floor as if the world is ending. Luckily, he hasn't hurt himself or anyone else . . . yet. But I'm concerned. His tantrums are occurring more frequently than ever. What can I do?

Tantrums in children with ASDs can be much more dramatic than those of typical children because they occur more frequently and are often accompanied by self-injurious behaviors such as head banging or unusual vocalizing such as grunting or shrieking.

My first piece of advice is that you not panic or overreact. Raising your voice or outright yelling will only escalate the tantrum. Try to remain calm and use a quiet but stern voice. Use as few words as possible, such as "No!" or "Stop!" If the tantrum does become cause for concern, protect siblings by removing them from the room and move furniture so that your child does not hurt himself.

Parents sometimes think excessive outbursts are merely symptoms of ASDs and allow their children to throw them. But children with ASDs can throw tantrums for the same reason that typical children do—to get attention. If your child is having difficulty communicating what he wants and becomes frustrated, a tantrum may be his way of telling you that you just don't understand. A child may also throw tantrums to avoid having to do certain tasks.

Be careful that you're not unintentionally reinforcing your child's tantrums. Sometimes these outbursts are used as avoidance behaviors. For example, if your child throws a tantrum every time he goes to the grocery store, and every time you end up leaving before you get even one item in your cart, you have taught your child that throwing a tantrum equals getting to leave the grocery store. One mother found that each time she asked her daughter to pick up her toys, she had a tantrum. The mother ended up picking up her toys. Her daughter had learned that throwing a tantrum equals not picking up toys. In these cases, you may have to wait out the tantrum and proceed with the task—grocery shopping or picking up toys—even as the child continues to protest. Don't give up or give in.

Figure out what sends your child into a tantrum. Is it something sensory in the environment, like overstimulating lights or large, noisy crowds? If so, be careful not to put your child into these situations or at least prepare your child in advance for them.

Note the behaviors your child exhibits just before throwing a full-blown tantrum so that you can try to ward it off. This is called the *rumbling stage*—think of it as the rumbling that occurs just before a volcano erupts. Warning signs can include facial grimacing, vehement refusal to cooperate, unusual noises, or intense stimming behaviors at a more rapid pace than usual. Children with Asperger's may show less obvious, more classic signs of discontent such as nail biting, a lowered voice, or muscle tension.

According to *Aperger Syndrome and Difficult Moments: Practical Solutions for Tantrums, Rage and Meltdowns* by Brenda Smith Myles and Jack South-wick, here are some techniques to follow to avoid your child from throwing a full-blown tantrum during the rumbling stage.

- Antiseptic bouncing: In a nonpunitive way, remove your child from the environment that is causing difficulty (e.g., the kitchen, the classroom, birthday party, or other social gathering). Sometimes a child just needs some downtime to regroup. For instance, if a child has a tantrum in the classroom, simply having him take a walk down the hall to get a drink from the water fountain may provide that downtime.

- Touch control: If a child is loudly tapping his hand or foot or displaying a behavior that is a precursor to a full-blown tantrum, gently touch his hand or leg to make him aware of the behavior so he can stop on his own.

- Proximity control: At home, you can simply sit or stand near your child to offer your child reassurance. At school, a teacher can do the same. This can make children feel safe and calm their anxiety.

- Signal interference: You and/or your child's teacher can set up secret codes to alert the child that the disruptive behavior is occurring.

- Home base: Sometimes children with ASDs need a chill-out zone where they can calm down and regroup. At home, this may be the child's bedroom. At school, this could be someplace quiet such as the library.[3]

What do you do if your child has already gotten past the rumbling stage and is having a full-blown tantrum? Try the interrupt-and-redirect method. The more attention you give to the tantrum, the more you encourage it. Shift your focus away from the tantrum and focus on something else, like doing a puzzle or art project. Try to pretend the tantrum is not even happening, and start talking to the child about other things, like the day's schedule. This may seem difficult, but it is amazing how well this strategy can pay off.

One mother reported that every time she took her son to a restaurant, his tantrum was accompanied by vomiting. After a few rounds of this, just when she was about to give up, she tried the interrupt-and-redirect method. She took her son to a restaurant during off-peak hours, sat through his wails and vomiting, and just as he was going into round two of wailing, she interrupted and said, "Okay, now let's clean this up." She took him to the bathroom to collect paper towels, and brought him back to the table, and they both cleaned up the mess together. She talked calmly over her son's muffled sobs about what special thing they would do after they ate at the restaurant, as if nothing had happened. Sure enough, the boy stopped crying, sat, and ate his meal. His mother was both stunned and thrilled that she could finally eat in a restaurant with her son. But was this a one-time deal? No. After that, his tantrum and vomiting cycle never recurred in restaurants.

Sometimes tantrums just happen. Even if we do our best to intervene during the rumbling stage or the rage cycle, our child may have an outburst anyway. But as you know, there is always an end in sight. This is the final phase of a tantrum, known as the *recovery stage*. During this stage, your child may feel physically and emotionally exhausted. Don't use this time to discuss his behavior or discipline him. Stay calm and take time to regroup yourself.

At a later time, if your child is old enough (usually by adolescence), you can discuss what happened and teach your child self-management strategies; help her recognize signs of impending anxiety that may set off a tantrum and offer relaxation techniques. With younger children, the best strategy is to continue to interrupt and redirect the tantrum until the child learns that it will not get her what she wants.

If you find that your child's tantrums continue despite your best efforts, I advise you to hire a behavioral consultant, who can help you with techniques on how to get the tantrums under control. (Behavioral consultants can be found through your local autism organizations or through ABA schools).

When my son is frustrated or upset, he scratches the side of his face—sometimes to the point where he bleeds. What can I do to make him stop?

As discussed in Part I of this book, self-injurious behaviors can be a result of physiological and/or social causes. Dr. Lorna Wing suggests that either you or a professional perform a functional analysis to determine when the behavior occurs so that you can take a behavioral approach to reducing or eliminating your child's self-injurious behaviors. For example, if you realize that your child begins banging his head or scratching to avoid a situation, such as right before a particular treatment session, you can teach the child more appropriate behaviors and reward them. If your child is using self-injurious behaviors to avoid a task, such as getting dressed, interrupt and redirect him to complete the task. Be careful that you are not inadvertently rewarding self-injurious behaviors by allowing your child to miss that treatment session or get out of doing a task. If your child is just trying to communicate with you, teach your child other ways to show you his needs, such as pointing to a desired object.

Sometimes medication (such as beta-endorphin inhibitors) is used to help decrease self-injurious behaviors. If you suspect that your child's self-injurious behavior is the result of a subclinical seizure (which is not associated with typical seizures but are characterized by abnormal EEG patterns), your child must see a specialist for an extensive EEG workup. If you suspect that the behavior may be the result of illness or pain (e.g., excessive and constant ear swatting may be the result of a chronic ear infection), bring your child to see the pediatrician.

If your child's self-injurious behavior is a form of extreme self-stimulation, you can use behavioral techniques to reduce or eliminate it. For example, if your child scratches incessantly, you can interrupt the behavior by taking the child's hand away from his face, redirect him by putting a puzzle in his hand, and do the puzzle with him. If you sense that your child is reacting as a result of hypersensitivity to sensory stimuli, you can use behavioral treatment and sensory integration treatments.

In more serious cases, protective clothing such as headgear is used to prevent injuries. But Dr. Wing warns that if you must use protective clothing, do so only for short periods of time, as it can really restrict children's movements and make it difficult for them to engage in activities. In some instances, protective clothing can actually increase self-injurious behaviors; a child may actually want to wear the clothing and engage in self-injury just to be able to wear it.

I know that I let our son with an ASD get away with things that I'd never let our typical daughter get away with, but I feel guilty about disciplining my son, and I'm not even sure how to do it. Any suggestions?

Parents should be consistent and fair in their child-rearing practices. Many parents let their children with ASDs get away with behaviors that they would never let their typical children get away with. For example, if their children with ASDs throw a toy, parents may ignore it. But if their typical children do the same thing, parents may say "No!" and take away the toy. Discipline should be consistent for all of your children and that includes your child with an ASD. Even if he doesn't fully understand the consequences of his behaviors, it's important to demonstrate fairness if for no other reason than to show your typical children that they are all being treated equally.

Some discipline techniques that work for typical children may work for children with ASDs as well, such as sending the child to his room or giving him a time-out. These techniques work well for some children, but you must be aware of your child's specific needs to determine whether or not the techniques will be effective. Sending a child with an ASD to his room may be exactly what he wants to avoid social interaction. A time-out may encourage stimming behaviors. The best way to find out what is right for your child is to try different techniques and observe your child's resulting behavior. For example, if you notice that your child is no longer hitting his sister, or that his misbehavior has decreased, you have found the right discipline strategy. Other strategies include removing a reward or a special treat such as TV or computer privileges, dessert, or anything else that your child values. Be aware that, over time, you may have to reconsider which reward gets withheld. For instance, witholding TV privileges may work for your child as a toddler, but as his interests and motivations change, you may have to switch to withholding computer privileges.

Timing is also an important factor in discipline. Be sure to discipline your child as soon as she misbehaves. Immediate discipline is the most effective way for your child to make the connection between the misbehavior and its consequences.

Whether your child's misbehavior is a form of getting attention, avoidance, stimming, or a result of miscommunication, there's usually a reason for it. In all cases, work on decreasing or eliminating the inappropriate behaviors. Ask your child's treatment therapists for suggestions. An effective strategy is to replace an inappropriate behavior with an appropriate one. For example, if your child hits you to get your attention, teach her to either say or signal "Help!" by tapping you on the shoulder instead. If you don't teach your child a new appropriate behavior, she will likely find another inappropriate behavior to replace the old one.

If your child continues to misbehave, be careful to not engage in negative attention. Just as the typical class clown in school gets most of the teacher's attention, your child may be misbehaving to keep getting your attention. In this case, you need to ignore it. If she hits you to get your attention, just walk away and pretend it didn't happen. If your child hits her sister, teach the sister to walk away as well. Ignoring the misbehavior can be an extremely effective technique, provided that your child is not putting herself or others in danger. If she's putting anyone in danger, you need to discipline immediately.

I find myself constantly disciplining my son. Although it seems to be working, I feel like I'm constantly expending a lot of negative energy. What can I do?

When I used to teach corporate seminars on how managers could effectively motivate their employees, I'd borrow a phrase from management guru Ken Blanchard—"Catch me doing something right!"

Most managers in the corporate world are great at catching their employees doing the wrong things but are not so great at catching their employees doing the right things. When I'd discuss the importance of giving positive reinforcement, I was often told, "Why do I have to tell them they're doing a good job? That's what I pay them for." Here's why: If you don't give your employees positive reinforcement in the form of praise or incentives on a continuous basis, they won't feel appreciated, and they'll lose their motivation.

This same commonsensical advice can also help you and your child. Reward the behavior you want repeated. If you want your child to stop tapping on the table or throwing a tantrum, go one step beyond just disciplining him for his misbehavior. When your child is sitting at the table quietly or playing appropriately with a puzzle—in other words, when he's *not* tapping and *not* throwing a tantrum—tell him what a great job he's doing. "Great job sitting quietly!" or "I like the way you're doing that puzzle!"

So catch your child doing something right. Actively seek out moments when he or she is doing all the right things, rather than constantly harping on all the wrong things.

Praise can give someone an immediate lift. Think about how it makes you feel when someone praises you. It feels terrific. You have the power to make your child feel terrific, too. When you praise your child, be specific. Don't just say, "You're doing a good job." Instead, say, "I like the way you're sitting with your hands so quietly in your lap" or "Great job rolling the ball to your sister." You can also model good behavior for your child. For example, you may sit next to your child and show him how to play quietly at the table.

Sometimes you can even turn a potentially negative situation into a positive one. For example, I became attuned to the times when Jake was about to lie down on his stomach and push a toy car back and forth in front of his face. This enabled me to stop the behavior, change it, and reward him for the appropriate behavior. The moment I saw him starting to slide his body down onto the floor, I'd catch him midslide, lift him up, place him in a seated position, put the train in his hand, and say, "Good sitting like a big boy!" Then I'd guide his hand to help him push the train appropriately, and when he'd continue on his own, I'd say, "Great playing with your train!" Sometimes I'd accompany the verbal praise with a treat, like a cookie or a hug. Other times, the verbal praise was enough—a big smile would spread across Jake's face, and I'd sense that he felt proud.

All of these positive reinforcements and reward systems make up a form of behavior modification that's used in ABA and other behavioral treatments for ASDs. Yet, people have been using these techniques in the corporate world for years. We all respond to praise and incentives. In this regard, your child with an ASD is no different.

I've always assumed that I'm supposed to do everything for my son. People say that I spoil him. What should I do?

Many parents assume that they have to do everything for their children with ASDs because of their disorder. They spoil their children because it doesn't occur to them that their children can do certain things by themselves. Helping a child with an ASD to be self-sufficient can be a wonderful way to boost self-confidence. One popular way to help children feel self-sufficient around the house is to show them how to prepare their own snacks and create opportunities for success. Place snack foods in a kitchen cabinet or shelf in the refrigerator that your child can reach. Find a low shelf for plastic plates, bowls, and utensils. Put snack foods in easy-to-open boxes, containers, or plastic bags. Break down the task into small steps and walk your child through them, using pictures, words, and actions. Take your child by the hand and lead him through the steps of getting a plate, going to the food cabinet, taking out the box of crackers, and so on. Even though you may have to practice this behavior over and over, it will be worth it. The simple act of making his own snack can do wonders for your child's self-esteem.

Children with ASDs can also help with household chores. They can learn to set the table, water the plants, or take out the garbage. These kinds of activities can also make them feel like a more valued part of the family.

My five-year-old son wandered right out the front door and across the street while I was unloading the dishwasher. Thankfully, he arrived home safely with the help of a neighbor. What can I do to help protect him?

Many children with ASDs require extra measures to keep them safe. While most parents baby-proof their homes for the first few years of their children's lives, parents of children with ASDs may have to maintain safety systems in place as their children get older.

There are many things that you can do in your home to ensure safety. The most effective way to keep a child from wandering off is to install locks from the inside. There are also security systems that beep to alert you that a door is being opened. If necessary, you can install a special lock on your child's bedroom door to prevent him from wandering off at night, but make sure you have immediate access to the room in case of fire or another emergency. Windows can also be safeguarded with special locks. Outside of the home, you can have your child carry an identification tag in his pocket or backpack or wear clothing with iron-on nametapes and/or a medical identification bracelet.

When safeguarding your home, first secure the areas that present the most potential danger for your child. Consider your child's behaviors to help you decide. For example, Nathan, who you'll recall was diagnosed with Autistic Disorder, had a propensity for breaking windows. His parents decided to replace the window glass with Plexiglas. Another child was a climber, so his parents made sure there were no heavy bookcases that could be tipped over or medicine cabinets that could be opened. They installed safety locks on all kitchen and bathroom cabinet doors and drawers. Another child was prone to running hot water, so his parents modified the faucets in the kitchen and bathrooms.

After you have identified your child's most likely sources of danger, take other safety precautions. Children with ASDs who are both curious and unaware of potential dangers may not be able to distinguish between juice and laundry detergent or pills and candy. Lock up all medicines and chemicals such as cleaning supplies, pesticides, and detergents. Cover electrical outlets. Conceal electrical cords. Keep electrical appliances such as toasters or power tools and knives, scissors, and sharp objects out of reach or safely locked up. Use a rubber mat on the bottom of the bathtub so your child won't slip, and replace open bottles with pump bottles to prevent accidental ingestion. For fire safety, lock up matches and lighters, put safety covers on gas stoves and oven knobs, and put tot-finder stickers (available from the local fire department) on bedroom windows to alert firefighters in case of a fire.

Parents come up with creative solutions to help their children sit through a meal without endangering others by throwing cups or utensils. One mother makes sure her son sits in the corner seat, so that it's difficult for him to jump up and run around during meals. Another mother used fishing string to tie her child's knife, fork, and spoon to the chair so that he can't throw them very far. She also switched to plastic plates and bowls and used Velcro to secure them to the table.

Modify the safety precautions in your home according to your child's skill level. For example, if your child can label or read, put large red stop signs on items or areas that are off-limits. Create Social Stories—short personalized stories—with pictures, words, or music, to teach your child about safety issues.

How do I cope with common activities outside the house that used to seem so simple, such as going to the grocery store or waiting in line at the bank?

Everyday errands that you used to be able to accomplish without even thinking can be a challenge if you're doing them with a child with an ASD. The first rule of thumb is to plan your outing and explain it to your child. Know where you're going, what you'll be doing, and how long the trip will take. Let your child know that he will return home or at another location at the end of the outing.

Make sure to give your child enough warning before you leave the house.

Be careful about saying things like, "We're leaving in five minutes!" Some children with ASDs have no concept of time, while others are obsessed with time and will be upset if you do not leave in exactly five minutes.

Before you venture out of your house, think about what may trigger your child's inappropriate behaviors, sensitivities, or tantrums and how you can minimize them. If large, crowded stores are too stimulating, you may choose to shop at a smaller grocery store. If you want to help your child adapt to a certain environment, work on ways to desensitize the experience to make it more manageable. Here are some helpful tips.

- **Grocery Store**: Be well-organized and structure the time. Keep your grocery list short so that you're not spending too much time in the store. Don't cruise every aisle. Involve your child in the shopping process by adding photos or drawings of the items on the list. Show your child how to retrieve items from the shelf and put them in the shopping cart. Make the last item a special treat, which can be a reward for your child's good behavior. Older or high-functioning children can also help carry groceries to the car and unload them at home.

- **Waiting in Line**: Go to the store or bank at an hour of the day when you know there will be a short waiting time. Bring toys, games, or snacks that will help your child pass the time in an enjoyable way. For a scheduled appointment such as a doctor's visit, call ahead to make sure the doctor is running on time. Or try to schedule an early morning appointment to ensure less waiting time and explain to the receptionist that your child has an ASD. If waiting produces anxiety or stimming, take a break and walk outside or try to redirect your child's attention with a game. If your child is old enough, you can bring along a visual schedule and a timer to show how long the wait will be.

- **New Situations**: Prepare your child for new experiences by showing pictures or photographs of where he is going. Make a visual and/or written schedule using pictures from books or magazines or even draw pictures of your own to demonstrate the sequence of events. For example, if you are going to the zoo, you can include pictures of the family in different scenarios, such as in the car, paying the entrance fee, looking at the animals, and so on. Visual schedules can also be used for vacations, birthday parties, and other unfamiliar situations.

Another way to ease a child's transition to a new place is to make up your own story about a family going there. Describe the situation so that your child will know what to expect and how to respond. When writing a social story, write it in the first or third person point of view, using positive language, descriptive sentences, and a clear format that includes an introduction, main body, and conclusion.

– **Religious Services or Ceremonies**: Arrive close to the beginning of the service to avoid waiting time, but make sure to allow some time for your child to get settled in. Choose a seat at the end of an aisle or close to the exit door to make it easier to leave. Speak to the rabbi, priest, minister, or other religious leader to inform him or her that your child has an ASD and any inappropriate behavior that may occur. Bring snacks or toys to help your child get through the service. Keep initial visits to services short and gradually increase the length of your visits over time. Special accommodations can be made for children with ASDs to have bar or bat-mitzvahs, receive confirmation, or take part in other religious rites.

– **Haircuts**: Prepare your child in advance by talking him through the steps at home, demonstrating with your own hands what is going to happen at the barbershop, and showing what items will be used, such as shampoo, a comb, scissors, or a blow dryer. You can also make up an individual schedule or calendar for your child that shows a photo of the barbershop, indicating when and where the haircut will take place. Use a more detailed picture schedule (known as an embedded schedule) as a visual aide to show each step of the visit: driving to the salon, sitting in the chair, having the robe put on, shampooing, combing, cutting, blow drying, getting a lollipop, and driving home. You can cut pictures out of a magazine or take your own photographs. Schedules can help remove anticipatory anxiety by providing structure, which is often comforting to children with ASDs.

– **Birthday Parties or Celebrations**: Make sure the party is appropriate for your child before accepting the invitation. If you fear that a party with loud music or a circus theme will be overstimulating for your child, decline the invitation. If you accept the invitation, use visual schedules to prepare your child for the party. If you have a video of a previous party, show that to your child and explain the sequence of events and what he

or she will be doing at the party. Sit with or near your child, and if necessary, limit your time there. Bring snacks or toys if you feel that they may
comfort him and make the experience more enjoyable.

–**School Bus**: Use a visual schedule or pictures and/or words to break
down exactly what will happen (e.g., waiting for the bus, climbing up the
steps onto the bus, sitting in the bus, and getting off the bus). Give your
child a snack, toy, or game for the ride. If it's your child's first time, you
can walk your child onto the bus and lead him to a seat. Try to choose a
seat near a window and near the bus driver. Let the bus driver know that
your child has an ASD and how to handle any inappropriate behaviors
that may arise.

We used to go out to eat as a family, but now it's difficult because our daughter with an ASD can't seem to handle it. Are there tips on how all of us can go to a restaurant together?

Try to set your child with an ASD up for success when you go out to eat at a
restaurant. First, make sure the restaurant is kid-friendly. A four star restaurant that requires children to be perfectly well mannered is not a good choice.
Second, make sure there is food on the menu that your child likes and that the
environment is conducive to your child's sensitivities. Will the noise level
bother him? Are there too many bright lights? Is it too crowded? Third, if this
is a family dinner, make sure the entire family is included in making the decision about which restaurant to go to. By making a unilateral decision based on
your child's special needs, you may cause unnecessary friction between siblings. Narrow down your options and give the siblings a choice.

If you are bringing a young child with an ASD to a restaurant, make sure to
bring toys and/or crayons and paper. If the child is old enough and can understand explanations, tell him where you are going and what he can expect—no
surprises. The more prepared your child is, the more comfortable he will be. If
your child has Asperger's or another form of ASDs where he doesn't understand
social nuances, you can explain the unwritten rules before you go to the restaurant. For example, you can write out the steps: When the hostess greets you, say
hello. When she shows you to your table, say thank you. Sit down at the table.
When the waiter gives you a menu and asks what you'd like to drink, tell him
what you want. When he brings you your drink, say thank you, and so on.

The first time we took Jake out to a restaurant after he was diagnosed, he was clearly not happy to be there, and we were totally unprepared for what was going to happen. Jake shrieked, hurled himself onto the floor, hid under the table, and continued to shriek. I crawled under to get him, which made him shriek louder. By the time I made it up from under the table (Jake still remained under), I noticed the stares—or more like glares—from other diners around me. I'd been in this situation with Jake before, feeling helpless in the midst of one of his outbursts and sensing that people were judging me as this bad parent for not being able to control my son. I wanted to shout at them that my son couldn't help it and that I really was a good parent. But the truth was that in these situations, I didn't feel like one. Needless to say, Franklin was more successful at extricating Jake from under the table, and we mumbled a few apologies to the management and patrons as we made a quick exit.

Determined to overcome this hurdle, we tried our restaurant outings two more times, but had the same experiences. Then one of our ABA therapists said that it was possible that Jake was learning that all he had to do was scream, and he'd get to leave the restaurant. She said to try it again, only this time to try to ignore or wait out his shrieking and reward him for being quiet.

So we tried another restaurant, purposely choosing an early dinner seating when we were the only ones there. Jake screamed, and Franklin and I sat there and tried to pretend that nothing unusual was happening. It was excruciating. But after a while, Jake seemed to be onto us. When we didn't dive under the table, Jake crawled out, and his shrieking subsided. But it wasn't over yet: He then began using Franklin as a jungle gym, climbing onto his back and trying to lie on top of his head. It took all of my self-restraint not to burst out laughing while trying to have a conversation with Franklin while Jake was draped over his head. But Franklin and I hung in there. Sure enough, when Jake was not getting the negative attention that he seemed to want, he stopped and sat down. In that split second that his butt hit the chair, Franklin and I loaded on the praise—"Good sitting like a big boy!" Out came the raisins, and Jake was rewarded. It got easier after that. Rewarding his positive behaviors and ignoring his negative behaviors made our restaurant experiences better. Were all of them perfect after that? Nope. But they were certainly more tolerable.

One mother reports that when her family goes out to a restaurant, "sometimes our son is very social and appropriate. Sometimes it's hard for him to sit still in a chair. He'll start to bang his head with both fists. I know he needs to stand and walk around. So I walk around with him. His behavior no longer embarrasses me—it is what it is. I've come to accept it. As long as he is not too loud or disruptive, he can act how he acts, and I'm not stressed out."

Another mother says that whenever she takes her son to a restaurant, she first tells the hostess or manager that her son has an ASD and requests a table that is quieter and apart from the others. If there are people seated close by, she apologizes to them if he is inappropriately vocalizing or throwing food. "I am proud of my son and honest about his disorder. I find people to be very understanding as long as I am quick to explain the situation."

My son engages in stimming behavior much more often when we're out in public than when we're at home. He flicks his fingers and makes odd faces. Sometimes I feel helpless when it happens. What can I do?

As discussed in Part I, stimming (or self-stimulatory behavior) can include hand flapping, finger flicking, eye tracking, or myriad inappropriate, repetitive behaviors that offer a child with an ASD some form of sensory stimulation or sensory reduction.

Since stimming may be a response to increased stress, one strategy is to remove the child from the situation that is causing the stress or change the situation. If your child starts stimming in a noisy and crowded area of the mall, go to a quieter area. If your child is reacting to a loud radio, turn the volume down. Another strategy to reduce or stop stimming is what we mentioned earlier: interrupting and redirecting the behavior. For example, if your child is flapping his hands, interrupt him by offering an appropriate distraction, such as playing a game or going for a walk. At the playground, instead of allowing Jake to lie facedown in the sandbox and gaze at nothing (another form of stimming), we learned to anticipate this situation and brought along a plastic pail and shovel that we showed him how to use. Each time Jake engaged in a new, nonstimming behavior, he received lots of positive reinforcement, either in the form of verbal praise ("Great playing with your truck!") or verbal praise coupled with a favorite treat (such as pretzels or raisins, which I always carried with me).

Of course, there are those days when you're stuck on a long line or a crowded mall and you've tried absolutely everything to get your child to stop stimming, but your child continues to stim anyway. Don't beat yourself up. Either bring your child to a place where he can stim in private, or else just let him stim. It's okay to take an occasional breather, just make sure you don't do this too often. Even though it may require a lot of effort to reduce the stimming, it will pay off in the long run. More work now will mean less work later.

Why bother reducing or eliminating stimming behavior if it's not physically harmful and may just be an annoyance? Because stimming can adversely affect a child's ability to learn and have a detrimental impact on a child's social life. Stimming can draw unnecessary negative attention from peers and cause a child to be stigmatized and left out of social activities. This situation generally happens in school, when neither you nor your other children are around to help.

If your child is in a special school for ASDs, the teachers will know how to handle stimming behaviors. In an inclusion classroom or in a general education school, teachers and aides can be taught how to help manage stimming behaviors so they do not disrupt the classroom. Explain what the stimming behaviors are and what may trigger them. Demonstrate how to redirect behaviors. Point out that recess and lunch periods may be especially difficult because that's when children are the most social and therefore more likely to tease or ostracize a child with an ASD. In these situations, your child may require additional prompting from a teacher or an aide to redirect stimming behaviors to more meaningful and appropriate activities, such as engaging in conversation or playing a game of tag. In fact, it has been shown that vigorous physical activity can help a child become more focused and stim less. It may be a challenge to add a formal exercise program to your child's already busy schedule, but you can encourage teachers to have the children play active games during recess. After all, physical exercise benefits all children. You can also incorporate exercise at home—by playing tag or jumping on a trampoline.

Children with ASDs who are old enough and advanced enough can be taught how to self-monitor their stimming. Because much of stimming occurs in private, it's largely up to a child to reduce or stop her stimming. There are ways to set up a reward system that can reinforce a child's self-management efforts. For example, one boy engaged in a tapping stim. He'd tap any surface he was near—a desk, table, or wall—the more resonant, the better. But his tapping became annoying and disruptive at school. A self-management program was put into place in which he was allowed to listen to jazz music (his favorite) through a headset during designated recess periods if he did not engage in stimming. This seemed to reduce his need to tap on random surfaces.

Through treatment intervention, stimming can be reduced and eventually disappear altogether. It's up to you and your child's treatment providers, teachers, and family members to help make this happen.

How can we make family vacations manageable? The last time we went to the airport, our flight was delayed, and our son had a major meltdown. He was so upset that we couldn't get him on the plane. Please help! We love our family vacations and don't want to give them up.

Vacations can be a challenge for a child with an ASD, but you can avoid many of the potential mishaps by doing one important thing: planning ahead. Now, you're probably thinking that you've planned ahead for vacations in the past, but there are very specific issues you need to consider when traveling with a child with an ASD.

Some aspects of vacations are stressful for even the most seasoned traveler—such as waiting at airports or finding that your prereserved rental car is not available. But there are subtler things that we seem to adjust to automatically, such as a change in routine or structure or just being in a new environment. While these are relatively easy adjustments for most people, they can become monumental hurdles for children with ASDs.

Keep in mind that the goal of your vacation is to have fun. Here are some tips to help you and your family have a good time.

- *Make sure your destination is right for your child*. Call the hotel in advance and find out if it's kid-friendly. Are there activities that your child may like? If your child likes to swim, make sure there's a pool. For video-game enthusiasts, make sure there's a game room. Some hotels offer mini-camps or special child care services. What kind of food is served? Ask if special foods can be prepared or else stash some of your child's favorite foods in your suitcase (such as jars of peanut butter and jelly and snack foods). What size is the hotel? Be careful of inns or hotels that are too small or too large. An intimate bed-and-breakfast may not be appropriate if your child has a tendency to be loud, and a very large hotel with lots of screaming children in the pool may be overstimulating.

- *Make sure the journey to your destination is right for your child*. Consider different options, such a flying, taking the train, going by boat, or driving by car, bus, or RV.

- *Prepare your child*. Get brochures, videotapes, or pictures of where you'll be going. You can even create a scrapbook. Use a monthly calendar to show the child when the vacation is approaching so that she begins to get used to the idea of going away and can prepare mentally and emotionally. You can also use an embedded schedule to break down the vacation into steps, starting from the airport and boarding the plane to ending at your destination. If you anticipate certain aspects of the trip may produce anxiety, you can use a sandwich approach when you show your picture cards. That is, sandwich an anxiety-producing event between two positive events. For example, if your child is afraid to board the plane, you can show him a picture of that favorite snack that he'll get to eat before boarding, and a picture of those great headphones he'll get to use once he sits down in his seat on the plane.

– *Ask for special considerations when you are flying*. Request a special meal for your child that takes into account dietary considerations, such as food allergies or sensitivities when you make your reservation. Let the gate and flight crews know that your child has an ASD and ask to board or exit the plane before or after other passengers. Request seating that will take into account your child's needs: Ask for a seat near the back of the plane if your child makes frequent bathroom visits, a seat in the bulkhead if your child needs extra legroom, a seat away from the wing if your child is sensitive to noise, or a seat near a window so that she can watch the view. Explain to your child that screeners may be checking inside his carry-on luggage to avoid unnecessary upset. Because of heightened airport security, you should alert screeners or airport security of that your child has an ASD, especially if your child has echolalia and may read a warning sign and begin to repeat "Bomb! Bomb! Bomb!" By law, in the case of a pat-down inspection, you can offer suggestions to airport personnel on how to touch your child so as not to upset him. You can also request that assistive devices, such as a communication board, not be counted as an extra carry-on item. When on the plane, tell passengers sitting near you that your child has an ASD, so they can be more understanding if your child misbehaves. Remember, some parents even have business cards printed up with brief explanations of ASDs to hand out to help promote awareness and compassion.[4]

– *Bring a babysitter or therapist*. We brought our babysitter/newly trained ABA therapist Anna with us on every vacation while Jake was still doing extensive ABA therapy. It required an extra suitcase filled with Jake's

ABA materials, but it was worth it. Jake was able to practice and maintain his skills in new settings, including the beach, and Franklin and I
were able to have some quality time just for us. You can also check to
see if the hotel offers child care or if there is a nearby center for autism
where you can receive specialized help or respite care.

– *Ease transitions*. When you arrive at the hotel, make minor adjustments
to the room that will make your child feel more comfortable. Move the
bed near a wall, put that favorite blanket or teddy bear on the bed, plug
in the nightlight from home, and add whatever other creature comforts
will make your child feel better. Take it slow at first. Rushing around unpacking and throwing on bathing suits the moment you enter the room is
not the best strategy for easing your child into the vacation.

– *Try to create some kind of routine*. For some of you, establishing a routine
defeats the whole purpose of vacation. I understand that. But there are
some parents who actually like falling into the same pattern every day:
having breakfast around the same time, going for a swim, and playing on
the beach. If this will work for you, that's great because it will benefit
your child with an ASD. If this doesn't work for you, read on.

– *Know when family vacations just aren't right for your family.* It's okay for
you to take a vacation without your child with an ASD. Sometimes, you
may need to vacation to reconnect with your other children or your
spouse. Your child with an ASD may be perfectly happy staying home doing his daily routine with people he feels comfortable with, such as a
close relative or your regular babysitter.

12

BROTHERS AND SISTERS: COPING WITH SIBLING ISSUES

We have other children besides our son with an ASD. How do we explain the diagnosis to them so that they can accept their brother's condition?

If there are siblings in the family, they need to be told about their brother's or sister's ASDs in an appropriate way. Don't be afraid to tell them, but also keep in mind that they may be overwhelmed. Often parents don't give siblings information about ASDs because they're trying to protect them. But this kind of thinking can backfire, and siblings can become frustrated, impatient, and nonaccepting of their brother or sister who cannot play with them, seems to ignore them, or throws horrific tantrums. Also, if siblings are not told the truth about ASDs, they tend to develop their own misconceptions. One child believed that he caused his brother's condition because he secretly hated him when he was born. Another child was afraid to be in the same room with his sister because he thought her condition was contagious, and he might catch it. One little boy kept trying to force a baseball cap onto his brother's head "to keep his brains from falling out any more."

How do you talk to siblings about ASDs?

First of all, be aware of your own feelings about the disorder; you're a role model for your children, and they'll be sensitive to your reactions. Are you feeling upset or angry or having trouble accepting the diagnosis? If so, this may be reflected in the way that you talk to your other children, either in your tone of voice, your mannerisms, or in the words that you use to explain the differences of your child with an ASD. If you are still struggling to sort out your own feelings, keep negative feelings in check when you tell siblings about ASDs. Your overall goal is to encourage a bonding relationship among siblings. With that in mind, explain your child's ASD in a way that is compassionate and clear. Siblings may not know how they are supposed to feel when they hear the news of a brother or sister's diagnosis and are likely to follow your lead. Help your children feel comfortable with the diagnosis.

When explaining an ASD to siblings, make sure to take into account their age and comprehension level. Because a two- or three-year-old sibling will not understand the phrase *autism spectrum disorder* or even the word *autism*, it's not necessary that you offer an explanation. But he or she can be taught how to play with a brother or sister in ways that won't cause unnecessary upset. For example, a two-year-old can learn to clap her hands rather than pull her brother's hair to get his attention and learn to roll a ball to her brother to interact with him. In fact, siblings of any age can learn appropriate ways to act and interact with a brother or sister with an ASD.

A four-year-old sibling is likely to ask many "why" questions when you explain that a brother or sister has an ASD. "Why can't my brother speak?" "Why won't he play?" "Why does he flap his hands?" Simple answers are required here. "Your brother hasn't learned how to speak or play," or "He flaps his hands when he feels upset." Make sure the sibling understands that certain inappropriate behaviors are unintentional. "I know you're upset that your brother knocked over your tower of blocks. He didn't mean it." Then help the sibling rebuild the tower.

With siblings who are six or seven years old, you can use appropriate, simple terms to explain ASDs. In *Siblings of Children with Autism: A Guide for Families*, Sandra Harris and Beth Glasberg describe a creative solution for explaining ASDs to this age group. You can create a book with your child and illustrate it with photos. In their example, seven-year-old Joe wrote a book about his brother Jack, who has an ASD.

> Joe and Jack are brothers. Joe likes to play, but Jack doesn't know how to play. Jack has autism. That makes Joe sad because he wants to play ball with Jack. Mommy says maybe Jack can learn to play with Joe. Dad will teach Jack how to play ball with Joe. This is a true story. The End.[1]

You can also read some of the wonderful children's books on ASDs that are available for this age group. Because children this age may not be ready to tell you how they are feeling, you can initiate conversations about emotional situations. For example, a sibling may be fearful when your child with an ASD throws a tantrum. You can reassure the sibling by saying, "It's okay to be afraid, but I will protect you and keep you safe."

Siblings ages nine to twelve can understand that ASDs are a problem in the brain, and that's why their brother or sister can't play, talk, or relate to them. You can model the behaviors that you want them to emulate when dealing with their siblings with ASDs. Siblings will look to their parents to see how they should react in situations that make them feel helpless or as if they have no control. For example, if the child with an ASD throws a block at a sibling, should the sibling yell at him? Demonstrate to the sibling that yelling is not the best solution and that a stern "No" is what may be required. Then explain that the behavior was not intentional and explore any feelings the sibling may have. Always let siblings know that they can come to you for help. It's crucial that children know their parents will support and protect them. At this age, they may have to field questions from their peers about ASDs. Therefore, let them know that they can come to you with any questions. Siblings this age should be encouraged to not only show compassion toward their brother or sister, but also to pursue their own interests outside of the home.

If the siblings are teenagers, you can explain ASDs in more detail and how it affects their brother or sister on different levels—socially and behaviorally. But remember that even if they understand the disorder on an intellectual level, they'll still need your support in dealing with feelings surrounding the diagnosis. Don't be discouraged if your once loving and attentive child has morphed into a teen who ignores his brother with an ASD and acts aloof, preferring to hang out with his friends. This is a typical developmental stage during which peer pressure may take precedence over family matters. Encourage your teen's independence, but at the same time, discourage a total rejection of the child with an ASD. Offer your teen coping strategies. If another teen makes fun of the fact that he has a brother with an ASD, teach him how to respond so that he can maintain his self-esteem. "My brother has an ASD—that's why he can't talk. But he's a computer whiz. You wouldn't believe what he can do." On some days, teens may feel embarrassed by a sibling with an ASD, especially when there are public displays of inappropriate behaviors, such as flapping or grunting at the mall. On other days, teens may feel pride in taking responsibility for their sibling with an ASD. Whatever feelings emerge, it's important for you to acknowledge and discuss them. Don't let an embarrassed teen feel ashamed about feelings of guilt or anger. Acknowledge these feelings and come up with ways to deal with them. Sharing your own feelings can also encourage your child to communicate and feel less alone.

Although parents may feel anxious about sharing the diagnosis of ASDs with siblings of any age, ironically, children and teens can often be much more accepting of the diagnosis than adults simply because they don't have any preconceived notions or biases about ASDs. By taking the mystery out of ASDs, siblings have the potential to be understanding, accepting, and supportive of their brothers or sisters with ASDs—and of all people with disabilities.

Here's what one mother says about explaining her son's diagnosis of an ASD to his brother.

I am the mother of a child on the autistic spectrum—a beautiful, funny, and mysterious eight-year-old named Max. When asked by friends or by other parents to try to explain what autism is, I often think about the way I try to describe Max's disorder to his younger brother, Tyler. I tell them, "When a person is autistic, it means that something in their brain is different than in other people's." To Tyler, age five, I explain that his brother Max's brain works differently from ours, so that it's hard for him to communicate what he's thinking or feeling. "That's why Max doesn't really want to play with other kids—except you—because he has his own very special ways of doing things, and it upsets him when they get disrupted."

Then Tyler points out: "But mom, Max taught himself Italian on the computer and is the smartest boy in his class—so how can he be autistic?"

I try my best to explain to Tyler that while every person is different in his or her own way, a person with autism has a uniquely different way of seeing and experiencing the world. Of course, I can't even begin to explain to him why Max is completely fascinated by the letters of the alphabet, or why he loves to count the numbers hidden on lampposts (numbers that most people never even notice), or why he needs to play the same song over and over and over again, or why Max knows the capital of every state or could read by the time he was barely eighteen months old, or how he achieves prodigious feats of memory that we now take for granted.

Tyler already knows I don't have those answers. Yet, even at five, Tyler already instinctively puts out his hand to make sure his older brother doesn't run across the street and grabs onto Max's shirt at the museum so he won't sprint off or get lost. He feels the need to look out for Max any way he can. He's even taken to making wishes in wishing wells for him.

Tyler's reaching out to his brother is just one of the ways that the mystery of autism has grabbed our family, the way it grabs all families it touches. To live with a child with autism is an often painful, but always inspiring journey that has forced us to hold together with love and commitment. It is a disorder that brings profound perspective and, yes, even a deep sense of joy. And that, perhaps, is the greatest mystery of all.

Our son's siblings know that he has an ASD, but we still haven't told our son that he has an ASD. Should we tell him?

In the beginning while you're trying to sort out your own feelings about the diagnosis, it's not necessary for you to tell your child about her condition. In fact, in most cases, your child will be too young to understand.

How to explain ASDs to your child depends on your child's age and her level of understanding. Children with ASDs who have average or above average intellectual ability can be told about their conditions, but in a way that they can understand and with sensitivity to their feelings.

Telling your child about her ASD is a personal decision. If you do decide to talk to your child about it, do it earlier rather than later. It's better that your child hears about ASDs from you rather than from her siblings or from other family members or friends. School-age children with ASDs often begin to develop an awareness that they are different, and self-esteem issues can arise if you're not honest with them about their diagnosis.

Some parents report that telling their children about their conditions made it easier for them to accept themselves. Understanding the reason why they had trouble in certain situations, like paying attention in noisy classrooms or finding buddies on field trips, helped these children feel more empowered. Giving them a reason for their challenges actually enhanced their self-esteem.

If you don't feel comfortable telling your child that she has an ASD, that's okay, but you may want to explore the reasons for your decision. Is it because of your own discomfort with the diagnosis? Is it a desire to protect your child? If so, from what? Some parents seem to perpetuate the stigma of ASDs by not telling their children. While parents may have good intentions in keeping the diagnosis a secret, they need to realize that other people will know, and there's nothing worse than a teenager finding out from someone else that she has an ASD.

Here's what some parents had to say.

> We didn't have a formal conversation with our daughter to tell her she had autism. We just never hid it. We talked about autism around the house from when she was young so that she and her brother and sister would know about it. It was always a part of our lives, and we wanted them all to accept it and not to be ashamed. Why hide the truth?

> Our son is pretty severely autistic, and I'm not sure if he would understand it even if we told him. I guess I like to fantasize about telling him. Just having that conversation would be great.

> I'm an adult with Asperger's, and I have a son who has the same diagnosis. I wish my parents had told me about my diagnosis when I was younger, so I wouldn't have had to wonder why I felt so different from the other kids. I told my seven-year-old son recently, and he was okay with hearing it. I used some books to help me tell him.

I've explained my son's diagnosis of an ASD to his siblings, and his sisters are okay, but his brother is not. He used to be so well behaved, and now he's acting out. What can I do?

Siblings who act out may be experiencing feelings of jealousy, resentment, or being left out because your child with an ASD requires more attention or receives special treatment. While there is no denying that your child with an ASD does require more attention, be careful about how you choose to deal with the sibling. Your typical son may tell you he's angry that you're not paying enough attention to him. Instead of giving into feelings of guilt and immediately jumping to the defensive, you can apologize, tell him how much you love and value him, and show empathy. "I'm sorry that I haven't spent as much time with you. You have every right to be angry with me. I'd feel the same way if I were in your shoes." Then ask questions and work together to figure out ways to reconnect and make him feel more special. Let him know you appreciate that he shared his feelings.

Sometimes, siblings may be acting out because they are afraid. You can come up with strategies for protecting a sibling from potentially hurtful situations—both emotional and physical—such as finding a hiding place for a child's special treasures, so they will not be destroyed, building a tower in a private place, or removing a sibling from the room if the sibling with an ASD is having a physical and emotional outburst.

If you don't encourage your children to express their feelings, their repressed feelings may manifest in other ways. Children may develop physical ailments, such as stomachaches or ulcers; emotional difficulties that result in depression; or behavioral problems, such as acting out in school. Also, siblings who may appear okay on the outside may not be okay on the inside. One mother had no idea how much her typical twelve-year-old daughter, a straight-A student, was affected by her brother having an ASD until she brought home C's on her report card. Her daughter explained that she'd been struggling with her schoolwork but had felt guilty about asking her parents for help. Children will often hold in their feelings to protect their parents because they can see how difficult it is for the parents to support a child with an ASD. It's important for you as a parent to let them know that you are there to protect them, not the reverse.

Siblings may also act out because they feel unduly burdened with the responsibility of being caretakers to their brothers or sisters with ASDs. Parents are often tempted to delegate caretaking responsibilities as soon as the sibling is old enough to take some of the pressure off them. Be careful. The child with an ASD is already demanding much of your attention, and siblings may have mounting resentment if they feel that they need to focus all their attention on their brother or sister as well. This can have a negative impact on the child's development, as well as strain sibling relationships.

Responsibilities must be divided up in a fair way. Household chores can include the child with an ASD, who can help by setting the table or feeding the dog. A sibling should not be required to be a disciplinarian. With the exception of mild reprimands, it is the parents who are responsible for discipline. Siblings should not have to be full-time babysitters either, although some child care responsibilities are appropriate, in much the same way that an older sibling would take care of a younger typical sibling.

You can make a difference in encouraging and guiding sibling relationships. Research indicates that the majority of siblings learn to handle and adapt to the experience of growing up with siblings with ASDs without negative effects. In fact, they often feel more positive about themselves and their situations.

Sometimes our daughter's siblings feel embarrassed by her behaviors, like when she's stimming in public. What can I do to help?

Sometimes siblings may feel uncomfortable or embarrassed when a child with an ASD stims in their presence in public. It's important to acknowledge their feelings of embarrassment and teach them strategies to deal with difficult behaviors, both on an emotional and practical level. Be a role model. Demonstrate how to express feelings appropriately. Show siblings what to say and what to do when their brothers or sisters with ASDs are engaged in self-stimulatory behaviors.

On a practical level, be aware of how you are behaving toward your child with an ASD when she is stimming. If you yell at her, you can bet that a sibling will do the same thing when the situation arises again. If you stress out, a sibling will probably react the same way. Also, your stress may further exacerbate the stimming behavior. You hold a tremendous amount of power. Make sure you are demonstrating appropriate behavior.

On an emotional level, you can model how to express feelings. It's okay for you to admit, "Your sister's behavior sometimes makes me feel anxious." In fact, it's healthy for siblings to know that you're human, too, and sharing your feelings can help relieve any guilt or shame they may have about their own reactions. It's important to teach siblings to differentiate between having feelings and acting on them. Siblings have every right to feel frustrated but do not have the right to act on their frustrations by yelling at or hitting the child with an ASD.

How do I help my daughter form a relationship with her brother with an ASD? She's tried to interact with him, but he's just not responding. I don't want her to give up, but I know she's discouraged. Is there anything I can do to help?

Just as parents dream of what it would be like if their child didn't have an ASD, siblings dream of having a typical brother or sister. Siblings generally want to bond with their brothers or sisters with ASDs but may not know how. Don't let them become discouraged when their efforts to play are ignored. You can teach them simple interactive skills. Find out what games or exercises the child is doing in treatment sessions and teach the sibling how to play them. For example, a young sibling can be taught how to roll a ball to her brother, blow bubbles, and help assemble a puzzle. An older sibling can be taught how to play games, as well as how to give praise ("Good job throwing the ball!") and give simple instructions ("Go get your cup").

Siblings can also be included in a child's therapy session as peer models who demonstrate play skills or social skills. Being involved in this way can make them feel special and important. Some siblings feel jealous that their brothers or sisters with ASDs are getting all the attention by going to therapy and are therefore happy to take part in the process.

Teaching siblings how to interact with their siblings with ASDs can make a big difference; it encourages the bonding process as well as boosts their self-esteem. One study compared before and after videos of siblings interacting with brothers and sisters with ASDs. The after videos, where the siblings had been taught certain play skills, showed that they were generally happier and played with their brothers or sisters more often and for longer periods of time.

I know it's difficult for our daughter to handle having a brother with an ASD all the time. I realize that so much of my time is devoted to him. How can I show his siblings how much I love them?

Your child with an ASD should be made to feel like a part of your family, not the center of it. No child, typical or with an ASD, benefits from *all* of his parents' attention.

Parents need to spend special, individual time with each of their children. While you may find it difficult to cram one more thing into your already busy schedule, this is crucial for your other children's development and self-esteem.

Carve out an evening or weekend day to focus on the sibling, rather than on your child with an ASD. Watch TV together, go to a movie, or play a game of cards. Just being together and sharing something between the two of you can go a long way in letting the child know how much you care.

Don't feel compelled to do everything as a family. Sometimes, it's okay to attend a sibling's soccer game or dance recital without bringing your child with an ASD, who may not only have trouble sitting through these events but also take the focus away from his sibling.

How can I maintain a sense of "normalcy" in our family for all of our children?

Here are a few simple tips.

- *Provide consistency.* Your child with an ASD and your other children need you to establish and stick to a routine—even if it's a new routine as a result of your child's diagnosis. Routines can provide comfort and a sense of normalcy for everyone.

- *Set realistic expectations for your children, your spouse, and yourself.* If you set goals that are beyond everyone's reach, you set everyone up for failure. Rather than piling on more and more responsibilities, adjust priorities. For example, it may be more important that an older sister is helping her brother with an ASD have breakfast rather than keeping her room neat. You may also want to lessen her current load of responsibilities for a while if you sense that she is having a difficult time adjusting to her brother's diagnosis.

- *Be patient and show compassion.* The diagnosis can be rough on everyone and, even though your own distress may cause you to feel impatient or short-tempered, it's important that you don't take your frustrations out on your children.

- *Demonstrate love and respect to all of your children.* Siblings can often feel left out and may need extra hugs and some special attention.

- *Focus on positives.* Minimize the focus on misbehaviors and comment on positive aspects of all your children.

- *Say thank you.* Thank your children for taking care of their brothers or sisters with ASDs and for making the necessary adjustments and accommodations in their own lives to help support their siblings with ASDs.

SOME THOUGHTS FROM SIBLINGS

Here are some letters from the siblings of children with ASDs with whose families I consult. This first letter was written by an eleven-year-old boy about his five-year-old sister with an ASD.

> We mostly include my younger sister in everything like going out to dinner and going to family stuff. But once we went to Florida for a long weekend without her. She stayed home with Grandma. I guess once in a while we go to the movies without her. I think that's normal. My friend Pete told me his sister doesn't always go with him when he goes out with his parents and his sister doesn't have autism.

The following is a joint letter from the brother and sister of an eleven-year-old boy with an ASD who recently went into a respite facility.

> We kids have a little bit of trouble having an autistic sibling. The autistic child gets more attention than the others just because he needs more help. Our names are Diane and Scott, and we have an autistic brother that no longer lives with us. Scott and I were not doing as well as we could have in school when my brother was here. This was because our parents were always chasing after our brother in the neighbors' yards, getting him ready, cleaning up the food he threw on the floor, and a lot of other things. So we were never able to study. This gave us no time for what we had to do. For example, studying for tests, or playing games, or going somewhere. We love our brother very much and were sad he left, but it has also made him and my family happier. Now he gets to go swimming daily, and he's lost quite a few pounds, and he is with people his level and people like him. Now our parents are able to help us study for tests, play games, and also they can attend our sports games. Life is different here, but we still are a happy family, no matter how close or how far, we still love each other.

This letter was written by a seven-year-old girl about her nine-year-old brother.

> Dear Santa,
>   Today I'm not writing about myself, I'm writing about someone else. I would like to ask you to please help my brother Michael. My brother has prob-

lems. He is autistic. He can't talk, so we can't understand him. When he wants something and we can't understand him, he starts to cry. If my family could hear him speak one word, it would be a miracle. If you do anything to help him speak, my family, friends and Michael would be very happy. So please, he needs your help. Thank you. And let him have a happy Christmas . . .

Sincerely yours,

Darcy

P.S. Merry Christmas . . .

Siblings deal with their own special issues surrounding ASDs, and it's important that their emotional needs are met so that they don't feel isolated. There are wonderful support groups that exist for siblings, both live and online. You can also be proactive by setting up a support group at your child's school. One mother spoke with the school psychologist who organized weekly meetings for siblings of children with special needs. It became a great way for her daughter to connect with other children who were dealing with similar issues so she could feel less alone. The school psychologist led the group in games and discussions. The group provided a safe space for the kids to vent their frustrations and talk about private issues that they didn't feel comfortable sharing with their parents. "It's like a private club," one sibling said. "It's been a great way to make new friends and talk to other kids who understand what I go through." You can contact your local ASA chapter for locations of sibling support groups near you in the United States or find your local international organization in Appendix E. You can also check Appendix F for online sibling support groups.

13

KEEPING IT PERSONAL: COPING WITH YOUR FRIENDS, YOUR MARRIAGE, AND YOUR SELF

How do I maintain my friendships when my friends have typical children and my child has an ASD?

The nature of your friendships may change after your child is diagnosed. Part of this is a result of time constraints. Much of your time is devoted to your child, with little left over to nurture friendships. Additionally, you may feel that your friends who have typical children really can't relate to your situation and that you can't relate to theirs.

After Jake was diagnosed, I had trouble trying to muster up feelings of joy upon hearing about a friend's daughter who sang in the school play or a friend's son who excelled at baseball, while my own son couldn't even speak let alone hold a baseball bat. I confided in my closest friends about how I was feeling, but even then I felt somewhat disconnected. They were compassionate and caring, yet I got the sense that they didn't really understand what I was going through. And so, I pulled away. I kept isolated. I understood my feelings, even if no one else did, and so I rationalized that I could work out my feelings by myself. But my strategy didn't work out the way I planned. I sank into a depression. I became more anxious. It took me months to realize that this was not the best strategy, and it wasn't a realization that I came to on my own. I had friends who did not give up on me, who kept coming after me even after I rejected their efforts to help. And I had a really good therapist who encouraged me to maintain my friendships.

Through my consulting work with families of newly diagnosed children, I've been able to collect stories from other parents about how their friendships were affected.

> We've maintained our friendships. My husband and I have always said that we wouldn't let our son's condition define us, so we actually don't purposely seek out other parents of autistic children. Initially, right after the diagnosis, I had a hard time being out with my friends. If they complained about their children, I resented that. How dare they complain about these trivial things their children were doing? Their children could speak, couldn't they? They had a perfectly normal life ahead of them, didn't they? I wanted to scream that out to them, but didn't want to come off as being self-righteous and indignant. This was an initial reaction, and it was based on hurt. I am so fortunate to have my best friend from when I was three years old as a support. I don't know what I'd do without her— we've been through a lot of tears together and I truly feel I'm not alone. I would have felt differently if I didn't have her.

> It's amazing how many new friendships we've formed as a result of autism. It's like a whole new community. At first I found it difficult to share what we were going through with my old friends who had typical children, so we really relied on the friendships we made in the support groups. Now we're more comfortable speaking with and spending time with our friends who have typical children. It's like we have two sets of friends, and they're all special.

> My friends were surprised about the diagnosis but have been my saving grace. They bring their kids over for play dates and give our son special attention.

My friends constantly remind me that typical kids do crazy stuff too. They tell me stories about how their kids have tantrums and have screaming fits in the mall. When my son bit his teacher once and I was nearly in tears, one of my friends told me about the time that her kid bit the teacher. I know it isn't exactly the same, but I love that my friends want to share their experiences with me, so I won't feel so bad. They support me as a parent and as a person, and they see my son for who he is— a kid with quirks who also has his strengths. One night my friends came to get me for a "reverse intervention." They said I wasn't having fun anymore and so they took me to a bar where we sat and drank cosmos and laughed and cried. I don't know what I'd do without them.

Here's my advice. You don't have to maintain all of your friendships after your child is diagnosed, but you should maintain some, make new ones, or at least have one friend in whom you can confide. It's so important to your well-being. Parents often find that by virtue of being part of the community of ASDs, they make new friends. There are wonderful support groups available for parents of children with ASDs. In addition to providing emotional support, these new friends, having walked in your shoes, may offer valuable practical advice on treatments, resources, service providers, and conferences in your area.

My marriage was fine before our son was diagnosed, but now it seems to be under stress. All of our focus is on our son with an ASD. What can I do to keep my marriage together?

An ASD has an impact on every aspect of a family's life, especially a marriage. An ASD can either be the glue that holds the couple together or the stress that pulls the marriage apart.

Marriage and childbirth are supposed to be happy moments in our lives, and we await the birth of a healthy child with great anticipation. When our child is diagnosed with an ASD, that happy picture gets shattered. Parents have said it feels as if their child has been kidnapped by an ASD in the middle of the night. The picture of the child is replaced with a picture of an ASD. The diagnosis of an ASD becomes the newest member of the family.

One of the causes of stress in marriages is the way parents react to the diagnosis. A grieving process may set in for one parent and not another. Highly charged emotions may be misunderstood or displaced onto one spouse, who becomes the scapegoat. The search for information about and appropriate treatments for ASDs could be a bonding experience, but teamwork is thwarted when one parent is in denial or chooses to not participate while the other parent is forced to do all the work. This trend can snowball, and resentments can build. In many cases, it is reported that the mother puts all her energy into the child with an ASD, while the father distances himself through work, creating a divide in the relationship.

Even if both parents do accept their child's diagnosis, there can still be undue stress on the marriage. Parents often devote all their energy to helping their children with ASDs and have none left to devote to their marriages. Romance becomes a thing of the past, and social lives and sex lives become nonexistent.

WHAT CAN YOU DO TO HELP YOUR MARRIAGE?

- *Remind yourself what attracted you to your spouse in the first place.* Try to unearth those qualities from the layers of hurt and anger that may have built up as a result of the diagnosis.

- *Ask for what you need.* We often expect our spouses to know how we are feeling and what we are thinking without telling them, thus setting ourselves up for disappointment if they don't meet our needs. Instead of blaming your partner for your unmet needs, ask for support. Say, "I need for you to listen to how I feel—even if you don't agree," or "I need your help in taking care of our son," or simply, "I need a hug." In addition to asking for support, be open to receiving it. Some people think that accepting emotional support is a sign of weakness, when in fact it's the opposite. Accepting support comes from a position of strength. Accepting support from your spouse can help cement your relationship.

- *Listen openly.* Most of us are so consumed with our own feelings and points of view that we don't take the time to stop talking and just listen. Listen openly to your partner. Don't blame. Don't attack. Don't say, "You *always* do this" or "You *never* do that." Marriage counselors recommend a helpful exercise for active listening. Sit facing your spouse, and let him or her talk. Don't interrupt or formulate your next argument. Just focus on paying attention to what your partner is saying. Don't jump into your point of view until your partner is finished speaking. When your partner is finished, it is your turn to speak while your partner listens. Although this simple exercise can be difficult to do, it is an incredibly effective way to improve communication between partners.

- *Communicate on a daily basis.* Express your feelings. Talk about problems or issues as they arise. Many times we ignore or repress feelings toward our spouses for fear of hurting the relationship, when in fact our unexpressed feelings are driving a huge wedge into it. We put off talking about problems or issues because we don't want to rock the boat and become angry when these problems are not addressed. Don't wait to communicate your feelings and address problems. The longer you wait, the more they will fester.

- *Use "I" statements.* Rather than saying, "You make me feel stressed," say, "I feel stressed when you say (or do) that." Be specific about what upsets you. Take responsibility for your own feelings. Even if the other person is causing you to feel stressed, you are the one who is responding in that way. You're entitled to your feelings, but the use of "you" at the beginning of a statement can sound accusatory and may automatically put the other person on the defensive. Begin statements with "I" so that the listener will be more open to hearing what you are saying.

- *Make time for your marriage.* Get a babysitter, relative, or respite care for your child with an ASD and go out to dinner or a movie. If possible, try to take a weekend away for just the two of you. Carve out time in your busy day for each other. Call each other on the phone. Come home from work on time or even early. Turn off the computer and get away from the websites about ASDs and chat rooms so that you can spend time with your spouse when he or she gets home from work. Designate nights when you take a break from ASDs and make a pact not to talk about them. Discuss sports or world events or plan a vacation. Rekindle your romantic relationship.

- *Make a conscious effort to work on your relationship.* All marriages require work, and when a marriage involves a child with an ASD, it requires even more work. About three months after Jake was diagnosed, Franklin and I sat down on the sofa in the living room and discussed whether or not our marriage would survive; the diagnosis was clearly tearing us apart. I spent all my time researching ASDs, Franklin spent more and more time away from home at work. I'd go to bed early; Franklin would come home late. We barely spoke. What conversations we did have were about Jake's diagnosis of an ASD—and we seemed to speak *at* rather than *to* each other. We were growing estranged. In that one conversation in our living room, we made the conscious decision to work at our marriage together. We still loved each other and maintained a sense of good will underneath all of the anguish. Honestly, in some ways it almost seemed easier to give up on the marriage. I wasn't sure if I had any more energy to work at one more thing in my life. We sought out the help of a couples' therapist who helped us through our difficult time.

Success in anything requires practice and hard work. Marriage is no different. In his book *The Seven Habits of Highly Effective People,* psychologist Stephen R. Covey tells the story of a man who asked for advice on his marriage. "My wife and I just don't have the same feelings for each other we used to have. I guess I just don't love her anymore and she doesn't love me. What can I do?" Covey listened patiently and said, "Love her." The man didn't understand. Covey went on to explain. Love is a verb; it's an action. It's not something that magically takes over you. It's something you do. It is a value that is actualized through loving actions.[1] Like anything else in life, if you want to be good at it, you need to work at it. Make an effort to show your partner that you care. A couple who works as a team to raise their child with an ASD can actually strengthen their marriage. They truly can create a deep and meaningful bonding experience.

Sometimes, however, the stress of the diagnosis can be so overwhelming that even the most well-intended couples don't make it. The reality of marriage is that sometimes it just doesn't work out, whether or not you have a child with an ASD. If this is the case, as in any divorce, try to make sure the child doesn't feel responsible for the breakup. Work together to come up with financial solutions and caretaking responsibilities that will benefit the child with an ASD.

Cindy N. Ariel, Ph.D., and Robert A. Naseef, Ph.D., are psychologists who specialize in helping couples cope with special needs in their families. This is what they wrote about the reality of marriage for parents of children with disabilities.

For a relationship that is fragile or unstable, a disability can be "the last straw." On the other hand, challenging life events can serve as catalysts for change. Some families disintegrate while others thrive despite their hardships. People can emerge from crisis revitalized and enriched. Hope for relationships really can spring from the crises people experience when their child has a disability.[2]

My husband is out of the house and at work the entire day while I'm trying to manage all of our son's treatment needs. I'm growing resentful. My husband says he wants to help out and be more a part of his son's life, but he doesn't know what to do. Any suggestions?

While in some cases, fathers are the primary caretakers of children with ASDs, mothers are more often the primary caretakers. "Caring for an autistic child can be a relentless and labor-intensive task—one that is overwhelmingly performed by mothers," says Jennifer Elder, a nursing researcher at the University of Florida's (UF) Center for Autism and Related Disabilities. In studies at UF, it was found that fathers were frustrated because they didn't know how to relate with children with ASDs. Fathers in the study were taught how to interact with their children using building blocks, bubbles, puppets, and toy cars and trucks. Once they learned how to relate to their children—through communication and play skills—they felt more empowered and connected to them. The study also indicated that these children showed tremendous improvement in their communication skills. In fact, it was reported that there was a 50 percent increase in the number of intelligible words the children spoke once their fathers had established good relationships with them. While your child may or may not experience such dramatic results, one thing is clear: A father plays an important role in helping a child with an ASD.

"It is important for both the child's mother and father to be involved in parent training whenever possible," said Jaime Winter, a research scientist at the University of Washington Autism Center. "Potential benefits that may follow from father participation include increased frequency of interaction and quality of interaction between fathers and their child with autism, increased treatment time for the child, and support for the child's mother."[3]

For more information on how to become more involved in helping out your child, talk to the best resources you have: your child's treatment providers. They are familiar with his specific needs and can offer great tips on games and activities that both you and your spouse can do at home with your child.

I love my son so much, but I'm feeling disconnected from him. How can I feel more connected?

It's often difficult to feel connected to your child if he rejects your hugs or seems indifferent to affection. It's painful when you say, "I love you," and your child can't say it back. And it's difficult to not take all of this personally, even when you know that you shouldn't. But there are ways to connect with your child—you just have to tune into your child's specific needs.

One of the best ways to establish a connection with your child is through laughter and play. Figure out what makes your child smile. Is it a favorite toy? Playing peekaboo? Jumping on the trampoline? Being tickled? If your child is in school or treatment sessions all day, it may seem like there's no time for fun, so it's up to you to make time for fun. Tune into to your child's sense of playfulness.

One mother found that her son who was overly sensitive to gentle touch but loved to wrestle. He was a big ten-year-old boy who weighed almost as much as his petite mom. She discovered his love of wrestling one day when they were sitting on the sofa. Usually, he didn't like it when someone sat too close to him, so his mother kept her distance. But on this day, she happened to reach over him to get the remote control for the TV, and as she did, she accidentally nudged him. He nudged her back. She looked at his face and noticed that he seemed to be playing a game. She nudged him a little harder, he nudged back, and before she knew it, they were rolling around on the living room rug in a playful wrestling match. The two of them laughed. It was an emotional moment for the mom. She was finally able to hold her son and be held by him. It had been a long time since they had hugged. After that, her son would actually initiate the wrestling match. He would approach his mom and give her a nudge. This became a mom/son special bonding activity. The boy's father reports that his son didn't want to wrestle with him. So he found his own special way to bond. His son loved the trampoline, so the two of them would go out in the backyard and jump together.

One great way to connect with your child is to figure out his communication preference. For example, is your child a visual, auditory, or kinesthetic learner? All of us have each of these senses, but there's always one that emerges as the dominant one. Visual learners like pictures and storybooks. Auditory learners like music and sounds. Kinesthetic learners prefer hands-on, tactile activities, like sculpting with clay or playing with Play-Doh. Sometimes, if you're not sure what your child's communication preference is, you can get clues from their stimming behaviors. A boy who taps on windows and loves music is most likely an auditory learner; a girl who is mesmerized by bright lights or engages in eye tracking is most likely a visual learner; a boy who flicks his fingers is most likely a kinesthetic learner. Within each of these categories, tune into your child's sensitivities. A visual learner may love colors but not bright lights. An auditory child may love music as long as it's not too loud. A kinesthetic child may prefer roughhousing over a gentle caress.

If you're not sure which type of category you're child falls into, don't worry. Experiment with different toys and games. Introduce new activities. Just because a child doesn't enjoy an activity initially doesn't mean that he won't ever enjoy it. Jake was initially afraid of the swings at the playground, but when he learned how to swing in his OT sessions, he began to love swinging. "Mo! Mo!" he used to say, indicating that he wanted to swing more. So he and I would sit side by side on our swings, pump our legs, and sail into the air. That's how we connected on some days. On other days, when Jake seemed "off" or detached, I'd just sit down near him. Just being in the same room with him often made me feel more connected; even if he was gazing off into space, I liked to believe that he felt my presence and felt more connected to me.

People keep telling me to do something nice for myself for a change, but I don't feel like it. Besides, I'd feel too guilty taking time away from my child with an ASD.

Friends and loved ones will probably recommend that you make time for yourself. This may seem absurd to you, especially if you are inundated with the demands of helping your child. Making time for yourself may also seem selfish, but keep in mind what flight attendants tell you on an airplane: "In case of emergency, parents should put on their oxygen masks first, then their children's." Put on your oxygen mask first! Making time for yourself is not selfish. It's both necessary and practical. If the thought of taking time away from your child makes you uneasy and produces feelings of guilt, think about it in a different way. Carving out time for yourself can actually make you a better parent. In other words, helping yourself will help your child.

I often hear from parents, "But I don't have time for myself!" Then make time. Start out by setting aside ten minutes a day to do something that makes *you* feel good—and that has nothing to do with ASDs. If you're feeling guilty, remind yourself that you are doing the right thing and that attending to your own needs is ultimately good for your child as well. The last thing your child needs right now is a burned-out parent. Keep those daily ten-minute breaks consistent. Don't skip a day. Try to build up from the ten minutes to fifteen, then twenty, all the way up to one hour a day.

What kinds of things can you do with your time? Create a life outside of ASDs. Take up activities that renew you as an individual. You can take a bath, go for a walk, call a friend, do yoga, play tennis, watch a sitcom on TV, read a novel, or anything else that makes you feel good and renews your spirit. The following are some additional stress-reducing tips from parents of children with ASDs.

– *Don't try to do everything yourself.* One mom's advice: "You may think you're Super Mom but you're not. I thought I was, and I almost went crazy trying to manage the house, my other kids, my job, and my son's therapy. Ask other people for help. Shift around your priorities. So maybe the beds don't get made every day, and there are dishes in the sink from dinner the night before, but there are more important things right now." Another mom said, "If there's something you just can't do with your child, get someone else to do that. I couldn't teach Samantha how to use the computer mouse for one of her treatment programs. It drove me crazy! A sixteen-year-old babysitter had her pointing and clicking in an hour. Best twelve bucks I ever spent!"

– *Breathe.* Seriously, take a few good, deep, cleansing breaths throughout the day to lower your stress level. Believe it or not, most adults don't even know how to take a deep breath. If you ask adults to breathe deeply, you'll see their chests move. Watch how a baby breathes when he's sleeping, and you'll notice his belly moving up and down. That's the correct way to breathe. Put your hands on your abdomen and breathe from your belly. If you can't figure out how to do this at first, try a good old-fashioned yawn. Yawning can also be an effective way to reduce stress.

– *Focus on the here and now.* This is called mindfulness—the art of being in the present moment. Instead of rushing around, take moments throughout the day to calm down and be mindful of the present moment. For example, instead of making phone calls or reading the newspaper while you rush through eating your lunch, just eat. Take the time to smell, taste, and enjoy your food. A simple act like mindfully eating, looking out the window at nature, or taking a walk can help ground you and relieve stress.

– *Focus on what you can control in the moment . . . not on what you can't control in the future.* Don't allow yourself to say, "I won't be happy until my child speaks or plays or gets better." Find joy in everyday moments and little victories.

– *Remember that feelings are not facts.* Just because you feel a certain way doesn't mean you are that way or that you need to act on your feelings.

– *Find your sense of humor.* Although it may be buried away somewhere, you can sometimes find humor in the midst of everyday stress. The parents of the boy who repeatedly broke the windows in their house eventually reached the point where they had coffee brewing for the window repairmen when they arrived and knew them all by name. "See you next week, Joe!" the parents would say after he fixed another window. One mom who could not get her son to stop squealing loudly in the middle of the mall decided to squeal with him. "What the heck. If people are going to stare, let me double their pleasure. Besides, my kid was so happy! Those were squeals of joy. I wanted to have some of that joy, too!" she said.

I know I should make more time for myself and my marriage, but I feel uncomfortable and guilty about leaving my child with a babysitter.

Parents may feel guilty about leaving their child at all, but it's important to spend time focused on yourself and on your relationship with your spouse. You can teach a babysitter or relative how to take care of your child's special needs. You can also contact teachers at local special education schools or contact psychology departments at local colleges for students majoring in special education. Other contacts include your local autism organizations, chapters of ASA or the ARC (formerly known as the Association for Retarded Citizens).

In addition to babysitting services, you can also opt for respite services. The word *respite* means break or breather—which is exactly what many parents need to relieve their stress and recharge. Respite care refers to short-term, temporary care that is provided for people with disabilities. It can involve daily caretaking in or outside of the house or overnight care for more extended periods of time. Families use respite care when they need a few hours off during the day or to take vacations that may be inappropriate for their children with ASDs. Many respite programs also provide caretaking training for parents and family members so that you can learn more techniques and feel more competent about caretaking. If you receive Medicaid, you can access these services through Medicaid service approved providers. There are also free-standing respite houses and respite camps. State respite programs may cover 40 hours per month of respite care. You can find information on respite care in the list of resources in Appendix F.

14

ADVICE TO LOVED ONES: COPING TIPS FOR FAMILY AND FRIENDS

POSITIVE AND HEALTHY WAYS FOR LOVED ONES TO SHOW THEIR SUPPORT

Your friends and loved ones may also need advice on how to cope when your child is diagnosed. They, too, may be trying to sort out their own feelings of sadness or confusion. In addition, they may want to help support you and your family but feel powerless to do so. They may not know what to do or say. Here's some advice to all your loved ones, to help them help you when your child is diagnosed with an ASD. Let them read this list of tips on how to show their support in positive and healthy ways.

- *Try to avoid the clichés.* Speak from your heart. Tell the parents of a child with an ASD that you care and that you are there for them.

- *Reach a place of acceptance.* Acceptance is difficult for everyone who knows and loves the affected family. You may feel guilty or helpless. Deal with your personal acceptance issues on your own. It's enough for parents to have to deal with their own acceptance issues surrounding their child's diagnosis without the additional stress of taking care of you. Talk to your friends or a therapist to sort out your feelings.

– *Show the family that you accept them and their child with an ASD.* Visit. Call. Invite them over. Ask questions about the diagnosis, treatment, and what you can do to help.

– *Be careful about offering unsolicited advice.* It is not helpful to say, "If you would only do X, your son would be just fine." If you do have suggestions, offer them in a nonjudgmental way, such as, "I read an article about such and such a treatment that may be helpful." If your suggestion is turned down, let it go. Don't persist, and don't take it personally. The parent may not be ready to hear it.

– *Don't play the blame game.* One woman scolded her daughter-in-law for causing her grandson's autism: "If you'd only read to him more often, he wouldn't be in this state." Another in-law blamed the marriage: "I told you not to marry her in the first place." Blaming is completely uncalled for and can damage your relationship with the affected family.

– *Don't criticize.* If the parent chooses an intensive course of treatment that you disagree with, it's not helpful for you to say, "That's not what I would do. When I raised you, I made sure you had playtime. Why aren't you doing that for your own child?" If you want to communicate your point of view, do it in a constructive and appropriate way so that the parent does not feel criticized or rejected.

– *Offer hope but not false hope.* One grandfather of a child with an ASD said, "My grandson's perfect. Just give him some therapy, and he'll grow out of it." It's wonderful to be optimistic, but offering unrealistic expectations can be very difficult for a parent to hear, especially when facing the reality of how much hard work goes into treating their child.

– *Reflect feelings.* That is, when a parent says "I feel terrible," instead of saying "Cheer up, look on the bright side," try saying, "You must feel terrible. This is a really difficult situation." If the parent says, "Sam cried for an hour during his treatment session today," instead of saying, "He'll get over it" and offering tips on how to help the child get over it, simply say, "It sounds like that must have been emotionally draining for you." Then let the parent talk.

- *Listen to what the parent has to say.* Most of us like to talk, especially when we're trying desperately to help someone we love. Make sure to make time to listen. Sometimes, we need to absorb the words and tune into the parent's tone of voice. Other times, we need to go beyond the words and be sensitive to nonverbal behavior. If you're face-to-face with the parent, notice what his or her body language is saying. Notice facial expressions. (What do the eyes tell you? Is the brow furrowed?) Notice body posture. (Are the arms crossed? Fists clenched?) These nonverbal cues can signal to you how the parent is really feeling. Using either verbal or nonverbal cues, you can reflect feelings. You can say, "You seem tense" or "You sound anxious" and follow up with "How can I help you?" If the response is "I don't know" or "There's nothing you can do," then offer suggestions, but be specific. Offer to help out with errands, housework, or child care. All of these listening techniques show that you care.

- *Be there.* Leave a phone message saying that you're around to help even if you don't get a response. If nothing else, you can sit with the parent and not say a word—just let him or her cry. Drop off a tin of cookies with a note. One family's neighbors organized a meal delivery. Each neighbor was responsible for dinner one night a week and dropped it off in a cooler that was left at the front door.

- *Don't take it personally.* Accept the parents for where they are emotionally. If a parent maintains that he or she doesn't want to talk, reacts angrily to something you say, or rejects your offer to help, don't take it personally. But don't just let it go at that, either. Let them know that you're there for them in the future. Don't be afraid to follow up again. Just because the parent can't accept your help at that moment doesn't mean they will never want your help. Keep in touch.

Showing that you care during this time can be a challenge. Just do what you can and know that your support means a lot. These tips will help make things easier for you and the parents you love.

HOW LOVED ONES CAN CONNECT TO A CHILD WITH AN ASD

Family and friends may feel awkward or anxious around your child because they want to make a connection but don't know how to go about it. I remember when my friends began having babies while I was still single. I'd visit them in the hospital, ooing and ahhing at their newborns from a distance, and pray that they wouldn't ask me to hold their babies or do anything that brought me within three feet of the darling but intimidating creatures. I'd had absolutely no experience with babies and was not planning on having one of my own for years. It wasn't until one of my friends, so sleep-deprived that she had no awareness of my anxiety, walked over to where I was sitting and just put her baby in my arms. I held my breath. What was I supposed to do? I was slouched down in the chair. Could I move? If I moved, would I hurt this tiny, defenseless being? "Here's how you do it," my friend said, and gently adjusted the baby so that her head was supported by the crook of my arm and her tiny feet remained swaddled in her blanket. I began to breathe again. It wasn't so difficult. After that, I actually looked forward to baby visits.

Much of our discomfort in life stems from feeling a lack of control and helpless. This feeling escalates when the stakes are high, especially in situations that involve someone we love. Sometimes, out of fear, family or friends pull away from us after our child is diagnosed, convincing themselves that they're being protective, by shielding the child from their ignorance of ASDs—when in reality, they're hurting the ones they love. Some pull away because they feel rejected; the child doesn't respond when they call her name or doesn't let them hug her.

You can teach your family and friends how to approach your baby, toddler, or child of any age with an ASD. You can teach them what to say, what to do, and how to respond to your child in different situations. Making your family and friends feel comfortable around your child will benefit everyone. It will make them feel more supportive and make you feel more connected.

Explain what the diagnosis means so they can understand your child's symptoms and behaviors. Explain treatments and how they work. Show them how to act around your child. We explained to Jake's grandparents how to interrupt and redirect his behavior when he engaged in self-stimulatory behavior; they learned how to stop Jake mid-cycle while he was spinning and get him to do a puzzle. We showed our family and friends how to hug Jake (firmly and quickly), told them what to avoid in his presence (loud voices and loud noises), and how to interact with him (hold your hand up and say "Give me five!" then wait for a response). They learned how to crouch down to his eye level to help Jake establish eye contact, guide his hand when he was doing a puzzle, and model social questions and answers that Jake was learning in his treatment sessions ("How are you?" "How old are you?" "What's your name?").

Here are some simple tips to pass onto friends and family who want to connect with your child.

- *Crouch down or sit so that you meet the child at eye level.* This will make it easier for the child to establish eye contact. Encourage eye contact when you are communicating with him. Gently guide the child's face toward yours, or move your head into his field of vision. If your child does not like to be touched, you can create blinders with your hands around the child's face so that the child will look straight ahead at you. You can also find something that will attract the child's attention, such as a favorite toy or food treat, and hold it in front of your eyes so that the child will look at you (then lower it slowly while praising the child for looking at you).

- *Be aware of how close you sit or stand to the child.* What is the child's comfort zone? If you're not sure, ask the parents. Some children need to be very close to a person, whereas others need distance.

- *Make sure the child is paying attention to you when you speak to him.* Help the child look at you, either by using a verbal prompt (saying the child's name) or adding a manual prompt (gently placing your hands as blinders on the sides of the child's face and moving his head so that his eyes are looking at you).

- *Keep it simple!* Speak in simple and clear language, using brief phrases that are specific, such as "Look at me" rather than just "Look." Use real words rather than cute made-up words, such as "Look at Grandma" rather than "Lookee at Nanna you silly-billy boy." Use phrases that are familiar to your child. For example, if he is learning to respond to "Do this" in his treatment sessions, don't say "I want you to do something for me now." Avoid using ambiguous phrases such as "Let's call it quits" or adding unnecessary words at the ends of sentences, such as "Do this, sweetie pie."

– *Respect the parents' wishes and the child's needs.* If a parent tells you that Jonathan doesn't like being hugged, don't hug him. If he doesn't like being patted on the head, don't pat him on the head. Unfortunately, friends and family members sometimes feel a sense of entitlement: "But I always hug all my grandchildren!" Be careful about overstepping boundaries. This may push you away from both the child and the parents.

– *Be persistent and patient.* You won't get the same quick response from a child with an ASD as you would from a typical child. Rolling a ball to a child with an ASD and expecting it to come right back to you may be unrealistic. You may have to follow that ball, put it in the child's hand, and guide the child through the entire process of rolling the ball. With most typical children, you'd only need to show them once, and they'd get it. This is not the case for most children with ASDs. You may have to show them again and again.

– *Don't act on your hurt feelings.* If you feel rejected because the child is not responding to you, don't give up. Don't take it personally. Just because a child doesn't look at you doesn't mean she doesn't love you. Hang in there. Ask the parent for guidance. Parents may also feel rejected if you give up on trying to connect with their child. They need to see that you are trying and that you care.

– *Find and join a support group.* There are wonderful groups that help extended families and friends of children with ASDs. They can be a great place for you to share what you're going through with others who are in similar situations. You can contact your local autism organizations for information (see Appendix D).

PARTING THOUGHTS ON COPING

Coping with ASDs is in some ways like training for a marathon. Franklin is a marathon runner. He actually just took up running again a few years ago after not having run since college. When Franklin started training, he was fiercely determined. He wanted so much to reach his end goal that he didn't pay much attention to the process of getting there. On his practice runs, he ran too hard and too fast and consequently got leg cramps, sustained a knee injury, and even vomited after one twenty-one-mile practice run. But none of this deterred Franklin. He kept on going. He overtrained—rarely taking the recommended days off between practice runs. On his first 15K race, he started out sprinting and ended up "hitting the wall" much too early. It wasn't until he had to drop out of the race from exhaustion that the realization hit him: If he wanted to succeed, he'd have to pace himself. So he slowed down—just enough to regroup, heal, and get himself organized—and he began to practice again. Since then, he has successfully run four marathons over the past four years.

Many parents have similar experiences when they enter the world of ASDs. It's like they've barely tied their shoes before they're off and running, breaking into a sprint before they've even had a chance to warm up or chart their course. Their determination gets the best of them, and they experience early burnout.

I'm not suggesting that "slow and steady" wins the race because in the case of ASDs, it doesn't. Be aware that the clock is ticking to get your child help, but remember that *working hard* is not the same as *working smart*. If you're just beginning your journey now, try to take a deep breath and get yourself centered before you make the important decisions. If you've already begun your journey, remind yourself to breathe along the way. Give yourself breaks. Keep up your spirits. Surround yourself with people who are going to help you stay positive. Remember that the beginning is the most difficult part. Ask any parent who's been there—the process of coping does get easier over time. You will figure out how to run your own personal marathon and find victories along the way.

PART IV:
HEALING

There are only two ways to live your life. One is as though nothing is a miracle. The other is as though everything is a miracle.

—ALBERT EINSTEIN

15

THOUGHTS ON HEALING . . .

The word *healing* can mean different things to different people. Before Jake was diagnosed, I thought about healing in an entirely different way—in the more traditional sense of the word. I thought of healing as getting better or being cured—as the endpoint to an illness. But not anymore. In fact, my vision of healing doesn't imply illness at all. And it's not some passive state where you wait for something to happen. Rather, I now think of healing as an active process: an energetic and constantly evolving process that encompasses hope and acceptance.

What I'm really talking about in this chapter is self-healing: accepting ourselves, our spouses, our families, and our children with ASDs. It's about accepting ourselves and our loved ones for who we are. Right now. Not two years ago before the diagnosis when life was different or two years from now when life may be different, but today.

If you're reading this and your child has just been recently diagnosed, you may not be ready for the self-healing step. Parents who've been through this know that right after your child is diagnosed most of your energy is focused on helping your child as you immerse yourself in the new world of autism spectrum disorders. You're on a mission to keep up-to-date with the latest research and treatments, attend autism conferences, read autism books, seek out autism professionals, and absorb anything that relates to autism. In the beginning, that's okay. Self-healing is not a priority when you're overwhelmed by the news of your child's diagnosis and hurrying to find the right treatment. But at some point, even if you choose to devote your life to helping your child with an ASD, you need to heal yourself—if for no other reason than to be a better parent to your child.

You may remain immersed in the world of ASDs for the rest of your life (many of us do), but your perspective will change over time. Suddenly, you find that this strange new world you've entered isn't so new anymore. It starts to feel familiar. You begin to integrate treatment sessions and specialists' visits into your everyday life. It's when you allow yourself to settle into your new life and your new role that the acceptance and healing process can take place.

Real acceptance doesn't happen automatically. Rather, acceptance is a process that you must consciously choose. You have the choice to accept yourself, your child, and your loved ones, imperfections and all.

The first step toward healing is learning to adjust your expectations, to accept what you are feeling under the circumstances, whether you're manic or depressed, driven or deflated, working too much or not working enough. There are good days and not so good days. There are the days when you feel like "parent of the year" for following through on all of the homework assigned to you by your child's therapy team, and days when you feel like "worst parent of the year" because your child is having a tantrum, you're exhausted, and you're not following through on anything. In fact, you may just find yourself on the floor having your own tantrum right alongside your child.

But it's all okay. Whether you're feeling like a great parent or a terrible parent, it's just a part of this process of acceptance. If you insist on being a perfectionist who must always have everything under control, you'll never win. As much as you may want to make everything perfect by controlling every situation and every one of your child's behaviors, constantly pushing for your child's treatment to work better and faster, you can't. If you want to set yourself up for success, just try to do the best you can and know that's enough. Let go of trying to be perfect all the time and trust that you're making the right decisions along the way, even if they don't always turn out the way you planned.

When parents call me for consultations, they tell me they want to do the very best and be the very best for their children. I know what that feels like. The stakes are different when you're making a decision for your children. Sometimes, parents come to me with stories of how they didn't choose the right treatment plan or the right treatment providers or agree to the right IEP. If you've been in that situation, you're not alone. I'll tell you what I tell the parents I work with: Give yourself a break. Forgive yourself. Accept that you made mistakes and don't allow them to hold you back. Pick yourself up and move forward.

You have the power to make changes if things don't go as planned. So, before you go off and make decisions about your child's treatments that may not be perfect, choose treatment providers who may not be perfect, or have days that are far from perfect, let me welcome you to the "imperfect club."

Self-acceptance also extends to accepting those around you, such as accepting your spouse even if he or she doesn't agree with every treatment decision or has a different point of view about your child; or accepting your parents, in-laws, and loved ones even if they're expressing unsolicited opinions out of a desire to help. It takes an enormous amount of energy to keep pushing against the people you love. It's often when you ease up on the pushing that you realize all of you are on the same team—your child's team—even if all of you are not speaking the same language yet.

One of the most important parts of the healing process is accepting your child for who she is right now. If you dwell on the past or focus all your energy on the future, you'll miss out on the joy that's right in front of you. You'll miss out on your own beautiful child who is being exactly who she is supposed to be and who loves and accepts you for who you are. Whether your child speaks or remains nonverbal, engages with others or continues to be disconnected, attends a general education school or a special school for autism, your child needs your acceptance and unconditional love.

It's amazing what can happen when we really accept our children. We learn to experience life in the moment. Our perspectives change. We value the things we used to take for granted. We learn to celebrate little victories. In fact, little victories become monumental events—our child waves or claps for the first time; we get our first real hug from our four-year-old; we have a family outing, and there's not one tantrum. Allowing ourselves to embrace these moments is part of the healing process. One parent of a child with an ASD described it like this.

> This is not going to sound like a big deal unless you know where we were in the beginning. Our four-year-old daughter didn't speak. Last night we put her to sleep in her new "big girl" bed, which is pretty high off the ground. About half an hour later she started yelling "Daddy! Daddy! Daddy!" I remember wondering about a year ago, "When will my daughter call out for me?

Every child with an ASD develops at her own pace. I've had the opportunity to follow three of the children I wrote about at the beginning of book and they have all grown in different ways. Nathan's parents accept and adore him for who he is and how far he's come. He still doesn't speak, but he has learned to use picture cards to point out what he wants. Now, at age eleven, Nathan attends a special school for autism. He has learned to be much more independent; he can help himself to snacks and take part in family chores (his favorite is sweeping). He loves to swim. He can now swim in the deep end of the pool and has learned to jump even higher than his brother and sister on the trampoline in their backyard.

Sam is no longer hyperactive now that she's taking new medication. At age five, she is in a special needs classroom at her local public school, where she also receives speech therapy and occupational therapy. Her favorite class is music, in which she's discovered her love for singing and playing the tambourine. Her teacher reports that she is always smiling.

Michael is still the most talkative one in his family. At seven years old, he attends public school where he is in a regular classroom with an aide. Michael is learning how to hold conversations with his classmates through a social skills group run by the psychologist at his school. At his most recent show-and-tell, his butterfly collection got the biggest round of applause from his classmates. Michael is excited about playing his first role in a school play.

Jake is now nine years old and attends a local private school. He and his three best friends play soccer, basketball, and baseball together—along with Super Mario and Star Wars video games. Even though we seem to be out of the woods, as a mom, I must confess that I still worry. I know that social pressures change and present their own challenges as kids get older. That's why we continue with Jake's social skills support on a monthly basis. Even though I can't predict his future, I want to make sure our son is as prepared as possible as he continues to forge his own way in the world.

Each one of these children has his or her own story—just like your child. All of us have our own personal experiences as we go through the process of healing. Along the way, what unites us all is the discovery that our children touch our hearts in ways that we could never have imagined.

No matter where our children with ASDs are now or end up, we are forever changed by our journeys with them. If you talk to most parents of children with ASDs, they'll tell you that their children become their teachers. I called Jake my "little guru." In many ways, we helped save each other. Had it not been for his diagnosis, I probably would have continued on my corporate fast track to the point where I may have lost perspective on what was really important to me. Jake taught me how to live in the moment and redefine my priorities and my preconceived notions of perfection. He taught me how to be a better mother and trust my instincts. Now that Jake is in school and I have the opportunity to go back to the corporate life that I had found so fulfilling before his diagnosis, I don't want to go back. I want to continue to fight for autism advocacy and help other parents fight to save their children.

Parents frequently tell me that their children with ASDs have taught them invaluable realizations. Here's what one couple said about their son.

> Our son Dov is now eleven. We watched with a mixture of joy and sadness as his eight-year-old sister surpassed him, and again as his six-year-old little brother has overtaken him and become his helper. I cannot even imagine what life is like for Dov—what he understands and what he doesn't. He is sweet and cheerful, but sometimes it seems as if Dov is in prison. And if you want to spend time with him, you have to get in that prison too. You have to get very small and very slow and maybe—just maybe—for an instant you get to connect with him. Dov is so forgiving as we struggle to understand him. By example, he has taught us so much about patience and tenacity and the enduring power of love.

This was written by Jonathan Shestack and Portia Iversen, who are among the many parents who feel passionate enough to take on the cause of ASDs as their life's work. Jonathan and Portia founded the organization Cure Autism Now (CAN), which provides information for parents, funds research for scientists, and advocates for the rights of people with ASDs. As you make your way into the world of ASDs, you'll find that there are other exceptional people like Jonathan and Portia. Karen and Eric London are parents who founded NAAR. Bob and Suzanne Wright are grandparents who founded Autism Speaks. Shelley Hendrix Reynolds and Jeana Smith, both parents, along with grandmother Nancy Cale, founded Unlocking Autism. Dr. Bernard Rimland is a father who founded ASA. And the list goes on.

If you're just beginning your journey, it may be difficult to imagine that you'll ever get involved with anything outside your immediate focus of attending to your child's needs. If you don't, that's okay. But know that there are parents out there who can relate to what you're going through. They know what it's like to have hopes and dreams. Jonathan and Portia said the following:

We still dream of the day when we will walk into Dov's room and hear him say, "I love you." And then because I know my knees will give out, I will have to cling to him for support, and he will say, "And I know you've loved me all these years.

You will find your way. Parents have this incredible strength that emerges when their children are diagnosed. I've seen it again and again. When I came across the following story, I thought of all the parents I work with. It's called "The Mountain," by Jim Stovall.

> There were two warring tribes in the Andes, one that lived in the lowlands and the other high in the mountains. The mountain people invaded the low-landers one day, and as part of their plundering of the people, they kid-napped a baby of one of the lowlander families and took the infant with them back up into the mountains.
>
> The lowlanders didn't know how to climb the mountain. They didn't know any of the trails that the mountain people used, and they didn't know where to find the mountain people or how to track them in the steep terrain.
>
> Even so, they sent out their best party of fighting men to climb the mountain and bring the baby home.
>
> The men tried first one method of climbing and then another. They tried one trail and then another. After several days of effort, however, they had climbed only several hundred feet.
>
> Feeling hopeless and helpless, the lowlander men decided that the cause was lost, and they prepared to return to their village below.
>
> As they were packing their gear for the descent they saw the baby's mother walking toward them. They realized that she was coming down the mountain that they hadn't figured out how to climb.
>
> And then they saw that she had the baby strapped to her back. How could that be?
>
> One man greeted her and said, "We couldn't climb this mountain. How did you do this when we, the strongest and most able men in the village, couldn't do it?"
>
> She shrugged her shoulders and said, "It wasn't your baby."

I present this story of "The Mountain" for all the mothers—and the fathers—and for all the loved ones of children with ASDs who have demonstrated enor-mous strength and courage in the face of adversity. I've had the privilege of meeting some extraordinary and loving parents, grandparents, uncles, aunts, cousins, and friends of children with ASDs who would have managed to get that baby down the mountain. I've also had the privilege of working with some extraordinary, bright, caring, and compassionate professionals, who love the children they work with so much that they could just as easily have been the ones who carried that baby down the mountain.

You're not alone. You will discover this cycle of healing if you haven't already. I didn't see it at first, but it slowly unfolded through my own experience with Jake. In the beginning, just after Jake was diagnosed, I reached out and called parents for help and advice. A year into the process, parents began calling me for advice. Whenever anyone asked how they could repay me, I said, just extend the same courtesy to the next parent who calls you. When you're on the receiving end of the line in the beginning, you just can't imagine what it's like being on the giving end. But you get there. It happens before you know it. All of a sudden you find yourself becoming the expert, and you're the one helping that parent with the newly diagnosed child. You discover there's this whole community of loving and giving people who embrace you. Once you're a part of it, it stays with you. Through your child, you're connected to this large extended family who understands and accepts you and knows what you're going through.

Even if you're only beginning your journey and this book is your first glimpse into the larger community of ASDs, you've already become a part of it.

Welcome to your new family.

MODIFIED CHECKLIST FOR AUTISM IN TODDLERS
(M-CHAT)

Please fill out the following about how your child <u>usually</u> is. Please try to answer every question. If the behavior is rare (e.g., you've seen it once or twice), please answer as if the child does not do it.

1. Does your child enjoy being swung, bounced on your knee, etc.?   YES NO

2. Does your child take an interest in other children?   YES NO

3. Does your child like climbing on things, such as up stairs?   YES NO

4. Does your child enjoy playing peek-a-boo/hide-and-seek?   YES NO

5. Does your child ever pretend, for example, to talk on the phone or take care of dolls or pretend other things?   YES NO

6. Does your child ever use his/her index finger to point, to ask for something?   YES NO

7. Does your child ever use his/her index finger to point, to indicate interest in something?   YES NO

8. Can your child play properly with small toys (e.g., cars or bricks) without just mouthing, fiddling, or dropping them?   YES NO

9. Does your child ever bring objects over to you (parent) to show you something?   YES   NO

10. Does your child look you in the eye for more than a second or two?   YES   NO

11. Does your child seem oversensitive to noise? (e.g., plugging ears)   YES   NO

12. Does your child smile in response to your face or your smile?   YES   NO

13. Does your child imitate you? (e.g., you make a face— will your child imitate it?   YES   NO

14. Does your child respond to his/her name when you call?   YES   NO

15. If you point at a toy across the room, does your child look at it?   YES   NO

16. Does your child walk?   YES   NO

17. Does your child look at things you are looking at?   YES   NO

18. Does your child make unusual finger movements near his/her face?   YES   NO

19. Does your child try to attract your attention to his/her own activity?   YES   NO

20. Have you ever wondered if your child is deaf?   YES   NO

21. Does your child understand what people say?   YES   NO

22. Does your child sometimes stare at nothing or wander with no purpose?   YES   NO

23. Does your child look at your face to check your reaction when faced with something unfamiliar?   YES   NO

M-CHAT SCORING INSTRUCTIONS:

A child fails the checklist when 2 or more critical items are failed OR when any three items are failed. Yes/no answers convert to pass/fail responses. Below are listed the failed responses for each item on the M-CHAT. Bold capitalized items are CRITICAL items.

1. No	6. No	11. Yes	16. No	21. No
2. **NO**	7. **NO**	12. No	17. No	22. Yes
3. No	8. No	13. **NO**	18. Yes	23. No
4. No	9. **NO**	14. **NO**	19. No	
5. No	10. No	15. **NO**	20. Yes	

Not all children who fail the checklist will meet criteria for a diagnosis on the autism spectrum. However, children who fail the checklist should be evaluated in more depth by the physician or referred for a developmental evaluation with a specialist.

Please note:
The M-CHAT was not designed to be scored by the person taking it. In the validation sample, the authors of the M-CHAT scored all checklists. If parents are concerned, they should contact their child's physician.

APPENDIX B

DIAGNOSTIC CRITERIA FOR THE FIVE PERVASIVE DEVELOPMENTAL DISORDERS

(DSM-IV-TR: Diagnostic and Statistical Manual of Mental Disorders Fourth Edition, Text Revision)

299.00 AUTISTIC DISORDER

A. A total of six (or more) items from (1), (2), and (3), with at least two from (1), and one each from (2) and (3):

> (1) qualitative impairment in social interaction, as manifested by at least two of the following:
>
>> (a) marked impairment in the use of multiple nonverbal behaviors such as eye-to-eye gaze, facial expression, body postures, and gestures to regulate social interaction
>>
>> (b) failure to develop peer relationships appropriate to developmental level

(c) a lack of spontaneous seeking to share enjoyment, interests, or achievements with other people (e.g., by a lack of showing, bringing, or pointing out objects of interest)

(d) lack of social or emotional reciprocity

(2) qualitative impairments in communication as manifested by at least one of the following:

(a) delay in, or total lack of, the development of spoken language (not accompanied by an attempt to compensate through alternative modes of communication such as gesture or mime)

(b) in individuals with adequate speech, marked impairment in the ability to initiate or sustain a conversation with others

(c) stereotyped and repetitive use of language or idiosyncratic language

(d) lack of varied, spontaneous make-believe play or social imitative play appropriate to developmental level

(3) restricted repetitive and stereotyped patterns of behavior, interests, and activities, as manifested by at least one of the following:

(a) encompassing preoccupation with one or more stereotyped and restricted patterns of interest that is abnormal either in intensity or focus

(b) apparently inflexible adherence to specific, nonfunctional routines or rituals

(c) stereotyped and repetitive motor mannerisms (e.g., hand or finger flapping or twisting, or complex whole-body movements)

(d) persistent preoccupation with parts of objects

B. Delays or abnormal functioning in at least one of the following areas, with onset prior to age 3 years: (1) social interaction, (2) language as used in social communication, or (3) symbolic or imaginative play.

C. The disturbance is not better accounted for by Rett's Disorder or Childhood Disintegrative Disorder.

299.80 ASPERGER'S DISORDER

A. Qualitative impairment in social interaction, as manifested by at least two of the following:

> (1) marked impairment in the use of multiple nonverbal behaviors such as eye-to-eye gaze, facial expression, body postures, and gestures to regulate social interaction

> (2) failure to develop peer relationships appropriate to developmental level

> (3) a lack of spontaneous seeking to share enjoyment, interests, or achievements with other people (e.g., by a lack of showing, bringing, or pointing out objects of interest to other people)

> (4) lack of social or emotional reciprocity

B. Restricted repetitive and stereotyped patterns of behavior, interests, and activities, as manifested by at least one of the following:

> (1) encompassing preoccupation with one or more stereotyped and restricted patterns of interest that is abnormal either in intensity or focus

> (2) apparently inflexible adherence to specific, nonfunctional routines or rituals

> (3) stereotyped and repetitive motor mannerisms (e.g., hand or finger flapping or twisting, or complex whole-body movements)

> (4) persistent preoccupation with parts of objects

C. The disturbance causes clinically significant impairment in social, occupational, or other important areas of functioning.

D. There is no clinically significant general delay in language (e.g., single words used by age 2 years, communicative phrases used by age 3 years).

E. There is no clinically significant delay in cognitive development or in the development of age-appropriate self-help skills, adaptive behavior (other than in social interaction), and curiosity about the environment in childhood.

F. Criteria are not met for another specific Pervasive Developmental Disorder or Schizophrenia.

299.80 RETT'S DISORDER

A. All of the following:

  (1) apparently normal prenatal and perinatal development

  (2) apparently normal psychomotor development through the first 5 months after birth

  (3) normal head circumference at birth

B. Onset of all of the following after the period of normal development:

  (1) deceleration of head growth between ages 5 and 48 months

  (2) loss of previously acquired purposeful hand skills between ages 5 and 30 months with the subsequent development of stereotyped hand movements (e.g., hand-wringing or hand washing)

  (3) loss of social engagement early in the course (although often social interaction develops later)

  (4) appearance of poorly coordinated gait or trunk movements

  (5) severely impaired expressive and receptive language development with severe psychomotor retardation

299.10 CHILDHOOD DISINTEGRATIVE DISORDER

A. Apparently normal development for at least the first 2 years after birth as man-ifested by the presence of age-appropriate verbal and nonverbal communication, social relationships, play, and adaptive behavior.

B. Clinically significant loss of previously acquired skills (before age 10 years) in at least two of the following areas:

  (1) expressive or receptive language

  (2) social skills or adaptive behavior

(3) bowel or bladder control

(4) play

(5) motor skills

C. Abnormalities of functioning in at least two of the following areas:

   (1) qualitative impairment in social interaction (e.g., impairment in nonverbal behaviors, failure to develop peer relationships, lack of social or emotional reciprocity)

   (2) qualitative impairments in communication (e.g., delay or lack of spoken language, inability to initiate or sustain a conversation, stereotyped and repetitive use of language, lack of varied make-believe play)

   (3) restricted, repetitive, and stereotyped patterns of behavior, interests, and activities, including motor stereotypes and mannerisms

D. The disturbance is not better accounted for by another specific Pervasive Developmental Disorder or by Schizophrenia.

299.80 PERVASIVE DEVELOPMENTAL DISORDER NOT OTHERWISE SPECIFIED (INCLUDING ATYPICAL AUTISM)

This category should be used when there is a severe and pervasive impairment in the development of reciprocal social interaction or verbal and nonverbal communication skills, or when stereotyped behavior, interests, and activities are present, but the criteria are not met for a specific Pervasive Developmental Disorder, Schizophrenia, Schizotypical Personality Disorder, or Avoidant Personality Disorder. For example, this category includes "atypical autism"—presentations that do not meet the criteria for Autistic Disorder because of late age of onset, atypical symptomatology, or subthreshold symptomatology, or all of these.

TREATMENTS AND INTERVENTIONS FOR AUTISM SPECTRUM DISORDERS

Note to Reader: This is a comprehensive list of almost all of the current treatments that are available for ASDs. This list is not an endorsement. Its purpose is to provide you with information. If you see a treatment that interests you, you can do further research by reading books, articles, accessing the Internet, and speaking with parents and professionals. For the purposes of this list, the title "Treatments and Interventions" refers to treatment tools, methodologies, theories, and therapies.

ACTIVITY SCHEDULES

Activity Schedules are treatment tools that are used to help children with ASDs to be less dependent on adult prompting and more self-directed at home and in the classroom. Developed by Lynn McClannahan and Patricia Krantz of the Princeton Child Development Institute, Activity Schedules use a set of pictures or a simple written checklist to illustrate step-by-step how to accomplish a task or complete a social interaction. Activity Schedules can provide children with ASDs sequential cues for everything from making a sandwich to initiating a conversation with a classmate. McClannahan and Krantz's book *Activity Schedules for Children with Autism: Teaching Independent Behavior* (1999) provides parents and teachers with practical advice about how to create and use activity schedules to reduce the child's need for extensive adult supervision.

APPLIED BEHAVIOR ANALYSIS (ABA)

ABA is a treatment methodology that was pioneered by Dr. Ivar Lovaas and is based on theories of operant conditioning by B. F. Skinner. In 1987, Lovaas published a study showing that almost half of the 19 preschoolers involved in intensive behavioral intervention—40 hours per week of one-on-one therapy—achieved "normal functioning." ABA has more scientific research to support it than any other treatment for ASD. Hundreds of researchers have documented the effectiveness of ABA for building a wide range of important skills and reducing or eliminating problem behavior (e.g., stimming and self-injurious and disruptive behaviors) in individuals with ASD. The best known ABA procedure used for teaching new skills is Discrete Trial Training (DTT), during which tasks are broken down into small teachable steps so that they can be learned more easily (see Discrete Trial Training). A reward system is used to motivate and reinforce a child while he or she is learning new skills and behaviors. ABA programs incorporate both therapist-directed and child-directed interventions, known as *incidental teachings*. In addition to teaching children basic skills, ABA also teaches play skills, social skills, communication skills, and relationship-building skills through peer modeling, activity schedules, and inclusion support in the classroom. ABA progress is measured frequently, recorded in written reports, and reviewed so that treatment can be updated and customized to meet a child's specific needs. ABA can be taught in formal one-on-one treatment sessions at home or at school and in a variety of other community settings. Parents are encouraged to take an active part in the process to support their children's goals. One of the primary goals of ABA is to make learning fun and enjoyable for the child, by offering lots of positive reinforcement and positive interactions.

ACUPUNCTURE AND ACUPRESSURE

Acupuncture, a component of traditional Chinese medicine, has been used to stimulate energy flow (Chi) and restore energetic balance to the body for over 2,000 years. Some acupuncture treatments support the maintenance of general health, while others focus on specific symptoms. For children with ASDs who are hyperactive and have problems sleeping, acupuncture treatments may promote a calming effect. Acupuncture treatments employ thin needles inserted just under the skin at specific points on energetic pathways called meridians. For young children who may have a difficult time remaining still, acupressure is more commonly used than acupuncture; therapists apply pressure with their hands or press blunted needles on (not under) the skin. Parents usually stay with the child during treatments. The child may receive treatment on a therapy table or while held in a parent's lap.

ANTIFUNGAL TREATMENT

Antifungal treatment is used to help maintain a healthy gastrointestinal (GI) tract. Allergens and yeast (candida albicans) overgrowth or "leaky gut" contribute to an unhealthy GI tract; some believe that a leaky gut aggravates symptoms of ASDs. Because many children with ASDs have a history of ear infections, and antibiotics can cause yeast infections, it is believed that these children can benefit from a yeast-free, sugar-free diet, supplemented by antifungal drugs such as Nizoral and Diflucan (these drugs can cause liver damage and require regular testing to monitor liver function). Parents should be aware that, just as use of antibiotics can lead to bacterial resistance, there is a possibility that antifungal treatments can lead to fungal resistance.

AQUATIC THERAPY

The American Therapeutic Recreation Association recommends aquatic therapy as an effective intervention for children with ASDs. Many children with ASDs have sensory difficulties and are easily distracted; the hydrostatic pressure that surrounds a child in the water produces a calming effect, while at the same time providing sensory input. In water, body weight is reduced by 90 percent, making this an ideal environment for exercise or physical rehabilitation. For children with ASDs, aquatic activities can help to improve sensory integration, body awareness, balance, and mobility skills. Beyond being an enjoyable experience, aquatic therapy has been shown to have physical, psychosocial, and cognitive benefits.

ART THERAPY

Art therapy can help children with communication skills, relationship building, sensory integration issues, and developing a sense of self. Art therapy can be a vehicle for understanding a child's emotional state, identifying conflicts, and solving problems and has been used to help children with ASDs express feelings and ideas. Art therapists may mirror or engage in shared drawing tasks to establish a rapport with children. It can be especially helpful for children who are nonverbal or who have difficulty with verbal expression.

ASSISTIVE TECHNOLOGY

Assistive technology includes the use of simple or complex technology or equipment that helps people function more fully in their homes, schools, and communities. Assistive technology can include computers, visual and auditory aids, assistive listening devices, adaptive toys, augmentative communication, daily living aids, environmental controls, and modifications for home, school, and recreation.

AUDITORY INTEGRATION TRAINING (AIT)

Dr. Guy Berard, a French ear, nose, and throat specialist, developed Audio Integration Training (AIT). Originally intended to rehabilitate hearing loss, AIT is now used for auditory and sensory processing disorders commonly found in children with ASDs. The goal of AIT is to improve listening skills and language competency through the use of the Ears Education and Retraining System (EERS). During a typical AIT session, a child wears specialized earphones to listen to music with selected frequencies filtered out. Proponents claim that EERS exercises the brain and inner ear, reducing hypersensitivity to sound and improving overall auditory processing. AIT typically consists of twenty half-hour sessions for ten consecutive days. Treatment can be repeated every six months. As a result of AIT, some parents report that their children have decreased impulsivity and are less sensitive to loud noises.

CANINE COMPANION

A trained assistance dog can provide children who have physical or developmental disabilities with companionship and support. Working with and caring for a canine companion can help a child with an ASD establish an emotional connection, feel secure, and develop confidence and independence. The bond between the child and the dog can be a step in learning how to form positive, reciprocal relationships with others.

CHELATION OR DETOXIFICATION THERAPY

Chelation is a treatment that is administered either orally or intravenously to remove unwanted metals from the bloodstream. Some people believe that children with ASDs have extremely high levels of mercury (similar to mercury poisoning) that either occurred in utero as the result of a mother's high mercury-content diet or infant vaccinations which contained the preservative thimerosal. Chelation therapy includes extensive lab testing for mercury toxicity.

CHIROPRACTIC

Doctors of Chiropractic adjust and manipulate the parts of the body where bones are connected, emphasizing the spinal column. Supporters contend that chiropractic adjustments can improve the behavior of children with ASDs by restoring

APPENDIX C 289

optimal function to the nervous system. In addition to physical manipulation, chiropractic treatments may also utilize heat and ultrasound. Sessions take place in the chiropractor's office and typically last ten to thirty minutes depending on the procedures performed.

CRANIO-SACRAL THERAPY (CST)

Developed in 1970 by John E. Upledger, an osteopathic doctor, Cranial-sacral therapy (CST) is a hands-on treatment used to improve the functioning of the cranial-sacral system, which is made up of the cerebral spinal fluid and membranes that surround and protect the brain and spinal cord. Proponents of CST believe this therapy improves the immune system and relieves restrictions or tensions impeding proper functioning of the body. In a typical hour treatment session, a practitioner applies gentle pressure to the neck, jaw, sacrum, and feet.

DAILY LIFE THERAPY

Developed by the late Japanese doctor Kiyo Kitahara, Daily Life therapy is a holistic treatment for children with ASDs. Kitahara's approach utilizes group dynamics, sensory integration, modeling, and physical activity to help children develop intellectually and socially. In the United States, Daily Life therapy is practiced at Boston's Higashi School, an international program providing education, physical activities, arts appreciation, and vocational training for individuals with ASD, ages three to twenty-two. In addition to treating children, the Higashi School offers parent training and other family support services. The goal of Daily Life therapy is to prepare children with ASDs to lead productive, independent, and socially satisfying lives in their communities.

THE DENVER MODEL

Dr. Sally Rogers, developmental psychologist and one of the world's leading researchers of ASDs, developed the Denver Model in the early 1980s as a developmental treatment approach for children with ASDs. The Denver Model combines intensive teaching and intensive focus on the development of social-communicative skills. Guided by the premise that optimal development occurs when the child is able to form emotional connections, the Denver Model emphasizes relationship building and communication. This treatment includes highly focused one-on-one work in the home and support and teaching at school. In the preschool classroom, the child with an ASD is fully included with typically developing children and support is embedded within group activities. Everyone who interacts with the child, both at home and at school, is working on the same treatment objectives. The

Denver Model is family-based; parents take the lead in determining their child's treatment objectives, participate in all team meetings, and receive support and training to help their child to meet objectives.

DIETARY INTERVENTION

The most useful diet for children with ASDs is the gluten-free/casein-free (GF/CF) diet. This was developed on the observation that children with ASDs are more likely to have food allergies and higher levels of yeast, gastrointestinal problems, and an inability to break down certain proteins. There is evidence that children with ASDs have deficiencies in vitamins and minerals and cannot properly digest gluten and casein. The GF/CF diet eliminates all food containing gluten, including wheat, oats, barley, and rye, and all dairy products—a source of casein. The GF/CF diet is an important component of the DAN (Defeat Autism Now) protocol. Other diets for ASDs include the Feingold diet (to treat hyperactivity), the Ketogenic diet (for seizures), the Body Ecology diet, the Anti-yeast/Fungal diet, and the Specific Carbohydrate diet. Parents should receive nutritional counseling before beginning any dietary intervention with their child.

DISCRETE TRIAL TRAINING (DTT)

Discrete Trial Training (DTT) is a core feature of Applied Behavioral Analysis (ABA). DTT breaks down complex skills into small, manageable steps so that skills can be more easily mastered by the child with an ASD. Skills are presented in "trials" during which the therapist gives a brief instruction or asks a question, the child responds, and the therapist provides a consequence (e.g., a reward or a guiding hand). Then the therapist records the data. DTT begins by teaching simple *learning readiness* skills, such as sitting in a chair, learning to respond to one's name, imitating, and making eye contact. DTT also helps to reduce behaviors that may interfere with learning, such as stimming or throwing tantrums. As children master the basic skills, they learn more complex skills such as communication and social skills. The goal of DTT is for the child to learn to generalize the skills from the therapy sessions into the outside world. A child who learns to wave, clap, or initiate a conversation in the session should be able to do these same things at home or in school. Goals and objectives in DTT are individualized to meet your child's specific needs. In its initial phase, DTT is an intensive treatment; children usually work for 25 to 40 hours per week in one-on-one sessions with a trained professional. The time requirement may be unrealistic or intrusive for some families. Research on ABA and the use of DTT, however, have consistently demonstrated that these techniques are highly effective in teaching new skills and behaviors to children with ASDs.

DOLPHIN THERAPY

Introduced in the 1970s, Dolphin therapy has gained recognition for helping children with ASDs. Psychologist David Nathanson, dolphin expert Horace Dobbs, and Dutch therapist Richard Griffioen discovered that the gentle, intelligent, and playful disposition of dolphins help children with ASDs increase their functional skills. In Dolphin therapy, children swim and play with the dolphins; they are able to touch them, instruct them, and learn from them. Proponents claim the children also are learning how to concentrate, retain information, and learn more effective communication skills.

EAROBICS AUDITORY DEVELOPMENT AND PHONICS PROGRAMS

Earobics is a series of computer-based interactive programs that can be used at home or school to help children develop better auditory processing, phonological awareness, and phonics skills. Earobics Step 1 is designed for children ages four to seven, and includes activities and games that teach children how to match sounds to letters, decode unfamiliar words, and learn to read and spell. Earobics also develops cognitive skills such as attention and memory. Different Earobics programs are designed for different age groups, ranging from age four through adulthood.

ENERGETIC THERAPIES

Some energetic interventions include psychic therapy, crystal healing, feng shui, Reiki therapy, and therapeutic touch. Most of them employ noninvasive healing techniques. The goal of these treatments is to balance the child's energy on a physical, emotional, and psychic level so the child can be more open to communicate and build relationships. The practice of feng shui includes the arrangement of furniture and objects in a manner that stimulates the Chi, or energy in the child's physical environment that can affect him emotionally or psychologically. None of these interventions has solid scientific evidence to support them and may be criticized for being "too alternative."

FACILITATED COMMUNICATION (FC)

Facilitated Communication is an alternative form of communication used by some individuals who have limited or no speech. With this technique, a facilitator physically supports the arm, hand, or wrist of an individual with an ASD to help him or her use a computer keyboard or typewriter or to point to symbols or letters on a picture or letter board. FC is complex and requires physical and emotional support, as well as creative problem solving. FC has strong anecdotal support, but researchers claim that it is not scientifically valid because it is difficult to ascertain whether the FC user or the facilitator is the one communicating.

FAST FORWORD

Fast ForWord is a patented program published by the Scientific Learning Corporation. It was developed in response to research indicating that individuals with ASDs and other language and learning disabilities may have a split second delay in the brain's ability to process sensory input. Through the use of computer games that provide thousands of precise repetitions (discrete trials), the program is designed to help retrain the child's brain to process information more efficiently.

The creators of Fast ForWord state that the success of this program is dependent upon repeated and intensive practice and recommend strict adherence to a schedule of one hundred minutes a day, five days a week, for six weeks.

FLOORTIME

Also known as the DIR (Developmental, Individual Difference, Relationship Based)/Floortime approach, Floortime was developed by child psychiatrist Dr. Stanley Greenspan. Floortime is a one-on-one intervention that focuses on the child's individual strengths and his or her relationship to others. Floortime is based upon the premise that individuals learn best when they are emotionally engaged. Rather than focusing solely on a child's symptoms, Floortime focuses on helping children learn the building blocks of relating, communicating, and thinking. It creates a circle of interaction between the child and parent, professional, or peer. Parents and professionals follow the child's lead to encourage paying attention, relatedness, and two-way communication. By capitalizing on the child's interests and motivations, Floortime helps the child master interpersonal, emotional, and intellectual skills. In a Floortime session the parent, therapist, or teacher often gets down on the floor to interact and play with the child. The Floortime experience is a spontaneous, unstructured time that strives to create circles of communication that engage the child and gives him/her the opportunity to practice back-and-forth communication. For example, if a child is stacking red blocks, his mother may add a blue block to the tower, prompting the child to engage with her rather than remaining absorbed in a solitary activity. Back-and-orth play helps the child make the link between cause and effect and provides him/her the opportunity to engage in a personal interaction. In this intervention, parents play a particularly active and critical role. Sessions are typically 20 to 30 minutes long.

GENTLE TEACHING

Gentle teaching, based on the writings and work of John J. McGee, is a relational approach that focuses on helping the child to feel safe, engaged, unconditionally loved, and loving toward others. In Gentle Teaching the bond between the caregiver and the child is prioritized over the teaching of specific skills. This approach encourages the child to make choices and emphasizes errorless learning, where the child cannot make a mistake. The caregiver redirects the child from inappropriate, aggressive, or self-injurious behavior; punishments and verbal reprimands are never used as a means of controlling behavior.

THE HANDLE INSTITUTE (HOLISTIC APPROACH TO NEUROLOGICAL DEVELOPMENT AND LEARNING EFFICIENCY)

The HANDLE Institute views the diagnoses for ASDs as labels for individuals whose attentional priorities are limited from infancy or early childhood, caused by irregularities in systems that support the senses and their interactions. HANDLE treatments are individualized to meet the specific needs of the child and may include reducing extraneous sounds in the environment or increasing the range of the child's bodily movement through activities done in a specific developmental sequence.

HEMI-SYNC

Developed by the Monroe Institute, Hemi-sync is a patented audio technology that uses concentration and relaxation tapes to help individuals achieve desired states of either alertness or relaxation.

HIPPOTHERAPY

Hippotherapy is a treatment that literally means "treatment with the help of the horse." Hippotherapy uses horseback riding to help children achieve specific rehabilitation goals. A trained therapist guides the horse's movements to help the child improve motor skills, coordination, mobility, and muscle tone. Speech, occupational, and physical therapies can all be delivered in the context of a hippotherapy session.

HOLDING THERAPY

Holding therapy, developed by child psychiatrist Dr. Martha Welch, is used with children who have ASDs or attachment disorders. This therapy seeks to create a bond between the child and parent or therapist through close physical contact. In a therapy session, a child exhibiting tantrum behavior is held close and reassured verbally. Sessions have no set time limit and end when the child relaxes and establishes eye contact. While proponents believe that holding therapy can be reassuring for a child, others contend that forced holding may be abusive and produce feelings of fear, confusion, and anger.

HOMEOPATHY

Homeopathic medicine has its roots in ancient Greece and was refined by Samuel Hahnemann in the nineteenth century. Homeopathy treatment is completely individualized; what works for one child may or may not work for another. An initial homeopathic consultation may take one to two hours and, depending on symptoms, two or three follow-up visits may be required. Homeopathic herbal remedies are prescribed in either pill, liquid, granule, or tablet form.

HYPERBARIC-OXYGEN THERAPY

Hyperbaric-oxygen therapy (HBOT) is the treatment of the entire body with 100 percent oxygen at greater than normal atmospheric pressures. An individual receiving HBOT lies in an airtight, pressurized chamber. HBOT is used for a number of health conditions, including brain injury, stroke, cerebral palsy, multiple sclerosis, and ASD.

IMMUNOTHERAPY

Some current research indicates that ASDs may be autoimmune disorders. Elevated levels of gamma interferon, alpha interferon, interleukin 6 and 12 in children with ASDs suggest excess immune activity that is directed at the self. Immunotherapies seek to restore balance in the child's immune system. Clinical trials are being conducted on the use of immunoglobulin with children with ASDs. This therapy has been shown to benefit individuals with chronic viral, bacterial, and fungal infections, as well as other immune deficiencies. Some children treated with immunoglobulin have experienced improvements in attention span, social interaction, and communication. Other immune enhancing therapies include steroid therapy, autoantigen therapy, vitamin C, and anti-inflammatory fatty acids. A complete immune evaluation should precede any therapy, and all immunotherapy should be overseen by a physician, preferably a clinical immunologist, allergist, or hematologist.

INTEGRATED PLAY THERAPY

Dr. Pamela J. Wolfberg pioneered integrated playgroups to create an environment where children with ASDs are able to grow and learn by playing with typical kids, using toys and games that promote social interaction and imagination. The playgroup usually consists of three to five children, the majority of whom do not have ASDs. An adult facilitates the playgroup and encourages children with ASDs to expand their communication and cognitive skills through play. In addition to benefiting children with ASDs, the playgroups help other children to be more accepting of those who play and communicate differently. Integrated play works best in those environments where kids naturally play, such as homes, schools, or community settings. Integrated playgroups come together for six months to a year, typically meeting twice a week for a half hour to an hour.

INTENSIVE INTERACTION THERAPY

Intensive Interaction therapy is designed to be a practical and fun approach to developing better communication skills. In this intervention, individuals who have difficulty with communication or social interaction are paired with a communication partner. The partner, typically a caregiver, therapist, or teacher with special training in this approach, supports the person to become more confident and successful as a communicator.

THE IRLEN LENS SYSTEM

The Irlen Lens System addresses visual sensitivities and perceptual problems with prescriptions for precision tinted glasses and through the use of colored transparencies placed over written text.

LADDERS (LEARNING AND DEVELOPMENTAL DISORDERS EVALUATION AND REHABILITATION SERVICES)

Affiliated with Massachusetts General Hospital for Children and Spaulding Rehabilitation Center, LADDERS is a comprehensive treatment and evaluation program that serves individuals with ASD and a wide variety of other conditions. Founded in

1981 by Dr. Margaret Bauman, LADDERS uses an interdisciplinary team approach for diagnosis, intervention, and referral to appropriate resources and services. The program has a strong commitment to families and provides parents with training and education to help them transfer learned skills to home, school, and community settings. Located in a teaching hospital, LADDERS involves physicians and other professionals in training to further research on the causes of ASDs and other developmental disorders and explores effective interventions for these conditions.

LINWOOD METHOD

The clinical staff at the Linwood Center in Maryland uses the Linwood Method to treat children with ASDs and provide consultation to school systems. Founded by Jeanne Simons and Sabine Oishi, the Linwood Method focuses on the child's strengths and interests with the goal of positively motivating students to learn. The staff act as models for students and create learning activities that are fun and exciting. This teaching method is designed to develop behaviors and skills that can be translated into more varied and functional activities. Teachers use whatever the child is interested in (string, keys, cartoon characters, etc.) to build an individualized educational and communication program. For example if a student is fascinated by string and has few other interests, string would be incorporated into his or her programs. The child would learn colors by using different colored strings and numbers by counting strings, and string would be used to reinforce the child's communication program.

MEDICATIONS

While there is no medication that "cures" ASDs, there are a number of medications that can be prescribed to alleviate specific symptoms associated with ASDs. Medication may be used to treat behavioral problems, attention disorders, anxiety, and depression. It can play an important role in helping improve social and communication skills for individuals with ASDs. Research shows that medication can help reduce hyperactivity, impulsivity, aggression, and obsessive preoccupations. In addition to targeting symptoms that interfere with a child's ability to participate in educational, social, and family settings, medications can also help increase the benefits of other interventions.

Medications most frequently used for children with ASDs include selective serotonin reuptake inhibitors (SSRIs), neuroleptics, stimulants, mood stabilizers, and antipsychotics (particularly the newer atypical forms which have fewer side effects). Sedatives may be used in rare situations for occasional sleep problems. Because children with ASDs do not always respond to medications in the same way that typically developing children do, it is critical that parents consult with a physician who treats children with ASDs. Any treatment plan should be regularly monitored to assess a medication's effectiveness and toxicity.

Children with ASDs often present other medical conditions and may be seen by more than one physician and treated with multiple medications. As all medications have side effects and interact with other medications, the child's doctor(s) must be well informed about all treatments. Parents should keep written records of all the medications that their children are taking, their reactions to these medications, and objective data about their symptoms (e.g., number of tantrums per day, sleep patterns, ability to focus, self-injurious behaviors, and so on).

THE MILLER METHOD

Developed by Arnold Miller and Eileen Eller-Miller, the Miller Method theorizes that some children with autism have "system-forming disorders," which impair the child's ability to organize, understand, and engage in their environment, and "closed system disorders," which allow the child to only interact with the environment in a repetitive and ritualistic manner. Using special equipment, such as a platform called the Miller square, large swinging balls, and Swiss cheese boards, children may learn to be more focused and convert stereotypic behaviors into functional ones. Assessments and treatment sessions also can be administered via satellite, over the Internet, or by telephone with the Millers and their staff.

MUSIC THERAPY

Music therapy encompasses a variety of performance and listening experiences. In clinical settings, music therapy has been shown to reduce blood pressure, alleviate pain, ease muscle tension, and promote movement during physical rehabilitation. Music can promote feelings of security and calmness and counteract depression. Music therapy can improve a child's physical, mental, and social functioning. Sessions can be both instructional and child-directed. For example, if a child begins banging on a drum, the therapist may also bang on the drum and create a rhythm for the child to follow. Music therapy can help to improve coordination skills, attention and focus, and relatedness skills.

NEUROFEEDBACK

Neurofeedback, also referred to as EEG Biofeedback, can be described as exercise for the brain. It is a direct training of brain function by which the brain learns to perform more efficiently. Neurofeedback sessions utilize sensors affixed with gel to the child's scalp and ears to monitor and provide feedback that can help a child with an ASD self-regulate and control brain waves. During a session, a child is seated in front of a video game; to play the game, the child must increase the activity of frequency bands displayed on the screen. This requires the child to be in an alert and attentive state; when the child loses focus, the video game slows down. Neurofeedback is a noninvasive treatment that supporters claim can alter brainwave activity of children with ASDs, so they become more like typically developing children of the same age and gender. An evaluation for neurofeedback takes approximately two hours. Typical neurofeedback sessions are 40 to 60 minutes long and take place one to five times per week. A therapist monitors treatment and remains in the room with the child during the session.

OCCUPATIONAL THERAPY (OT)

Occupational therapy, or OT, does not have to do with job skills, as its name may imply. Rather, OT is used to help children with ASDs achieve competence in all areas of their lives, including self-help, play, socialization, and communication. OT provides support for children who have difficulty with sensory, motor, neuromuscular, and/or visual skills. Through OT, children can learn such skills as how to balance their body weight, respond to touch, communicate with others, and accomplish daily tasks. OT sessions are usually held in a clinician's office or in a school setting with the aid of special equipment. Occupational therapists may use swings, trampolines, climbing walls, and slides to help a child with gross motor coordination and sensory issues. OT also addresses fine motor skills, such as writing and drawing. Depending on the child's needs, therapists may use a variety of treatments. Many OT techniques used in therapy sessions—such as brushing, wearing a weighted vest, deep pressure, and joint compressions—can be reinforced at home or in other settings. OT may also incorporate sensory integration techniques (Sensory Integration therapy is described in more detail in this section).

PEER MEDIATED INTERVENTIONS

Peer Mediated Interventions help children with ASDs gain social skills and make positive connections with their peers. Participation in small playgroups and partnering with another child provide opportunities for the child with an ASD to learn from peer modeling. A teacher or other adult helps facilitate interactions and encourages the children to work through any problems. Research studies with preschoolers found that Peer Mediated Interventions increased social interactions for children with ASDs; those who learned to initiate social interaction demonstrated a decrease in disruptive behaviors. Schools report that Peer Mediated Interventions not only build social competence in children with ASDs, but help children without disabilities to be more tolerant and accepting of others.

PEER MODELING

Many children with ASDs do not naturally observe, imitate, and interact with their peers. Peer modeling provides a structured setting where children can improve play and social skills. A behavioral therapist or trained adult facilitates play sessions that engage children in age appropriate games and activities and incorporate typical peers as models. Initially the activities are tailored around the interests of the child with an ASD to increase his or her motivation to participate. For example, if a child likes to jump on the trampoline, the therapist may create a game where the children take turns copying each other's actions while jumping, this helps to increase the child's attention span and observational skills. The length of the sessions depends on the age and cognitive level of the children involved. Peer modeling is also used in schools to help the child with an ASD learn classrooms routines and tasks. The child's teacher, school psychologist, or guidance counselor usually facilitates peer modeling in school.

PICTURE EXCHANGE COMMUNICATION SYSTEMS (PECS)

The Picture Exchange Communication System, or PECS, helps children acquire and initiate functional communication skills. Developed in 1985 and first used at the Delaware Autistic Program, PECS is an augmented communication system that uses pictures and ABA methods to teach children with ASDs or other communication disorders. Pictures are used to help children learn colors, numbers, and specific words. PECS can be used to help children form sentences, regulate behavior, and learn scheduled activities. For example, posting pictures next to the bathroom mirror of a child brushing his or her teeth and combing his or her hair can help a child with an ASD remember the morning routine. A child can hand his or her mother a picture of an apple to indicate what he or she wants to eat. PECS is helpful in laying a foundation for language, as well as providing a means for nonverbal children to communicate.

PHYSICAL THERAPY

Physical therapy (PT) is prescribed for children with ASDs to enhance their physical abilities by treating impairments of movement that interfere with developmentally appropriate functioning. Some children with ASDs have low muscle tone, as well as poor posture, balance, and coordination. Physical therapists help children increase endurance and develop motor control and motor planning. PT sessions include training in functional skills, as well as passive, active, resistive, or aerobic exercises. Therapeutic exercises are often used in combination with equipment such as weights, exercise balls, and balance boards to increase muscle strength and endurance and to facilitate body awareness and coordination. Aquatic exercises, whirlpools, and orthotics may also be part of a child's treatment. A physical therapy session, in which the therapist works one-on-one with the child, typically lasts 45 minutes. PT can take place in a therapist's office, at home, or in school. Physical therapists are professionally trained and licensed.

PIVOTAL RESPONSE TRAINING (PRT)

Doctors Robert and Lynn Koegel, cofounders of the Autism Research Center at the University of California, Santa Barbara, have expanded upon the principles of Applied Behavioral Analysis to develop PRT. In Pivotal Response Training, specific behaviors known as *pivotal behaviors* are seen as central in affecting general areas of functioning. By changing these pivotal behaviors, it is believed that other associated behaviors will change without specifically targeting the associated behaviors. Pivotal response techniques include positive reinforcement, changing and correcting behaviors, and child choice. PRT focuses on teaching children communication and language skills, and how to have effective social interactions. Most significantly, PRT helps children learn the skills they need to enjoy positive social interactions and to make friends. Unlike more clinical treatments, PRT is designed to fit into the child's everyday life. It is an intervention that uses natural learning opportunities at home, in school, or in any inclusive setting. Because PRT encompasses the child's whole world, parent involvement is critical to the success of this treatment. As partners in the process, parents learn PRT strategies and train teachers, family members, and others on how to use this approach with their child.

PLAY THERAPY

Play Therapy, facilitated by a child psychiatrist or psychologist, can promote emotional growth and help children acquire and practice specific play skills. Some children with ASDs have rigid and ritualistic behaviors that make it difficult to form positive, reciprocal relationships. Play therapy helps these children develop the skills they need to engage in interactive play. During the session, the therapist uses toys and activities as a springboard to more appropriate play. Play therapy can also help children to better understand and express their emotions. The therapist and the child discuss and act out ways to cope with emotions and create better outcomes in social situations. For example, a therapist may use puppets to act out a bullying situation, allowing the child to express his or her feelings about bullies and the therapist to introduce effective strategies for dealing with them. The therapist works one-on-one with the child in sessions that usually last 45 minutes.

PRAYER

In its 2002 National Health Survey, the Centers for Disease Control and Prevention found prayer to be Americans' most commonly used "alternative medicine." Numerous scientific studies have documented the effects of prayer or spiritual healing. Prayer has been shown to inhibit the growth of cancer cells, protect red blood cells, and promote healing. Additional studies have found that individuals who participate in an organized religion have lower blood pressure, fewer incidences of heart disease, stroke, and depression, and are less likely to be substance abusers or commit suicide. Increasingly, modern medicine is recognizing a link between spirituality and health.

PROMPT SPEECH THERAPY

Prompt Speech Therapy is an intervention provided by speech therapists specially trained in this technique. During a Prompt Speech Therapy session, the therapist uses his or her fingers to elicit the correct sound. For example, to help a child generate an "m" sound, the therapist places an index and middle finger on top of the child's lips and presses the lips to make the shape needed for the "m" sound. Each time a sound is practiced, the placement of the therapist's fingers reminds the child where the sound is made. The therapist also works with the child to strengthen the muscles needed for speech.

RAPID PROMPTING

Soma Mukhopadhyay developed the Rapid Prompting method as a tool to expand vocabulary and eventually teach conversational skills to nonverbal children with ASDs. Mukhopadhyay created rapid prompting as a way to help her son Tito who was diagnosed with a severe ASD; today Tito is a published poet and writer. This low tech method teaches children with ASDs, who either do not speak or whose speech is difficult to understand, to communicate by pointing to letters on a piece of paper arranged either in alphabetical order or in the same order as a typing keyboard. Initially, the teacher sits with the child and asks yes or no questions. Over time, more detailed questions are introduced and the child, with assistance from the teacher, spells out the answers by pointing to the letters. As the child becomes proficient, he or she independently responds to questions.

RELATIONSHIP DEVELOPMENT INTERVENTION (RDI)

Relationship Development Intervention (RDI) is a developmental program that employs specific exercises and activities to teach relationship skills. The program provides clear objectives and follows a step-by-step curriculum to help children systematically master skills. At the novice level, a coach (typically a teacher, therapist, or parent) works directly with the child. As the child progresses, the coach is replaced by a peer partner who facilitates the exercises. Guided by the principle of *joyful collaboration*, the child is invited—not forced—to interact. While the use of fun activities and engaging coaches are effective motivators for participation, supporters believe that is the shared enjoyment and collaborative aspect of the program that help children learn how to develop meaningful relationships.

RHYTHMIC ENTRAINMENT INTERVENTION (REI)

Founded by Jeff Strong in the 1980s, Rhythmic Entrainment Intervention (REI) claims that music can be used to stimulate the central nervous systems and improve brain functioning for children with ASDs. Parents are interviewed and complete a detailed survey about their child's functional level. Based on this information, Strong creates two individually tailored compact disks with percussion rhythms; one designed to have a calming effect and the other to help the child focus. Parents are advised to play the appropriate CD once a day for approximately ten weeks.

SAMONAS (SPECTRAL ACTIVATED MUSIC OF OPTIMAL NATURAL STRUCTURE METHOD)

Spectral Activated Music of Optimal Natural Structure, or SAMONAS, is an intervention designed to help individuals with a variety of disabilities (including ASDs) develop their auditory processing skills, lessen hypersensitivity to sound, and improve neurological functions. The SAMONAS method uses compact discs with electronically tailored classical music and nature sounds. This treatment takes place in the home, with the child listening to the SAMONAS compact discs 15 to 60 minutes a day, 5 days a week, for 4 to 7 months.

SCERTS (SOCIAL COMMUNICATION, EMOTIONAL REGULATION, AND TRANSACTIONAL SUPPORT) MODEL

The Social Communication, Emotional Regulation, and Transactional Support, or SCERTS Model, is an eclectic approach made up of three components: social communication, emotional regulation, and transactional support. Social communication seeks to enhance spontaneous language and social interactions for children with ASDs. Using everyday activities and daily routines, such as teaching opportunities, a communication partner helps the child with an ASD express emotions and encourages communication about those things that interest the child. To help these children learn to regulate their emotions, SCRETS employs a variety of strategies including deep pressure, music, opportunities for activity and movement, and a calm soothing environment. Interfering behaviors are prevented or lessened by supporting a child's emotional regulation across all settings. Finally, SCRETS provides transactional support to families and staff to assure a smooth team process and reduce stress. SCERTS supports the child to meet goals across home, school, and community settings.

SECRETIN

Secretin, a hormone produced by the small intestines, is used in the diagnosis of gastrointestinal problems. In 1996, a young boy with an ASD who received Secretin for an endoscopy showed improvements in some of his autistic symptoms. Other parents whose children have received Secretin have reported improvements in eye contact, attention, language skills, and sleeping problems. The NICHD has studied this phenomenon and found no statistically significant improvements in autistic symptoms for children who received Secretin when compared to children who received a placebo. In addition, FDA approves Secretin only in a single dose; no research has been done on the safety of repeated doses.

SENSORY INTEGRATION THERAPY

The goal of Sensory Integration Therapy is to help the child better absorb and process sensory information. Sensory integration involves taking in information through the senses and organizing and integrating this information in the brain. Sensory integration therapy focuses on the basic senses: tactile (touch), auditory (hearing), vestibular (sense of movement), and proprioceptive (body position). A child can have a dysfunctional sensory system in which one or more senses is overly responsive or under responsive to stimulation from the environment. For example, a child may overreact to certain sounds, textures, or visual stimuli, or underreact to pain. Sensory dysfunction can affect a child's posture or coordination skills. Therapy for sensory integration dysfunction is usually done by an occupational therapist, physical therapist, or speech therapist who provides sensory and motor activities, often in the form of games, exercises, and play. One popular form of sensory integration is called auditory integration training (AIT).

SOCIAL SKILLS GROUPS

Social Skills Groups provide direct instruction, practice, and generalization of interpersonal skills with age appropriate peers. Children with ASDs may have difficulty in reading social cues and need extensive training in social interactions. Social Skills Groups provide a structured, supportive environment where children can practice friendship skills and problem solving strategies. Social groups are led by a trained facilitator, often a psychologist or behavioral therapist. Role-playing, discussion, and cooperative games and activities help children develop empathy and improve interpersonal skills. Social Skills Groups meet in a variety of settings and may include community outings. Some schools provide social skills groups as a way to help children with ASDs interact better with their classmates. The school psychologist or guidance counselor usually runs these groups.

SOCIAL STORIES

In 1991, Carol Gray created Social Stories as a vehicle to teach social skills to children with ASDs. A story is developed about a specific situation or event, and the child is given as much information as possible to help him or her understand and figure out the expected or appropriate response. Social Stories usually have three sentence types: descriptive sentences (which address who, what, where, when, and why); perspective sentences (which teach the child how to take another person's point of view in order to read and understand others' thoughts and emotions); and directive sentences (which suggest a response). The Social Story is a short narrative presented in the first person that helps the child to learn to respond appropriately to a specific event or situation. For example, a story can teach children when to say thank you, when to wash their hands, how to share toys, or how to participate in classroom routines. Social Stories can be written by anyone—a parent, teacher, or even a child—and are customized to meet the individual needs of the child. Social Stories may be accompanied by pictures, photographs, or music.

THE SON-RISE PROGRAM

The Son-Rise Program, part of the Autism Treatment Center of America, uses a loving and nonjudgmental educational approach to help parents and caregivers make a connection with children with ASDs. The emphasis of the program is not to teach the child to master pre-determined skills, but to join in a child's repetitive, ritualistic behaviors and engage in interactive play in order to establish a rapport with the child. The Son-Rise Program believes that parents are their child's best resource and, therefore, teaches parents educational and attitudinal tools and techniques to help them become their child's teachers.

SPEECH AND LANGUAGE THERAPY

Speech and Language Therapy helps a child to communicate more effectively both verbally and nonverbally, using words and/or body language. The speech/language pathologist (SLP) provides appropriate interventions that help the child form words or communication systems, process information, and express him or herself. The SLP also teaches the child the pragmatics of language, such as how to initiate and sustain a conversation. Children may be taught to read body language and facial expressions, as well as how to organize their thinking. In a speech therapy session, the child is taught in individual and/or small group sessions, depending on the child's skill level. Sessions usually last 30 to 45 minutes and are run by a speech pathologist in his or her office, your home, or your child's school. Sessions may incorporate language-based exercises, games, and activities. For nonverbal children, the therapist may use prompted speech therapy or augmentative treatments such as American Sign Language, communication boards, voice output communication devices or Picture Exchange Communication Systems (PECS).

THERAPEUTIC HORSEBACK RIDING

Therapeutic Horseback Riding provides an enjoyable and beneficial experience for children with ASDs. Physical benefits include improved posture, balance, motor skills, and muscle tone. Therapeutic riding can help those with learning or emotional disabilities develop better concentration, patience, and interpersonal skills. Children can gain confidence and experience a sense of freedom through Therapeutic Horseback Riding. Even though Hippotherapy also uses horses, Therapeutic Horseback Riding differs from it in that its primary goal is to encourage children to ride independently.

THERAPEUTIC MASSAGE

Therapeutic massage involves manipulation of the body's soft tissue (muscles, tendons, and ligaments), which can improve blood and lymph circulation. Body-work therapies like therapeutic massage may help children with ASDs by reducing anxiety, hyperactivity, self-stimulatory behaviors, sleeping problems, and improving overall motor and sensory functioning.

TOMATIS METHOD

Developed by Dr. Alfred Tomatis, a French ear, nose, and throat specialist, the Tomatis Method is a form of auditory therapy similar to AIT (previously described). The Tomatis approach focuses on improving a child's listening and communication skills, while Bernard's AIT focuses on reducing hypersensitivity to sound. The Tomatis Method uses modified auditory feedback in a broad range of frequencies and vocal exercises to develop self-listening skills. This treatment has been used for children with ASDs who have auditory processing disorders, expressive and receptive speech and language difficulties, impaired social skills, and organizational problems. Parents report their children experience better listening skills, reduced tactile defensiveness, and improved language skills.

TEACCH (TREATMENT AND EDUCATION OF AUTISTIC AND RELATED COMMUNICATION HANDICAPPED CHILDREN)

TEACCH was developed in the 1970s at the University of North Carolina's School of Medicine; it is now used widely across the United States and internationally for the assessment and treatment of people with ASDs. Incorporating a variety of interventions including Applied Behavioral Analysis and developmental approaches, programs are developed to meet an individual's specific communication, social, and educational needs. TEACCH utilizes a highly structured physical environment and a thorough, ongoing assessment of skills to provide treatment that enables individuals to succeed at home, in the classroom, and in the greater community. Family involvement in treatment is encouraged and parents are considered partners on the treatment team. TEACCH has been replicated in different schools and classrooms in the United States and internationally (in Denmark, France, Norway, Sweden, and Switzerland).

VERBAL BEHAVIOR

In the 1950s, behaviorist B. F. Skinner developed an approach for parents to use in helping their children with ASDs develop better communication skills. His technique, Verbal Behavior, emphasizes repetition and the use of rewards to reinforce desired behavior. Verbal Behavior focuses on functional units of language, what Skinner termed *echoics, mands, tacts, and intraverbals*. Skinner believed that, in order to communicate, children need to learn imitative speech (echoics), how to request or obtain what they want (mands), to develop a vocabulary for what is in their environment (tact), and how to engage in conversational language (intraverbals). Skinner's work, along with the work done by Ivar Lovaas, provides the foundation for Applied Behavioral Analysis.

VIDEO MODELING

Video Modeling is used to teach specific skills, play sequences, and social exchanges. It also can be used to help an individual with an ASD gain perspective on a given situation. Children with ASDs often need repeated exposure and practice to acquire new skills. In this approach a peer or adult is videotaped performing a specific task or engaging in a social interaction. The child repeatedly views a video illustrating a specific skill that the child is attempting to learn. A behavioral therapist or trained caregiver, using the same gestures and language from the script of the video, teaches the child to perform the task or interaction. Videos can be homemade. For example, a child with an ASD who is learning to select clothes for school can watch a video of a peer or sibling going to the closet and picking out clothes, while talking about how to decide what to wear. Video Modeling can be used for teaching basic skills, such as how to wash hands or more complex skills such as how to hold a conversation. Studies have shown that Video Modeling is an efficient and effective teaching technique that helps children with ASDs to learn and generalize skills.

VISION THERAPY

In Vision Therapy, a behavioral optometrist prescribes special lenses and eye movement exercises to improve a child's visual system. Many children with ASDs have fleeting eye contact, poor spatial organization, and sensitivity to light. During the eye evaluation, children try on different lenses while performing a variety of activities like standing on a balance beam or catching a ball that is swinging on a string. Different lenses are prescribed to address specific problems. For example ambient lenses are used to improve spatial organization related to the child's body posture and movement through space. Eye movement exercises, to be practiced at home on a daily basis, are used in combination with prescribed lenses.

VITAMINS AND MINERALS

The megavitamin approach is based on evidence that some children with ASDs have metabolic errors that may be overcome by larger amounts of certain vitamins. The most popular supplement for children with ASDs is a vitamin B_6 and magnesium mixture that proponents believe increases concentration and eye contact, while decreasing interfering behaviors. Other recommended vitamins and minerals include cod liver oil supplements, calcium, and vitamins A, B_1, B_5, B_{12}, and C. Children vary enormously in their needs for various nutrients. Parents considering the use of vitamin and mineral supplements should speak first with a nutritionist or nutritionally informed physician.

YOGA

The ancient practice of Yoga may help some children with ASDs to improve motor, communication, and social skills. Success of this intervention is dependent upon a positive relationship between the child and the Yoga teacher, who may use music, dance, and stories to establish a connection with the child. Once there is a trusting relationship, the teacher can introduce Yoga poses (asana), breathing exercises (pranayama), and deep relaxation techniques. Yoga has been shown to strengthen the nervous system, develop body awareness, increase concentration, and improve overall health.

APPENDIX D

NATIONAL ORGANIZATIONS FOR AUTISM IN THE UNITED STATES

These organizations can provide a wealth of information about ASDs for parents and professionals. Many offer free newsletters, magazines, and resource information. You can either call them or log on to their websites to find your local chapter or to access more information.

AUTISM RESEARCH INSTITUTE (ARI)
4182 Adams Avenue
San Diego, CA 92116
Fax: 619-563-6840
Website: www.autismwebsite.com/ari/index.htm.

A nonprofit organization established in 1967, ARI is primarily devoted to conducting research and disseminating the results of research on the causes of autism and on methods of preventing, diagnosing, and treating autism and other severe behavioral disorders of childhood. This organization provides information based on research to parents and professionals throughout the world. Defeat Autism Now! (DAN!) is a project of ARI. DAN! is dedicated to educating parents and clinicians regarding biomedically-based research, appropriate testing, and safe and effective interventions for autism. DAN! offers conferences for parents and professionals.

ASSOCIATION FOR SCIENCE IN AUTISM TREATMENT (ASAT)
PO Box 7468
Portland, ME 04112-7468
Telephone: 207-253-6008
Fax: 207-253-6058
Website: www.asatonline.org

ASAT supports all scientifically sound research on the prevention, treatment, and cure of autism, as well as all treatments for autism that are shown to be effective through solid scientific research, regardless of discipline or domain. The website offers a good assessment of current treatment programs.

AUTISM SPEAKS
2 Park Avenue, 11th Floor
New York, NY 10016
212-252-8584
Website: www.autismspeaks.org

Autism Speaks' goal is to find answers for all who struggle with autism. It is committed to raising public awareness of autism and its effects on individuals, families, and society and to giving hope to all who deal with the hardships of the disorder. Autism Speaks also seeks to raise funds to facilitate research on autism and is dedicated to uncovering the biology of autism and developing effective biomedical treatments through research funding. Austim Speaks was founded in February 2005 by Bob Wright, chairman of NBC Universal, and his wife Suzanne, after their grandson was diagnosed with autism. The organization offers an extremely comprehensive website with daily news and information, expert interviews, and other important information for parents and grandparents of newly diagnosed children and anyone seeking to learn more about the autism epidemic.

AUTISM SOCIETY OF AMERICA (ASA)
7910 Woodmont Avenue, Suite 300
Bethesda, MD 20814-3067
Telephone: 301-657-0881 or 800-3AUTISM (toll-free)
Fax: 301-657-0869
Website: www.autism-society.org

Autism Society of America (ASA) was established as one of the first nonprofit organizations for autism. Its mission is to promote lifelong access and opportunity for all individuals within the autism spectrum and their families to be fully participating members of their community. ASA has local chapters all across the United States and offers a newsletter. ASA offers one of the most comprehensive websites for ASDs. ASA provides extensive information about autism causes, treatments, education, and education approaches, advocacy at state and federal levels, active public awareness, and federal and international resources. In both English and Spanish, the ASA website offers information and gives advice on learning to live with autism—such as coping with sibling issues, life after high school, and planning for the future. ASA has a fantastic, new way to find local resources (doctors, legal experts, educational programs, etc.) called AutismSource, which can be accessed through their main website.

CURE AUTISM NOW (CAN) FOUNDATION
5455 Wilshire Boulevard, Suite 715
Los Angeles, CA 90036-4234
Telephone: 323-549-0500 or 888-8AUTISM
Fax: 323-549-0547
Website: www.cureautismnow.org

CAN is an organization of parents, clinicians, and leading scientists committed to accelerating the pace of biomedical research in autism through raising money for research projects, education, and outreach. Founded by Jonathan Shestack and Portia Iversen, parents of a child with autism, CAN's primary focus is to fund essential research through a variety of programs designed to encourage innovative approaches toward identifying the causes, prevention, treatment, and a cure for autism and related disorders. CAN is one of the largest providers of support for autism research and resources in the United States. Since its founding, CAN has committed over $20 million in research, the establishment and ongoing support of the Autism Genetic Resource Exchange (AGRE), and numerous outreach and awareness activities aimed at families, physicians, governmental officials, and the general public. CAN works to bring families, scientists, and researchers together in order to increase understanding, promote collaboration, and facilitate research on a practical level. These efforts include information distribution, parent and professional conferences, and think tanks attended by top researchers in autism and other relevant fields. CAN works with local and national media, the United States Congress, and the National Institutes of Health to increase awareness and encourage more aggressive funding of biological research in autism. CAN holds events and walkathons around the country where families can participate to help raise money and autism awareness.

DOUG FLUTIE JR. FOUNDATION FOR AUTISM
PO Box 767
Framingham, MA 01701
Telephone: 508-270-8855 or 1-866-3AUTISM
Fax: 508-270-6868
Website: www.dougflutiejrfoundation.org

The Doug Flutie Jr. Foundation for Autism's mission is to aid financially disadvantaged families who need assistance in caring for their children with autism; to fund education and research into the causes and consequences of childhood autism; and to serve as a clearinghouse and communication center for new programs and services developed for individuals with autism.

FAMILIES FOR EARLY AUTISM TREATMENT (FEAT)
Families for Early Autism Treatment
PO Box 255722
Sacramento, CA 95865-5722
Telephone: 916-463-5323
Fax: 916-381-5029
Website: www.feat.org

FEAT is a nonprofit organization of parents, educators, and other professionals dedicated to providing world-class education, advocacy, and support. FEAT advocates for early and intensive treatment and has several chapters throughout the United States and Canada.

FOUNDATION FOR EDUCATING CHILDREN WITH AUTISM (FECA)
PO Box 813
Mount Kisco, NY 10549
Telephone: 914-941-FECA
Website: www.fecainc.org

FECA is a nonprofit organization dedicated to providing the appropriate educational opportunities for children with autism based on Applied Behavior Analysis (ABA), through the development of schools, inclusion and vocational programs, consumer advocacy, and community outreach. Through these activities, FECA enriches the lives of children with autism, helping them achieve their greatest potential. FECA partners with The Mount Sinai School of Medicine's Seaver Center brings medical and educational professionals together to advance research and treatment for children with autism, helping to provide them with the best learning environments.

NATIONAL ALLIANCE FOR AUTISM RESEARCH (NAAR)
99 Wall Street
Research Park
Princeton, NJ 08540
Telephone: 609-430-9160 or 888-777-NAAR
Fax: 609-430-9163
Website: www.naar.org

NAAR was the first organization in the United States dedicated to funding and accelerating biomedical research focusing on autism spectrum disorders. NAAR was established in 1994 by parents Karen and Eric London, who were concerned about the limited amount of funding available for autism research. NAAR was created in a spirit of optimism and excitement over the opportunities for accelerating the pace of autism research. This spirit continues to guide the organization today, enabled by recent advances in the neurosciences and other scientific fields. NAAR seeks to determine causes, prevention, effective treatments, and ultimately a cure for autism spectrum disorders. NAAR has now funded nearly $30 million in autism research worldwide, making it the largest private funder of autism research. The research initially funded by NAAR has made a dramatic impact on the autism research landscape in the United States, Canada, and Europe, and has been leveraged into more than $50 million in autism research awards by the National Institutes of Health (NIH) and other funding sources. "Walk F.A.R. for NAAR," the organization's signature fund-raising event, has attracted more than 170,000 walkers in walks throughout the United States and now in the United Kingdom and Canada, providing a wonderful community event for families, friends, and businesses to demonstrate their support of autism research and awareness.

NATIONAL AUTISM ASSOCIATION
PO Box 1547
Marion, SC 29571
Telephone: 877-NAA-AUTISM
Fax: 877-622-2884
Website: www.nationalautismassociation.org

The mission of the National Autism Association is to advocate on behalf of those who cannot fight for their own rights, raise public and professional awareness of autism spectrum disorders, and empower those in the autism community to never give up in their search to help their loved ones reach their full potential.

ORGANIZATION FOR AUTISM RESEARCH (OAR)
2111 Wilson Boulevard, Suite 600
Arlington, VA 22201
Telephone: 703-351-5031
Website: www.OAR@researchautism.org

Led by parents, grandparents, and relatives of children and adults with autism, OAR uses applied science to answer questions that parents, families, individuals with autism, teachers, and caregivers confront daily. OAR's website offers free online programs that can be downloaded for parents and professionals, including "A Parent's Guide to Research," which explains scientific research and treatment. It also provides "an Educator's Guide to Autism," which provides parents, teachers, and education professionals with a plan for teaching a child with autism in the general elementary classroom setting.

TALK ABOUT CURING AUTISM (TACA)
PO Box 12409
Newport Beach, CA 92658-2409
Telephone: 949-640-4401
Fax: 949-640-4424
Website: www.tacanow.com

TACA provides information and connections to improve the quality of the family life of people with autism. For all families affected by autism, TACA focuses on building the autism community by connecting people with each other and the professionals who can help them, allowing them to share stories and information. The TACA website offers resources, articles, support groups, and information on autism, biomedical intervention, dietary intervention, and behavioral based therapy.

UNLOCKING AUTISM
PO Box 15388
Baton Rouge, LA 70895
Telephone: 866-366-3361
Fax: 225-665-7547
Website: www.unlockingautism.org

The overall goal of Unlocking Autism is to bring the issues of autism from individual homes to the forefront of national awareness. The organization seeks to educate parents about pending legislation and existing laws, biomedical and behavioral treatments; raise funds for autism research; and assist parents of newly diagnosed children by providing direction through a parent-to-parent support hotline in an effort to network families across the United States. In 1999, Unlocking Autism launched the Open Your Eyes project, which is a collection of pictures of people with autism from all over the United States, as well as several other countries. It is their hope that the collection will put a face on statistics and will serve as an educational tool for the general public. In the first year, they collected over 3,500 pictures. Their ultimate goal is 58,000. The pictures were displayed for the first time at the Hear Their Silence 2000 Rally in Washington, DC. Unlocking Autism offers a parent-friendly website with current information on autism.

APPENDIX E

INTERNATIONAL ORGANIZATIONS FOR AUTISM

No matter where you live in the world, you can always access information about ASDs through the Internet, or through your local organization for autism. This list was compiled courtesy of the National Autistic Society.

THE NATIONAL AUTISTIC SOCIETY (NAS)
393 City Road
London, EC1V 1NG
Telephone: 020-7833-2299
Fax: 020-7833-9666
Website: www.nas.org.uk/

The National Autistic Society is the United Kingdom's foremost organization for people with autism and those who care for them, spearheading national and international initiatives and providing a strong voice for autism. The organization works in many areas to help people with autism live with as much independence as possible. The NAS exists to champion the rights and interests of all people with autism and to ensure that they and their families receive quality services appropriate to their needs. The NAS website includes information about autism spectrum disorders and support and services available in the United Kingdom. NAS has comprehensive services and resources that include: autism accreditation, diagnosis and assessment, training courses and conferences, NAS schools, services for parents and caregivers, services for professionals, and more.

THE INTERNATIONAL ASSOCIATION AUTISM EUROPE
Rue Montoyer 39 11 1000 Brussels
Belgium
Telephone: +32 (0) 2 675 7505
Fax: +32 (0) 2 675 7270
E-mail: wao.contact@worldautism.org
Website: www.autismeurope.arc.be

WORLD AUTISM ORGANISATION
Rue E. Van Becelaere 26 B
Bte 21 B-1170 Bruxelles
Belgium
Telephone: +32 (0) 2 675 7505
Fax: +32 (0) 2 675 7270
E-mail: contact@worldautism.org
Website: www.worldautism.org

WORLD AUTISM ORGANIZATION
c/o Autism Research Unit
School of Health Sciences
University of Sunderland
Sunderland, SR2 7EE, UK
Telephone: 0191 510 8922
Fax: 0191 567 0420
E-mail: contact@worldautism.org
Website: www.worldautism.org

ALBANIA
LINDJA E DIELLIT ASSOCIATION
Rr. Teli Ndini, no 19
Tirana
Albania
Telephone: +355-4-377-409
Fax: +355-4-347-047
E-mail: terri_karazi@hotmail.com

AUSTRALIA

AUTISTIC ASSOCIATION OF NSW
41 Cook Street (PO Box 361)
Forestville NSW 2087
Australia
Telephone: +61 (0) 2 8977 8300 or toll-free 1800 06 99 78
Fax: +61 (0) 2 8977 8399
E-mail: contact@autismnsw.com.au
Website: www.autismnsw.com.au

AUTISM ASSOCIATION QUEENSLAND
PO Box 363
437 Hellawell Road
Sunnybank Hills
Queensland 4109
Australia
Telephone: +61 (0) 73 273 2222
E-mail: mailbox@autismqld.asn.au
Website: www.autismqld.asn.au

AUTISM TASMANIA
PO Box 1552
Launceston
TAS 7250, Australia
Telephone: +61 (0) 363 443 261
E-mail: autism@autismtas.org.au
Website: www.autismtas.org.au

AUTISM VICTORIA
PO Box 235
Ashburton
Victoria 3147
Australia
Telephone: +61 (0) 3 98 85 0533
Fax: +61 (0) 3 98 85 0508
E-mail: autismav@vicnet.net.au
Website: http://home.vicnet.net.au/~autism/

AUTISM ASSOCIATION OF WESTERN AUSTRALIA (INC)
Postal Address: Locked Bag 9
Post Office
West Perth
WA 6872
Australia
Telephone: +61 (08) 9489 8900
Fax: +61 (08) 9489 8999
E-mail: autismwa@autism.org.au
Website: www.autism.org.au

AUSTRIA

ÖSTERREICHISCHE AUTISTENHILFE
Eßelinggasse 13/3/11
A-1010 Wien
Austria
Telephone: +43 1 533 96 66
Fax: +43 1 533 78 47
E-mail: office.autistenhilfe@nextra.at
Website: www.members.magnet.at/autistenhilfe

BAHRAIN

BAHRAIN SOCIETY FOR CHILDREN WITH BEHAVIORAL AND
COMMUNICATION DIFFICULTIES
PO Box 37304
Kingdom of Bahrain
Telephone: +973 17 730960
Fax: +973 17 737227
E-mail: autism@batelco.com.bh
Website: www.childbehavior.org
For direct contact within the United States, call or fax: 206-350-3256

BELGIUM

ASSOCIATION DE PARENTS POUR L'EPANOUISSEMENT DES
PERSONNES AUTISTES (APEPA)
Rue Château des Balances
3/27 B-5000 Namur
Belgium
Telephone: +32 (0) 81 744 350
Fax: +32 (0) 81 744 350
E-mail: apepa@guest.ulg.ac.be
Website: www.ulg.ac.be/apepa

VLAAMSE VERENIGING AUTISME
Groot Begijnhof 14
B 9040 Gent
Belgium
Telephone: +32 (0) 78 152 252
Fax: +32 (0) 92 188 383
E-mail: vva@autismevlaanderen.be
Website: www.autismevlaanderen.be

BRAZIL

ASSOCIAÇAO BRASILEIRA DE AUTISMO (ABRA)
Rua do Lavapes, 1123
Cambuci 01519-000
Sao Paulo, SP
Brazil
Telephone: +55 (11) 242 8822
Fax: +55 (11) 270 2363
E-mail: info@ama.org.br
Website: www.ama.org.br

BULGARIA

PARENT'S ASSOCIATION AUTISTIC CHILD SOFIA
Medical Academy
Department of Child Psychiatry
33 Prochlada str.
BG–1619 Sofia
Bulgaria
Telephone: +359 2 57 30 13

CANADA

AUTISM SOCIETY CANADA
PO Box 65
Orangeville
ON, L9W 2ZS
Canada
Telephone: +1 519 942 8720 or 1-866-874-3334 (toll-free)
Fax: +1 519 942 3566
E-mail: info@autismsocietycanada.ca
Website: www.autismsocietycanada.ca

AUTISM SOCIETY OF ALBERTA
#101, 11720 Kingsway Avenue
Edmonton, Alberta
T5G 0X5, Canada
Telephone: +1 403 453 3971
Fax: +1 403 447 4948
E-mail: autism@compusmart.ab.ca
Website: www.edmontonautismsociety.org

AUTISM SOCIETY OF BRITISH COLUMBIA
301-3701 East Hastings Street
Burnaby, British Columbia
V5C 2H6, Canada
Telephone: +1 604 434 0880 or 1-800-437 0880 (toll-free)
Fax: +1 604 434 0801
E-mail: info@autismbc.ca
Website: www.autismbc.ca

AUTISM SOCIETY MANITOBA
825 Sherbrook Street,
Winnipeg
Manitoba
Canada R3A 1M5
Telephone: +1 204 783 9563
Fax: +1 204 783 9563
E-mail: asm@escape.ca

AUTISM SOCIETY NEW BRUNSWICK
30 Ealey Crescent
Riverview NB
New Brunswick
Canada E1B 1E6
Telephone: +1 506 372 9011 or 888 354 9622 (toll-free)
Fax: +1 506 372 9011
E-mail: asnb@nbnet.nb.ca
Website: www.abj.nb.ca/autismnb/index.html

AUTISM SOCIETY OF NEWFOUNDLAND AND LABRADOR
44 Torbay Road, Nuport Building
St. Johns, Newfoundland
A1A 2G4, Canada
Telephone: +1 709 722 2803
Fax: +1 709 722 4926
E-mail: info@autismsociety.nf.net
Website: www.autism.nf.net/

AUTISM NORTH WEST TERRITORIES
4904 Matonabee Street
Yellowknife
North West Territories, X18 1X8
Canada
Telephone: +1 867 920 4206
Fax: +1 867 873 0235
E-mail: lynnelkin@hotmail.com

AUTISM SOCIETY OF NOVA SCOTIA
1505 Barrington Street
The Maritime Centre B2 Level
Halifax, Nova Scotia
B3J 3KS, Canada
Telephone: +1 902 429 5529
E-mail: society@autismcentre_ns.ca
Website: www.autismsocietynovascotia.ca/

AUTISM SOCIETY ONTARIO
1179A Kings Street West
Toronto, Ontario
M6K 3C5, Canada
Telephone: +1 416 246 9592
Fax: +1 416 246 9417
E-mail: mail@autismsociety.on.ca
Website: www.autismsociety.on.ca

THE AUTISM SOCIETY OF PRINCE EDWARD ISLAND
PO Box 75
York
Prince Edward Island
Canada C0A 1P0

FÉDÉRATION QUÉBÉCOISE DE L'AUTISME ET DES AUTRES
TROUBLES ENVAHISSANTS DU DÉVELOPPEMENT
65 rue de Castelnau Ouest, local 104
Montréal (Quebec)
Canada H2R 2W3
Telephone: +1 514 270 7386
Fax: +1 514 270 9261
E-mail: jean-claude.marion@qc.aira.com
Website: www.autisme.qc.ca/

AUTISM WORKING GROUP YUKON
1 Kokanee Place, Whitehorse,
YT, Y1A 5Y2
E-mail: fox-thompson@ykent.yk.ca

CHILE

DNG CORPORACIÓN ANDALUÉ
Serrano 317
San Francisco de Limache
Chile
Telephone: +56 (33) 412 160
Fax: +56 (33) 416 674
E-mail: andalue@ctcinternet.ci

ASOCIACION CHILENA DE PADRES Y AMIGOS DE LOS AUTISTAS
Gran Avenida José Carrera N° 2820
San Miguel, Santiago
Chile E-mail: jespindola@aspaut.cl
Website: www.aspaut.cl

CHINA
BEIJING REHABILITATION ASSOCIATION FOR AUTISTIC
CHILDREN (BRACC)
The No. 6 Hospital attached to Beijing University
No. 51 North Huayuan Road
Haidian District
Beijing
100083 PR China
Telephone: +86 (0) 10 6207 8248
Fax: +86 (0) 10 6202 7314
E-mail: barac@public.fhnet.cn.net
Website: www.autism.co.cn

CROATIA

CENTAR ZA AUTISM
Dvorniciceva 6
10 0000 Zagreb
Croatia
Telephone: +385 (0) 1468 3867
Fax: +385 (0) 1468 3867

CZECH REPUBLIC

AUTISTIC
Kyselova 1189/24
182 00 Prague 8
Czech Republic
Telephone: +42 858 4141
Mobile: 0605 400 865
E-mail: autistic@volny.cz
Website: www.volny.cz/autiskic

DENMARK

LANDSFORENINGEN AUTISME
Kiplings Alle 42, 2860 Søborg
Denmark
Telephone: +45 70 25 30 65
Fax: +45 70 25 30 70
E-mail: kontor@autismeforening.dk
Website: www.autismeforening.dk

EGYPT

THE EGYPTIAN AUTISTIC SOCIETY
9 Road 215
Degla, Maadi
Cairo
Egypt
Telephone: +202 754 2704
+2012 217 7766
Fax: +202 519 7055
E-mail: info@autismegypt.com
Website: www.autismegypt.com

ESTONIA

Estonian Autistic Society
Tamme pst. 45–1,
50405, Tartu
Estonia
Telephone: +372 (0)7 380 336

FINLAND

FINISH ASSOCIATION FOR AUTISM (FAAAS)
Junailijankuja 3
SF-00520, Helsinki
Finland
Telephone: +358 9774 2770
Fax: +358 (0) 9 772 7710
E-mail: henrietta.gyllenbogel@autismiliitto.fi
Website: www.autismiliitto.fi/

FRANCE

AUTISME FRANCE
1209 Chemin des Campelieres
06250 Mougins
France
Telephone: +33 (0) 493 460 177
Fax: +33 (0) 493 460 114
E-mail: autisme.france@wanadoo.fr
Website: www.autismefrance.org

GERMANY

BUNDESVERBAND HILFE FÜR DAS AUTISTISCHE KIND
Vereinigung zur Förderung autistischer Menschen e.V.
Bebelallee 141
22297 Hamburg
Germany
Telephone: +49 40 511 5604
Fax: +49 40 511 0813
E-mail: autismus-bv-hak@t-online.de
Website: www.autismus.de/

GHANA

AUTISM AWARENESS CARE AND TRAINING (AACT)
16B 1st Circular Road
PO Box OS 3043
Osu, Accra
Ghana
Telephone: +33 (0) 21 762 619
Fax: +233 (0) 21 762 619
E-mail: aact@ghana.com

GREECE

GREEK SOCIETY FOR THE PROTECTION OF AUTISTIC PEOPLE
2 Athenas Street
105 51 Athens
Greece
Telephone: +30 210 321 6550
Fax: +30 210 321 6549
E-mail: gspap@internet.gr

HONG KONG
SOCIETY FOR THE WELFARE OF THE AUTISTIC PERSON (SWAP)
Room 210-214, Block 19
Shek Kip Mei Estate
Kowloon
Hong Kong
Telephone: +852 2788 3326
Fax: +852 2788 1414
E-mail: swap@netvigator.com
Website: www.swap.org.hk

HUNGARY
AUTISTÁK ÉRDEKVÉDELMI EGYESÜLETE
Hungarian Autistic Society (HAS)
Kossuth Lajos utca 16
H-1161 Budapest
Hungary
Telephone: +36 1 405 4731
Fax: +36 1 405 3863
E-mail: mobil.autist@dpg.hu

ICELAND
UMSJONARFELAG EINHVERFRA
Hátuni 10 b
105 Reykjavik S: 1590
Iceland
Telephone: +354 562 1590
Fax: +354 562 1526
E-mail: einhverf@vortex.is
Website: www.einhverfa.is

INDIA
ACTION FOR AUTISM
T370 Chiragh Gaon, Third Floor
New Delhi 110 017
India
Telephone: +91 11 29256469
Fax: +91 11 29256470
E-mail: autism@vsnl.com
Website: www.autism-india.org

INDONESIA

AUTISM FOUNDATION OF INDONESIA
Jl. Buncit Raya no. 55
Jakarta Selatan 1270
Indonesia
Telephone: +62 21 797 1945
Fax: +62 21 799 1355
E-mail: mbudhiman@yahoo.com

IRELAND

IRISH SOCIETY FOR AUTISM
Unity Building
16/17 Lower O'Connell St.
Dublin 1
Republic of Ireland
Telephone: +353 (01) 874 4684
Fax: +353 (01) 874 4224
E-mail: autism@isa.iol.ie
Website: www.iol.ie/isa1

ASPERGER SYNDROME ASSOCIATION OF IRELAND (ASPIRE)
Carmichael House, North Brunswick Street
Dublin 14, Ireland
Telephone: +353 (0) 1 878 0027
Fax: +353 (01) 873 5737
E-mail: asperger@email.com
Website: www.aspire-irl.org

ISRAEL

ISRAELI SOCIETY FOR AUTISTIC CHILDREN (ALUT)
3 Habonim Street, Ramat-Gan 52462
Israel
Telephone: +972 (0) 3 612 6120
Fax: +972 (0) 3 612 6123
E-mail: Alut_il@netvision.net.il
Website: www.alut.org.il

ITALY

AUTISMO ITALIA
Via Spartaco, 30
20135 Milano
Italy
Telephone: +39 (0)2 5410 7499
Fax: +39 (0)2 5410 4154
E-mail: info@autismoitalia.org
Website: www.autismoitalia.org

JAPAN

AUTISM SOCIETY JAPAN
2-2-8 Nishi-Waseda,
Shinjuku-ku, Tokyo 162-0051
Japan
Telephone: +81 (0) 3 3232 6478
Fax: +81(0) 3 5273 8438
E-mail: asj@mub.biglobe.ne.jp
Website: www.autism.or.jp

KENYA

AUTISM FOUNDATION OF KENYA AND AUTISM RESOURCE CENTRE
PO Box 288-00502 Karen
Nairobi
Kenya
Telephone: +254 20 882650
Fax: +254 20 883783

KUWAIT

KUWAIT AUTISM CENTER
Al-Rodha, Block 2
Yousef Al-Abieh Street
PO Box 33425
Al-Rodha 73455
Kuwait
Telephone: +965 254 0351
Fax: +965 254 0247
E-mail: q8autism@ncc.moc.kw
Website: www.q8autism.com

LEBANON

LEBANESE AUTISM SOCIETY
Telephone/fax: +961 1 364 433
E-mail: autismlb@hotmail.com
Telephone: +961 3 612 581 (Contact: Moussa Charafeddine)
Fax: +961 3 866 519
E-mail: rhabab@inco.com.lb or mcharafeddine@hotmail.com
Website: www.autismlebanon.org, www.friendsfordisabled.org.lb,
    www.tawahud.com

LITHUANIA

AUTIST CARE SOCIETY "AUTISTA"
Melioratoriu 10-7
38187 Dembava
Lithuania
Telephone: +370 651 13629
Fax: +370 45 500326
E-mail: autista@takas.lt
Website: www.geocities.com/autista_lt

LUXEMBOURG

AUTISME LUXEMBOURG ASBL
Association des Parents de Personnes Atteintes d'Autisme de Luxembourg
    asbl
37, Rue Michel Welter
L-2730 Luxembourg
Telephone: +352 408 266
Fax: +352 298 039
E-mail: appa@appa.autism.lu

REPUBLIC OF MACEDONIA

MACEDONIAN SCIENTIFIC SOCIETY FOR AUTISM
Institute of Immunology and Human Genetics Institutes, Faculty of Medicine
PO Box 60
1109 Skopje
Republic of Macedonia
Telephone: +389 2 3110 55
Fax: +389 2 3110 558
E-mail: vladotra@hotmail.com
Website: www.mnza.org.mk

MALAYSIA
NATIONAL AUTISTIC CENTRE OF MALAYSIA
4 Jln Chan Chin mooi, Off Jln Pahang
53200 Kuala Lumpur
Malaysia
Telephone: +60 3 422 3744
Fax: +60 3 422 3744

MALTA
THE EDEN FOUNDATION
Bulebel, Zejtun ztn 08
Malta
Telephone: +356 895 612/677 319 (children) or +356 673 706/7 (adults)
Fax: +356 691 447/8 (children) or +356 662 260 (adults)
E-mail: info@edenfoundation.com
Website: www.edenfoundation.com

MOROCCO
ASSOCIATION DES PARENTS ET AMIS D'ENFANTS INADAPTES
68 Rue du Neuf, Avril
Maarif
Casablanca
Maroc
Telephone: +212 25 81 43/25 57 11
Fax: +212 2 25 57 11

NAMIBIA
AUTISM NAMIBIA
PO Box 5043
Windhoek
Namibia
Telephone: +264 61 224 561
Fax: +264 61 228 255
E-mail: petaut@africaonline.com.na
Website: www.autism-sa.org

NEPAL

NEPAL AUTISTIC SOCIETY
PO Box 7947, Gyaneswor-33
Kathmandu, Nepal
Telephone: + (0)977 1 417 140
E-mail: autisticsociety@hotmail.com

THE NETHERLANDS

AUTISM ASSOCIATION FOR OVERSEAS FAMILIES
IN THE NETHERLANDS
Van Beverningkstraat 20
2582 VH Den Haag
E-mail: mail@aaof.info
Website: www.aaof.info

NEDERLANDSE VERENIGING VOOR AUTISME
The Dutch Autism Society
Prof. Bronkhorstlaan 10
3723 MB Bilthoven
The Netherlands
Telephone: +31 (0)30 22 99 800
Fax: +31 (0)30 26 62 300
E-mail: info@autisme-nva.nl
Website: www.autisme-nva.nl

NEW ZEALAND

AUTISM NEW ZEALAND INC.
PO Box 7305, Sydenham
Christchurch 8002
New Zealand
Telephone: +64 (0) 3 332 0550
Fax: +64 (0) 3 332 1024
E-mail: autismnz@xtra.co.nz
Website: www.autismnz.org.nz

CLOUD 9 CHILDREN'S FOUNDATION (ASPERGER'S SYNDROME)
PO Box 30979
Lower Hutt
New Zealand
Telephone: +64 4 920 9488
E-mail: foundation@entercloud9.com
Website: www.withyoueverystepoftheway.com

NIGER

ASSOCIATION ESPOIR POUR L'AUTISME AU NIGER
BP 11509 Niamey
Niger

NIGERIA

NIGERIAN AUTISTIC SOCIETY
PO Box 7173
Wuse, Abuja
Nigeria
Telephone: +234 (0) 9 523 6670 or +234 (0)9 413 7769

NORWAY

AUTISMEFORENINGEN i NORGE
Postboks 4528, Nydalen
0404, Oslo
Norway
Telephone: +47 23 00 81 00
Fax: +47 23 00 81 09
E-mail: post@autismeforeningen.no
Website: www.autismeforeningen.com

PANAMA

PANAMANIAN SOCIETY FOR THE PARENTS OF AUTISTIC CHILDREN
Apartado 6
141-Zona 6
El Dorado
Panama
E-mail: vlathrop@msn.com

PHILIPPINES

AUTISM SOCIETY PHILIPPINES
47 Kamias Road
1102 Quezon City
Philippines
Telephone: +63 (2) 926 6941
Fax: +63 (2) 926 6941
E-mail: info@autismphils.org
Website: http://home.pacific.net.ph/~autism-phils

POLAND

KRAJOWE TOWARZYSTWO AUTISMU
National Autistic Society
c/o Professor Tadeusz Galkowski
Stawki 5/7
00-183 Warsaw
Poland
Telephone: +48 2 283 13211 ext. 51 or +48 2 284 77100

PORTUGAL

ASSOCIACÂO PORTUGUESA PARA PROTECCÂO AOS DEFICIENTES
AUTISTAS
Prolongamento Da Rua 1
Bairro Do Alto Da A Juda
1300-565
Portugal
Telephone: +351 21 361 2650
Fax: +351 21 361 6259
E-mail: appda.autismo@mail.telepac.pt
Website: www.appda.rcts.pt

ROMANIA
AUTISM ROMANIA-ASSOCIATION OF PARENTS OF CHILDREN WITH
AUTISM
Postal address: OP9 CP95 Bucharest
Street address: Apele Vii Street, 28
Sixth district, Bucharest
Romania
Telephone: +40 21 424 7388
Fax: + 40 21 230 3614
E-mail: contact@autismromania.ro or president@autismromani.ro
Website: www.autismromania.ro

SCOTLAND (SEE UNITED KINGDOM)

SERBIA

AUTISM SOCIETY OF SERBIA
Information Centar
Generala Horvatovica 26
Beograd 11000
Yugoslavia
Telephone: +381 11 444 3064
E-mail: autism@beotel.yu
Website: www.beotel.yu/~autism

SINGAPORE

AUTISTIC ASSOCIATION (SINGAPORE)
Block 381
Clementi Avenue 5
05-398, Singapore 120381
Telephone: +65 774 6649
Fax: +65 774 6957
E-mail: autism@singnet.com.sg
web.singnet.com.sg/~autism

AUTISM RESOURCE CENTRE (SINGAPORE)
PATHLIGHT SCHOOL
6 Ang Mo Kio Street 44
Singapore 569253
Telephone: +65 6323 3258
Fax: +65 6323 1974
E-mail: arc@autism.org.sg
Website: www.autism.org.sg

SLOVAKIA
SPOLOCNOST NA POMOC OSOBÁM S AUTIZMOM (SPOSA)
Fedakova 5
PO Box 8
841 02 Bratislava 42
The Slovak Republic
Telephone/fax: 004212/ 544 11 774
E-mail: sposa@pobox.sk
Website: www.sposa.sk

SOUTH AFRICA
AUTISM SOUTH AFRICA
PO Box 84209
Greenside 2034
Republic of South Africa
Telephone: +27 11 486 3696
Fax: +27 11 486 2619
E-mail:autismsa@iafrica.com
Website: www.autism-sa.org

SPAIN
ASOCIACIÓN DE PADRES DE NIÑOS AUTISTAS (APNA)
C/ Navaleno 9
28033 Madrid
Spain
Telephone: +34 91 766 22 22
Fax: +34 91 767 00 38
E-mail:apna@apna.es
Website: www.apna.es

ASOCIACIÓN ASPERGER ESPAÑA
Apartado de Correos 244
28080 Madrid
Spain
Telephone: +34 63 936 3000
Fax: +34 95 618 3662
E-mail: infor@asperger.es
Website: www.asperger.es

SWEDEN

RIKSFÖRENINGEN AUTISM (RFA)
The National Autistic Society
Hantverkargatan 87
112 38 Stockholm
Telephone: 08-702 05 80
Fax: 08-644 02 88
E-mail: info@autism.see
Website: www.autism.se/

FÖRENINGEN ASPERGER/HFA
The Asperger/HFA Society
c/o Marie Strega
Grevegårdsv. 206
421 61 Västra Frölunda
Sweden
E-mail: foreningen@ashfa.cjb.net
Website: ashfa.cjb.net

SWITZERLAND

AUTISMUS SCHWEIZ/AUTISME SUISSE
Rue de Lausanne 91
CH-1700 Fribourg
Switzerland
Telephone: +41 (0)26 321 36 10
Fax: +41 (0)26 321 36 15
E-mail: infodoc@autism.ch
Website: www.autismswiss.ch

AUTISMUS DEUTSCHE SCHWEIZ (GERMAN SPEAKING)
Fischerhöflirain 8
8854 Siebnen
Switzerland
Telefon und Telefax
Telephone: +41 (0)55 440 60 25
Fax: +41 (0)55 440 60 25
E-mail: info@autismus.ch
Website: www.autismus.ch

AUTISME SUISSE ROMANDE (FRENCH SPEAKING)
2, Avenue de Rumine
CH-1005 LAUSANNE
Tél. +41 (0) 21 341 93 21
Fax +41 (0) 21 341 90 79
E-mail: info@autisme-suisse.ch
Website: www.autisme-suisse.ch

TANZANIA
NATIONAL ASSOCIATION FOR CARE OF AUTISTICS (NACA)
Department of Psychiatry
Muhimbili Medical Centre
PO Box 65293
Dar es Salaam
Tanzania
Telephone: +255 51 43209
E-mail: bmutag@udsm.ac.tz

THAILAND
THE ASSOCIATION OF PARENT FOR THAI PERSONS WITH AUTISM
279/35-36 Pracha Uthit 17
Ratburana
Bangkok 10140
Telephone: + 66 (0) 2 427 1813, 868 1583
Fax: + 66 (0) 2 868 1584
E-mail: jackyy@pacific.net.th
Website: www.autismthaiparents.org

THE ASSOCIATION FOR THE PERSONS WITH ASPERGER SYNDROME
127 Sukhumvit Rd Soi 62 Yak 1
Prakanong, Bangchak
Bangkok 10260
Thailand
Phone: 662 332 1510 11
Fax: 662 332 2379
E-mail: apas@aspergerthai.org
Website: www.aspergerthai.org

TRINIDAD AND TOBAGO (WEST INDIES)
AUTISTIC SOCIETY OF TRINIDAD & TOBAGO
St. Helena Village Junction
Via Caroni Post Office
Trinidad
West Indies
Telephone: +1 868 669 0462
E-mail: autismtt@excite.com

TURKEY
TÜRKIYE OTISTIKLERE DESTEK VE EGITIM VAKFI (TODEV)
Erenköy Istasyon Cad. no 54
Kat 2, Daire 8
Erenköy—81070 Istanbul
Turkey
Telephone: +90 (0) 216 363 8372, 357 2623
Fax: +90 (0) 216 348 4432

UKRAINE
AUTISM SOCIETY OF UKRAINE
PO Box 47
Gorlovka 26
UKR-338026
Ukraine
Telephone: +380 6242 53009

UNITED KINGDOM

ENGLAND
THE NATIONAL AUTISTIC SOCIETY (NAS)
393 City Road
London EC1V 1NG
England
Telephone: +44 (0) 20 7833 2299
Fax: +44 (0) 20 7833 9666
E-mail: nas@nas.org.uk
Website: www.nas.org.uk

NORTHERN IRELAND
PARENTS AND PROFESSIONALS AND AUTISM (PAPA)
Donald House
Knockbracken Healthcare Park
Saintfield Road
Belfast BT8 8BH
Northern Ireland
Telephone: +44 (0) 28 9040 1729
Fax: +44 (0) 28 9040 3467
E-mail: info@autismni.org
Website: www.autismni.org

SCOTLAND
THE NATIONAL AUTISTIC SOCIETY IN SCOTLAND
Central Chambers, First Floor
109 Hope Street
Glasgow G2 6LL
Scotland
Telephone: +44 (0)141 221 8090
Fax: +44 (0)141 221 8118
E-mail: scotland@nas.org.uk

SCOTTISH SOCIETY FOR AUTISM
Hilton House, Alloa Business Park
Whins Road
Alloa FK10 3SA
Scotland
Telephone: +44 (0)1259 720 044
Fax: +44 (0)1259 720 051
E-mail: autism@autism-in-scotland.org.uk
Website: www.autism-in-scotland.org.uk

WALES

AUTISM CYMRU
6 Great Darkgate Street
Aberystwyth, Ceredigion
Wales, SY23 1DE
Telephone: 01970 625 256
Fax: 01970 639 454
E-mail: autismcmyru@btclick.com
Website: www.autismcymru.org

THE NATIONAL AUTISTIC SOCIETY IN WALES
Glamorgan House, Monastery Road
Neath Abbey, Wales, SA10 7DH
Telephone: 01792 825 915
Fax: 01792 815 911
E-mail: wales@nas.org.uk

UNITED STATES OF AMERICA

AUTISM SOCIETY OF AMERICA
7910 Woodmont Avenue, Suite 300
Bethesda, Maryland 20814
Telephone: +1 301 657 0881
Telephone: 1800-3AUTISM
Fax: +1 301 657 0869
E-mail: info@autism-society.org or chapters@autism-society.org
Website: www.autism-society.org

VENEZUELA

VENEZUELAN SOCIETY FOR CHILDREN AND ADULTS WITH AUTISM

Avenida Alfredo Jahn con Tercera Transversal

Quinta EMAUS

Urbanización Los Chorros

Caracas 1071.

Venezuela

Telephone: +58 212 2342536; 58-212-2371051

Fax: +58 212 2387339

E-mail: lnegron@cantv.net

Website: www.sovenia.com.ve

Please note: These organizations are provided for your help and information only. They are sites maintained by other groups, organizations, and individuals, and these links are provided in good faith. The presence of a link does not necessarily imply that the NAS endorses or supports the originator(s), nor does the absence of a group imply that the NAS does not support it. The NAS cannot be held responsible for any damage or loss caused by any inaccuracy or inconsistency in linked sites or pages, nor does it have any jurisdiction over the content of these resources or their accessibility. All sites are checked for autism relevance and information content prior to publication here, but given the nature of ease of updating on the Web, we cannot be held responsible for the quality of the information provided.

APPENDIX F
INTERNET RESOURCES

The following is a list of organizations and their website addresses to help you find additional information about ASDs.

AMERICAN ACADEMY OF PEDIATRICS: An organization of pediatricians committed to the attainment of optimal physical, mental, and social health and well-being for all infants, children, adolescents, and young adults. It offers an Autism Resource page and a Developmental Stages guide covering children's health topics, including autism.
www.aap.org

AMERICAN SPEECH-LANGUAGE-HEARING ASSOCIATION (ASHA): A professional, scientific, and credentialing association for members and affiliates who are audiologists, speech-language pathologists, and speech, language, and hearing scientists.
www.asha.org

ABA RESOURCES FOR RECOVERY FROM AUTISM/PDD/HYPERLEXIA: Provides comprehensive, worldwide, parent-friendly information about behavioral intervention, including service providers, articles on research, ABA resources, health insurance, advocacy, ABA support groups, and more. (See also Cambridge Center for Behavioral Studies.)
http://rsaffran.tripod.com/aba.html

ASPERGER SYNDROME EDUCATION NETWORK, INC. (ASPEN): Provides education about the issues surrounding Asperger's and ASDs to help individuals achieve their maximum potential. Offers advice on advocacy in areas of appropriate educational programs, medical research funding, adult issues, and increased public awareness and understanding.

www.aspennj.org

ASSOCIATION OF RETARDED CITIZENS (ARC): An advocacy group that works to include all children and adults with cognitive, intellectual, and developmental disabilities in every community. May direct you to other parents and professionals in your area.

www.thearc.org

AUTISMASPERGER.NET: Serves to build greater awareness of the autism spectrum and in particular, Asperger's Syndrome. This is the Web home of autism expert Stephen Shore.

AUTISM COACH: Offers comprehensive products and information on children with ASDs.

www.autismcoach.com

AUTISM CONNECT: International autism news, events, interviews with experts, online discussions, and much more.

www.autismconnect.org

THE AUTISM EDUCATION NETWORK: Information on autism education, advocacy, resources, special education law, and more. Offers Web-based training and support programs, as well as a Family Assistance Fund.

www.autismeducation.net

AUTISM-EUROPE: An international association whose objective is to advance the rights of individuals with autism and their families and help improve their quality of life. Autism-Europe plays a key role in raising public awareness and promoting rights of people with autism in thirty-one European countries.

www.autismeurope.org

AUTISM-INDIA: Legal, medical, and educational information about autism serving South Asia.

www.autism-india.org

AUTISMINFO.COM: Information about autism facts, treatment, state-by-state resources, up-to-date news on autism, upcoming conferences in the U.S. and more.

www.autisminfo.com/

AUTISMONLINE.ORG: The mission of AutismOnline is to connect the parents of newly diagnosed children with autism and professionals working with these children with critical resources, support, and research information in their own language. Includes information in Japanese, Spanish, Italian, Korean, Russian, and other languages.
www.autismonline.org/

AUTISM ONE RADIO: An online radio program for parents and professionals covering the recovery, care, and treatment of children with autism. Features expert hosts and guests and up-to-date news stories.
www.autismone.org/radio

AUTISM RESEARCH FOUNDATION: Information on the neurobiological underpinnings of autism and related disorders.
www.ladders.org

AUTISTIC SOCIETY: Offers information, news, and research on ASDs. Created a supportive worldwide community through online interactive forums for parents, siblings, and professionals.
www.autisticsociety.org

AUTISMSOURCE: A service of the Autism Society of America, AutismSource offers a comprehensive online directory of local resources that include ASA chapters, physicians, lawyers, camps, dentists, related services, and more.
www.autism-society.org

AUTISM SOURCES: Nationwide online directory of ASA chapters, professionals, government resources, diagnostic centers, and service providers.
www.autismsource.org

AUTISM TEACHING TOOLS: A resource to help parents and professionals find specific tools and teaching tips for working with children who have ASDs. Information on teaching specific skills, educational manuals, and hundreds of books, games, toys, videos, and more.
www.autismteachingtools.com

AUTISM TODAY: Comprehensive online source for the latest news, resources, and information on autism, with a question and answer section with experts in the field of ASDs. When you can't make it to a live course or conference, Autism Today offers online courses and teleclasses.
www.autismtoday.com

CAMBRIDGE CENTER FOR BEHAVIORAL STUDIES: Offers scientifically validated information about the causes of autism and comprehensive information about Applied Behavior Analysis (ABA).
www.behavior.org/autism

CENTER FOR DISEASE CONTROL AUTISM INFORMATION CENTER (CDC): Features general autism resources including an information center, an overview on developmental screening, and links to information concerning specific CDC programs related to autism spectrum disorders. CDC in is also available in Spanish. You can also access information about the Children's Health Insurance Program that provides free or low-cost health insurance for eligible children.
www.cdc.gov

CENTERS FOR MEDICARE AND MEDICAID SERVICES: Medicaid is health insurance that helps many people pay for some or all of their medical bills. This website gives information about qualification and state programs.
www.cms.hhs.gov/medicaid/consumer.asp?

CENTER FOR OUTREACH SERVICES FOR THE AUTISM COMMUNITY: A nonprofit agency providing information and advocacy, services, family and professional education, and consultation to New Jersey's autism community.
www.njcosac.org

CENTER FOR THE STUDY OF AUTISM: Affiliated with the Autism Research Institute, this center conducts research into treatments and provides information online for parents and professionals.
www.autism.org

CLINICALTRIALS.GOV: Provides regularly updated information about federally and privately supported clinical research in human volunteers. ClinicalTrials.gov offers information about a trial's purpose, participant eligibility, locations of trials, and phone numbers for more details.
www.clinicaltrials.gov

COALITION FOR SAFE MINDS: A private nonprofit organization founded to investigate and raise awareness of the risks to infants and children of exposure to mercury from medical products, including thimerosal in vaccines.
www.safeminds.org

CONSORTIUM FOR CITIZENS WITH DISABILITIES (CCD): A coalition of approximately 100 national disability organizations working together to advocate for national public policy that ensures the self determination, independence, empowerment, integration, and inclusion of children and adults with disabilities in all aspects of society.

www.c-c-d.org

COUNCIL FOR EXCEPTIONAL CHILDREN (CEC): The largest international professional organization dedicated to improving educational outcomes for individuals with exceptionalities, students with disabilities, and/or the gifted. CEC advocates for appropriate governmental policies, sets professional standards, provides continual professional development, advocates for newly and historically underserved individuals with exceptionalities, and helps professionals obtain conditions and resources necessary for effective professional practice.

www.cec.sped.org

COUNCIL FOR LEARNING DISABILITIES (CLD): An international organization that promotes effective teaching and research. CLD is composed of professionals who represent diverse disciplines and who are committed to enhance the education and lifespan development of individuals with learning disabilities. CLD establishes standards of excellence and promotes innovative strategies for research and practice through interdisciplinary collegiality, collaboration, and advocacy.

www.cldinternational.org

DISABILITY RIGHTS EDUCATION AND DEFENSE FUND (DREDF): A national law and policy center dedicated to protecting and advancing the civil rights of people with disabilities through legislation, litigation, advocacy, technical assistance, and education and training of attorneys, advocates, persons with disabilities, and parents of children with disabilities.

www.dredf.org

DIVISION TEACCH (TREATMENT AND EDUCATION OF AUTISTIC AND RELATED COMMUNICATION HANDICAPPED CHILDREN): This internationally acclaimed program provides interdisciplinary training in autism.

www.teacch.com

EDUCATIONAL RESOURCES INFORMATION CENTER (ERIC): A digital library of education-related resources, sponsored by the Institute of Education Sciences of the U.S. Department of Education. The library provides a comprehensive, easy-to-use, searchable, Internet-based bibliographic, and full-text database of education research and information that also meets the requirements of the Education Sciences Reform Act of 2002.

www.eric.ed.gov

EXPLORING AUTISM: Offers general information about the genetics of autism.
www.exploringautism.org

FIRST SIGNS: Comprehensive website dedicated to identification and intervention of children with developmental disorders by creating a national model for disseminating information about early warning signs, the need for routine screening, and treatment options.
www.firstsigns.org

GLOBAL AND REGIONAL ASPERGER SYNDROME PARTNERSHIP (GRASP): Run by individuals diagnosed with Asperger's Syndrome and high-functioning autism, this website offers an insightful perspective to increase public awareness of the unique challenges and strengths of people diagnosed with Asperger's Syndrome and high-functioning autism.
www.grasp.org

HARBOR HOUSE LAW PRESS: Publishes information about special education law and advocacy designed to meet the needs of parents.
www.harborhouselaw.com

THE HELP GROUP: A nonprofit organization serving children with special needs related to autism, Asperger's disorder, ADHD, learning disabilities, mental retardation, abuse, and emotional problems.
www.thehelpgroup.org/

INTERAGENCY AUTISM COORDINATING COMMITTEE: Coordinates autism research and other efforts within the Department of Health and Human Services (DHHS).
www.nimh.nih.gov/autismiacc/index.cfm

INTERNATIONAL RETT SYNDROME ASSOCIATION: Provides information, referrals, resources for families affected by Rett Syndrome.
www.rettsyndrome.org

KENNEDY KRIEGER INSTITUTE: An internationally recognized facility located in Baltimore, MD, dedicated to improving the lives of children and adolescents with developmental disabilities. They offer school, clinical, and professional training and research programs.
www.kennedykrieger.org

LOVAAS INSTITUTE FOR EARLY INTERVENTION: A research-based program that specializes in teaching children with autism using the Model of Applied Behavior Analysis created and developed under the direction of Dr. O. Ivar Lovaas.
www.lovaas.com

MAAP SERVICES FOR AUTISM, ASPERGER'S, AND PDD: A nonprofit organization dedicated to providing information and advice to families of more advanced individuals with autism, Asperger's syndrome, and Pervasive Developmental Disorder (PDD). Has a professional and parent support listings for every state.
www.maapservices.org

MEDLINEPLUS: On online service of the U.S. National Library of Medicine and the National Institutes of Health. Provides definitions and basic information about ASDs.
www.nlm.nih.gov/medlineplus/ency/article/001526.htm?AddInterest=1053

MIAMI CHILDREN'S HOSPITAL DAN MARINO CENTER: An integrated neurodevelopmental center specializing in the diagnosis and treatment of children at risk for developmental and psychological problems. The center also coordinates community outreach projects.
www.mch.com/clinical/neuroscience/dan_marino.htm

NATIONAL ASSOCIATION FOR THE EDUCATION OF YOUNG CHILDREN (NAEYC): Dedicated to improving the well-being of all young children, with particular focus on the quality of educational and developmental services for children from birth through age eight.
Website: www.naeyc.org

NATIONAL ASSOCIATION OF PROTECTION AND ADVOCACY SYSTEMS (NAPAS): This organization and the Client Assistance Programs comprise the nationwide network of congressionally mandated, legally based disability rights agencies They work in partnership with people with disabilities to protect and advocate for and advance their human, legal, and service rights.
Website: www.napas.org

THE NATIONAL AUTISTIC SOCIETY OF THE U.K. NAS: The National Autistic Society exists to champion the rights and interests of all people with autism and to ensure that they and their families receive quality services appropriate to their needs. This site includes information about autism and Asperger's syndrome and about support and services available in the United Kingdom.
Website: www.nas.org.uk

NATIONAL CENTER ON BIRTH DEFECTS AND DEVELOPMENTAL DISABILITIES (NCBDDD): A division of the Center for Disease Control that promotes the health of babies, children, and adults, and enhances the potential for full, productive living. Their work includes identifying the causes of birth defects and developmental disabilities, helping children to develop and reach their full potential, and promoting health and well-being among people of all ages with disabilities. As part of the Autism Information Center, their "Learn the Signs, Act Early" campaign provides milestones for child development and ways to measure your child's growth.
www.cdc.gov/ncbddd/dd/ddautism.htm

NATIONAL DISSEMINATION CENTER FOR CHILDREN AND YOUTH WITH DISABILITIES (NDCCYD): A central source of information on disabilities in infants; toddlers; children; and youth; IDEA, which is the law authorizing special education; No Child Left Behind (as it relates to children with disabilities); and research-based information on effective educational practices. The center provides information about disabilities to families, educators, and other professionals and also serves as a referral center. The center and its website offer services in Spanish, too.
www.nichcy.org

NATIONAL FRAGILE X FOUNDATION: Provides information, resources, and support for families of children with fragile X syndrome.
www.nfxf.org

NATIONAL INFORMATION CENTER FOR CHILDREN AND YOUTH WITH DISABILITIES: To find the name and number of the Early Intervention program in your state (NICHCY).
www.nichcy.org/states.htm

NATIONAL INSTITUTE OF CHILD HEALTH AND HUMAN DEVELOPMENT (NICHD): Part of the National Institutes of Health, the biomedical research arm of the U.S. Department of Health and Human Services. They conduct research into various aspects of autism, including its causes, prevalence, and treatments.
www.nichd.nih.gov/autism

NATIONAL INSTITUTE FOR MENTAL HEALTH (NIMH): Works to improve mental health through biomedical research on the mind, brain, and behavior. The autism page has booklets, fact sheets, and other publications and resources on autism spectrum disorders.
www.nimh.nih.gov/healthinformation/autismmenu.cfm

NATIONAL INSTITUTE OF NEUROLOGICAL DISORDERS AND STROKE (NINDS):
Conducts and supports research on brain and nervous system disorders. The institute has an autism page that reviews common signs of autism, how it's diagnosed, causes, treatments, and research. Also in Spanish.
www.ninds.nih.gov/disorders/autism/detail_autism.htm

NATIONAL INSTITUTE ON DEAFNESS AND OTHER COMMUNICATION DISORDERS (NIDCD): Provides information on how speech and language normally develop, the communication problems of autism, and how the speech and language problems of autism are treated. Also in Spanish.
www.nidcd.nih.gov/health/voice/autism.asp

NATIONAL PROTECTION AND ADVOCACY SYSTEM: Federally mandated network that protects the rights of persons with disabilities through legally based advocacy.
www.napas.org

NATIONAL RESEARCH COUNCIL OF THE NATIONAL ACADEMIES OF SCIENCE (NRC): Provides general information on autism and a link to "Educating Children with Autism (2001)," written by the Commission on Behavioral and Social Sciences and Education (published by the National Academies Press). This comprehensive report outlines an interdisciplinary approach to education and can be downloaded free.
http://lab.nap.edu/nap-cgi/discover.cgi?term=autism

NATIONAL REHABILITATION INFORMATION CENTER (NARIC): Collects and disseminates the results of research funded by the National Institute on Disability and Rehabilitation Research (NIDRR).
www.naric.com

THE NATIONAL RESPITE LOCATOR SERVICE: Sponsored by the ARCH National Respite Network, this site helps parents find respite services in their state and local area to match their specific needs.
www.respitelocator.org/index.htm

NATIONAL VACCINE INFORMATION CENTER: A national organization advocating reformation of the mass vaccination system.
www.nvic.org

THE NEURO IMMUNE DISFUNCTION SYNDROME RESEARCH INSTITUTE (NIDS): Consists of the *NIDS Parents Coalition* and the *NIDS Scientific Board* and is dedicated to increasing the public's awareness of the likely connection between neuro-immune and/or autoimmune dysfunction and conditions such as autism.
http://nids.net/index.htm

NEW YORK STATE DEPARTMENT OF HEALTH: Offers an *Early Intervention Program Clinical Practice Guideline Report of Recommendations on Autism.*
www.health.state.ny.us/nysdoh/eip/autism/autism.htm

ONLINE ASPERGER SYNDROME INFORMATION AND SUPPORT (OASIS): Provides general information on Asperger's Syndrome and related disorders, including resources and materials, events listings, and publications.
www.aspergersyndrome.org or www.udel.edu/bkirby/asperger

OFFICE OF SPECIAL EDUCATION PROGRAMS (OSEP): Dedicated to improving results for infants, toddlers, children, and youth with disabilities from birth through age twenty-one by providing leadership and financial support to assist states and local districts. The IDEA authorizes formula grants to states and discretionary grants to institutions of higher education and other nonprofit organizations to support research, demonstrations, technical assistance and dissemination, technology and personnel development, and parent training and information centers.
www.ed.gov/about/offices/list/osers/osep/index.html

OFFICE OF SPECIAL EDUCATION AND REHABILITATIVE SERVICES (OSERS): Committed to improving results and outcomes for people with disabilities of all ages. OSERS provides a wide array of support to parents and individuals, school districts, and states in three main areas: special education, vocational rehabilitation, and research.
www.ed.gov/about/offices/list/osers

PARENT INFORMATION AND RESOURCE CENTER (PIRC): Created by the U.S. Department of Education to provide parents, schools, and organizations that work with families with training, information, and technical assistance to understand how children develop and what they need to succeed in school.
www.pirc-info.net

PARENT TRAINING AND INFORMATION CENTER: These programs are funded by the Office of Special Education Programs in the US Department of Education. The purpose of these centers is to help provide training and information to meet the needs of parents of children with disabilities living in the area served by the center.
www.angelfire.com/ny/Debsimms/pti.html

PLAY PROJECT: A training and early intervention center helping parents and professionals learn effective, low-cost, and efficient ways to provide intensive intervention programming for young children with autism.
www.playproject.org

PRESIDENT'S COMMITTEE ON MENTAL RETARDATION (PCMR): Conducts forums, national awards programs, and conferences and produces relevant publications, while collaborating with public and private partners to further the inclusion of people with disabilities into the social mainstream.
www.acf.hhs.gov/news/facts/pcmrfspr.htm

PUBLIC AUTISM AWARENESS: Offers live autism news from around the world (updated every five minutes) and an online forum for information, help, and support.
www.paains.org.uk

THE STUDIES TO ADVANCE AUTISM RESEARCH AND TREATMENT NETWORK (STAART): Congress passed the Children's Health Act of 2000, legislation that mandated many activities, among them the establishment of a new autism research network—at least five centers of excellence in autism research. In response, the five Institutes of the NIH Autism Coordinating Committee (NIMH, NICHD, NINDS, NIDCD, and NIEHS) have implemented the Studies to Advance Autism Research and Treatment (STAART) network program. Made up of eight centers across the country, each center contributes to autism research in the areas of causes, diagnosis, early detection, prevention, and treatment. The website includes information about the centers and treatment studies.
www.nimh.nih.gov/autismiacc/staart.cfm

THE SCHAFER AUTISM REPORT: The most comprehensive and most widely read autism publication at no cost! The report monitors half a dozen of the larger autism-related e-mail lists, as well as larger dailies and websites, for important news and developments and sends out one posting per day to your e-mail account. The mission is to promote autism awareness and education with the goal of finding the best treatments, preventions, and cures for the range of disorders labeled as the autism spectrum.
home.sprynet.com/~schafer

SIBLING SUPPORT PROJECT: The Sibling Support Project is a national effort dedicated to the interests of over six million brothers and sisters of people with special health, mental health, and developmental needs. Based in Seattle since 1990, they have trained service providers in all 50 states, England, Ireland, New Zealand, and Japan on how to implement the award-winning Sibshop program for young brothers and sisters, resulting in over 200 replications in 8 countries. They sponsor the Internet's first and largest Listservs for young and adult siblings where participants share their issues with others who truly understand. They have provided leadership for similar sibling efforts in Japan, England, Ireland, Belgium, Croatia, Iceland, New Zealand, Australia, Greece, and Guatemala.
www.thearc.org/siblingsupport

SIBLINGS OF AUTISM AND RELATED DISORDERS: An online "safe haven" for siblings of children with ASDs to learn about ASDs and share their experiences with other siblings.
www.siblingsofautism.com

SUMMER CAMPS: Summer camps for children with ASDs or special needs can be a wonderful way for children to make friends, develop skills and abilities, and have fun in a safe, nurturing environment. Being surrounded by other children with ASDs or special needs can help foster a child's self-esteem and confidence and can offer an enjoyable retreat from their regular routines. Here are some resources that include directories of camps for ASD and special needs:
http://wmoore.net/therapy.html
www.campspecialists.com/special-needs-camps.htm
www.kidscamps.com *www.*mysummercamps.com/camps/Special_Needs_Camps/Autism

TALK AUTISM: Shares knowledge, information, and assistance about autism. The website offers a comprehensive interactive resource directory service called "Expert Find" to help parents find services, products, and experts in their area; a "Virtual Speaker" to access experts and specialty chats or distance learning online; and a "Help Wanted" section where parents can post autism-related questions about their child, a treatment or a product, and receive answers from specialists.
www.talkautism.org

TD SOCIAL SKILLS: Provides information on and resources for teaching social, communication, and play skills through video modeling techniques.
www.tdsocialskills.com

UC DAVIS M.I.N.D. INSTITUTE: Brings together parents, educators, physicians, and scientists in fields as diverse as molecular genetics and clinical pediatrics in treating and finding cures for neurodevelopmental disorders.
www.ucdmc.ucdavis.edu/mindinstitute

UNIVERSITY OF NORTH CAROLINA'S TREATMENT AND EDUCATION OF AUTISTIC AND RELATED COMMUNICATION-HANDICAPPED CHILDREN (TEACCH): This division focuses on the person with autism and the development of a program to enable these individuals to function as meaningfully and as independently as possible in the community.
www.teacch.com

UNIVERSITY OF WASHINGTON'S AUTISM CENTER: Provides diagnostic evaluations and multidisciplinary intervention services for children with autism spectrum

disorders from infancy through adolescence. Website offers information on research, advocacy, autism facts, and more.
www.depts.washington.edu/uwautism

UNIVERSITY OF CALIFORNIA AUTISM RESEARCH AND TRAINING CENTER: The goals of the center are to understand and treat autism through the use of pivotal response treatments, as well as the improve elementary and secondary education efforts for children with autism and other severe disabilities. Their primary interests lie in research and training (both pre-service and in-service), focusing on family support and on the education of children with autism in community environments and classrooms with their typically developing peers.
www.education.ucsb.edu/autism/index.html

VIDEO MODELING: Offers a complete listing of all Special Kids Video Modeling Therapy Programs, as well as ancillary teaching products.
www.special-kids.com or call 800.KIDS.153

WRIGHTSLAW: Up-to-date information about special education law and advocacy for children with disabilities. Includes articles, cases, newsletters, and resources in the advocacy libraries and law libraries.
http://wrightslaw.com

WRONGPLANET.NET: A Web community designed for individuals with Asperger's Syndrome, autism, and other PDDs. Provides a *forum* in which members can communicate with each other, an article section where members may read and submit essays or how-to guides about various subjects, and a chat room for real-time communication with other "Aspies."
www.wrongplanet.net

YALE CHILD STUDY CENTER: Offers comprehensive, multidisciplinary evaluations for children with social disabilities, usually focusing on the issues of diagnosis and intervention. The website offers frequently asked questions from parents of newly diagnosed children with ASDs.
www.info.med.yale.edu/chldstdy/autism

RECOMMENDED READING

Because many of you may not have much time for reading right now (especially if your child has been diagnosed recently), I've listed my top choices for books to get you started. They are listed in alphabetical order by title. Other recommended reading is listed below.

MY TOP CHOICES

Children with Autism: A Parent's Guide edited by Michael D. Powers, Psy.D. (Bethesda, MD: Woodbine House, 2000). This is a comprehensive reference book for parents and practitioners, with chapters written by various experts on child development, daily and family life, medical concerns, educational programs, early intervention, legal rights, advocacy, and more. It also includes parent statements at the end of each chapter and a list of state resources in the appendix.

Demystifying Autism Spectrum Disorders: A Guide to Diagnosis for Parents and Professionals, by Carolyn Thorwarth Bruey, Psy.D. (Bethesda, MD: Woodbine House, 2004). An excellent choice for parents, loved ones, or practitioners who want to further understand a child's diagnosis of ASD and written in language the layperson can understand.

Emergence: Labeled Autistic by Temple Grandin and Margaret M. Scariano (Novato, CA: Arena Press, 1986) and *Thinking in Pictures and Other Reports from My Life with Autism* by Temple Grandin (New York, NY: First Vintage Books, 1995). Temple Grandin offers a rare glimpse into the world of ASDs from the inside; she is autistic. She also has her Ph.D. in animal science and has a gift for writing with clarity, poignancy, and a sense of humor about her experiences. Her other books are wonderful as well (see "Other Recommended Reading").

Facing Autism: Giving Parents Reasons for Hope and Guidance for Help by Lynn

M. Hamilton. (Colorado Springs, CO: Waterbrook Press, 2000). A mother shares her story of coping with her son's autism and offers insight into different treatments, both scientifically proven and alternative, such as ABA, dietary intervention, immunotherapy, and sensory integration.

Healthcare for Children on the Autism Spectrum: A Guide to Medical, Nutritional, and Behavioral Issues by Fred R. Volkmar, M.D., and Lisa A. Wiesner, M.D. (Bethesda, MD: Woodbine House, 2004). The goal of this book is to help parents keep their children with ASDs healthy, which the authors acknowledge can be a challenge. There is comprehensive information on how to maintain your child's medical, nutritional, and behavioral well-being, including advice on how to manage sleep problems, dental care, eating habits, sensory issues, and more.

Let Me Hear Your Voice: A Family's Triumph over Autism by Catherine Maurice. (New York, NY: Ballantine Books, 1994). As a mother of two children with autism, Maurice relates a candid account of her family's struggles with the disorder and offers strength and hope to parents who are dealing with a newly diagnosed child. The book reads like a novel. I often recommend it to the parents and loved ones of a child with an ASD.

Overcoming Autism: Finding the Answers, Strategies, and Hope That Can Transform a Child's Life by Lynn Kern Koegel and Claire LaZebnik. (New York, NY: Viking Penguin, 2004). A parent-friendly book with tips on how to handle your child's meltdowns, self-stimulation, fears, and fixations and how to teach your child social skills and communication skills. It also includes a chapter on "Family Life: Fighting Your Way Back to Normalcy."

OTHER RECOMMENDED READING

The following books are also excellent. You'll be able to prioritize your reading selection by determining which titles are most relevant to your child's needs at any given time.

Abrams, Philip, and Leslie Henriques. *The Autistic Spectrum Parents' Daily Helper: A Workbook for You and Your Child.* Berkeley, CA: Ulysses Press, 2004.

Addison, Anne. *One Small Starfish.* Arlington, TX: Future Horizons, 2002.

Anderson, Johanna. *Sensory Motor Issues in Autism.* San Antonio, TX: The Psychological Corporation, 1999.

Anderson, Winifred, Stephen Chitwood, and Deirdre Hayden. *Negotiating the Special Education Maze: A Guide for Parents and Teachers,* 3rd ed. Bethesda, MD: Woodbine House, 1997.

Attwood, Tony. *Asperger's Syndrome: A Guide for Parents and Professionals.* London, U.K.: Jessica Kingsley Publishers, 1998.

——. *Why Does Chris Do That? Some Suggestions Regarding the Cause and Manage-ment of the Unusual Behavior of Children and Adults with Autism and Asperger Syndrome*. Shawnee Mission, KS: Autism Asperger Publishing Company, 2003.

——. *Exploring Feelings: Cognitive Behavior Therapy to Manage Anger*. Arlington, TX: Future Horizons, 2004.

Baker, Bruce L., and Allen J. Brightman. *Steps to Independence: Teaching Everyday Skills to Children with Special Needs*, 4th ed. Baltimore, MD: Paul H. Brookes, 2004.

Baker, Jed. *The Social Skills Picture Book*. Arlington, TX: Future Horizons, 2003.

——. *Social Skills Training for Children and Adolescents with Asperger Syndrome and Social-Communications Problems*. Shawnee Mission, KS: Autism Asperger Publishing Company, 2003.

Ballare, Antonia, Angelique Lampros (contributor), and Eileen G. Ciavarella (Illus-trator). *Behavior Smart! Ready-to-Use Activities for Building Personal and Social Skills for Grades K–4*. West Nyack, NY: The Center for Applied Research in Ed-ucation, 1994.

Band, Eve B., Sue Lynn Cotton, Emily Hecht, and Garby B. Mesibov. *Autism Through a Sister's Eyes*. Arlington, TX: Future Horizons, 2001.

Baron-Cohen, Simon. *The Essential Difference: The Truth About the Male and Female Brain*. New York, NY: Perseus Books Group, 2003.

Baron-Cohen, Simon, and Patrick Bolton. *Autism: The Facts*. Oxford, New York: Ox-ford University Press, 2003.

Baron-Cohen, Simon, Donald J. Cohen, and Helen Tager-Flushberg. *Understand-ing Other Minds: Perspectives from Developmental Cognitive Neuroscience*. Ox-ford, New York: Oxford University Press, 2000.

Barron, Judy, and Sean Barron. *There's a Boy in Here: Emerging from the Bonds of Autism*. Arlington, TX: Future Horizons, 2002.

Batshaw, Mark (Ed). *Children with Disabilities*, 5th ed. Baltimore, MD: Paul H. Brookes, 2002.

Beane, Allan L. *The Bully Free Classroom: Over 100 Tips and Strategies for Teachers K-8*. Minneapolis, MN: Free Spirit Publishing, 1999.

Begun, Ruth Weltmann (ed). *Ready-to-Use Social Skills Lessons & Activities for Grades Pre-K*. West Nyack, NY: The Center for Applied Research in Education, 1995.

Berkell Zager, Dianne E. (Ed). *Autism: Identification, Education, and Treatment*, 2nd ed. Mahwah, NJ: Lawrence Erlbaum Associates, 1999.

Bishop, Beverly, and Craig Bishop. *My Friend with Autism*. Arlington, TX: Future Horizons, 2002.

Blanchard, Kenneth, and Spencer Johnson. *The One Minute Manager Anniversary Ed: The World's Most Popular Management Method*. New York, NY: William Mor-row, 1982.

Bleach, Fiona. *Everybody Is Different: A Book for Young People Who Have Brothers or Sisters with Autism*. Shawnee Mission, KS: Autism Asperger Publishing Company, 2002.

Bondy, Andy, and Lori Frost. *A Picture's Worth: PECS and Other Visual Communication Strategies in Autism (Topics in Autism)*. Bethesda, MD: Woodbine House, 2002.

Brill, Marlene Targ. *Keys to Parenting the Child with Autism*, 2nd ed. Hauppauge, NY: Barron's Educational Series, Inc., 2001.

Brooks, Robert, and Sam Goldstein. *Raising Resilient Children: Fostering Strength, Hope, and Optimism in Your Child*. New York, NY: McGraw-Hill, 2002.

Buron, Kari Dunn, and Brenda Smith Myles (foreword). *When My Autism Gets Too Big! A Relaxation Book for Children with Autism Spectrum Disorders*. Shawnee Mission, KS: Autism Asperger Publishing Company, 2004.

Campbell, Pam, and Gary N. Siperstein. *Improving Social Competence: A Resource for Elementary School Teachers*. Boston, MA: Allyn and Bacon, 1994.

Cartalano, Robert A. (ed.), and Fred R. Volkmar (foreword). *When Autism Strikes: Families Cope with Childhood Disintegrative Disorder*. New York, NY: Plenum Press, 1998.

Charlton, James. *Nothing About Us Without Us: Disability Oppression and Empowerment*. 2nd ed. Berkeley, CA: University of California Press, 2000.

Christopher, Williams, and Barbara Christopher. *Mixed Blessings*. Nashville, TN: Abingdon Press, 1989.

Cihak, Mary K., and Barbara Jackson Heron. *Games Children Should Play: Sequential Lessons for Teaching Communication Skills in Grades K–6*. Santa Monica, CA: Goodyear Publishing Company, 1980.

Cohen, Donald J, and Fred R. Volkmar, eds. *Handbook of Autism and Pervasive Developmental Disorders*, 2nd ed. Hoboken, NJ: John Wiley & Sons, 1997.

Cohen, Shirley. *Targeting Autism: What We Know, Don't Know, and Can Do to Help Young Children with Autism and Related Disorders*, 2nd ed. Berkeley, CA: University of California Press, 2002.

Coleman, Jeanine. *The Early Intervention Dictionary: A Multidisciplinary Guide to Terminology*, 2nd ed. Bethesda, MD: Woodbine House, 1999.

Covey, Stephen R. *The 7 Habits of Highly Effective Families*. New York, NY: Franklin Covey, 1997.

——. *The 7 Habits of Highly Effective People: Powerful Lessons in Personal Change*. New York, NY: Free Press, 2004.

Crary, Elizabeth, and Marina Megale (illustrator). *I Want to Play*, 2nd ed. Seattle, WA: Parenting Press, 1996.

Cutler, Eustacia. *Thorn in My Pocket: Temple Grandin's Mother Tells the Family Story*. Arlington, TX: Future Horizons, 2004.

Davis, Bill, and Wendy Goldband Schunick. *Breaking Autism's Barriers: A Father's Story*. London, U.K.: Jessica Kingsley, 2001.

Dawson, Geraldine, and Kurt W. Fischer, eds. *Human Behavior and the Developing Brain.* New York, NY: Guilford Press, 1994.

Dillon, Kathleen. *Living with Autism: The Parents' Stories.* Boone, NC: Parkway Publishing, 1997.

Dowd, Tom, and Jeff Tierney. *Teaching Social Skills to Youth: A Curriculum for Childcare Providers.* Boys Town, NE: Boys Town Press, 1992.

Doyle, Barbara T., and Emily Doyle Iland. *Autism Spectrum Disorders from A to Z: Assessment, Diagnosis . . . & More!* Arlington, TX: Future Horizons, 2004.

Durand, V. Mark. *Sleep Better! A Guide to Improving Sleep for Children with Special Needs.* Baltimore, MD: Paul H. Brookes, 1998.

Elias, Maurice J., and Steven E Tobias (contributor). *Social Problem Solving: Interventions in the Schools.* New York, NY: Guilford Press, 1999.

Ernsperger, Lori. *Keys to Success for Teaching Students with Autism.* Arlington, TX: Future Horizons, 2002.

Featherstone, Helen. *A Difference in the Family: Living with a Disabled Child.* New York, NY: Penguin USA, 1981.

Feiges, Lynne Stern, and Mary Jane Weiss. *Sibling Stories: Reflections on Life with a Brother or Sister on the Autism Spectrum.* Shawnee Mission, KS: Autism Asperger Publishing Company, 2004

Fouse, Beth, and Maria Wheeler. *A Treasure Chest of Behavioral Strategies for Individuals with Autism.* Arlington, TX: Future Horizons, 1997.

Fovel, J. Tyler. *The ABA Program Companion: Organizing Quality Programs for Children with Autism and PDD.* New York, NY: DRL Books, 2002.

Frankel, Fred H., and Barry Wetmore (illustrator). *Good Friends Are Hard to Find: Help Your Child Find, Make, and Keep Friends.* Los Angeles, CA: Perspective Publishing, 1996.

Freeman, John, Drake Lorelei, and Eileen Vining. *Teach Me Language: A Language Manual for Children with Autism, Asperger's Syndrome, and Related Developmental Disorders.* Langley, BC: SKF Books, 1997.

Frith, Uta. *Autism: Explaining the Enigma,* 2nd ed. Malden, MA: Blackwell Publishing, 2003.

———. *Autism and Asperger Syndrome.* Cambridge, NY: Cambridge University Press, 1991.

Gagnon, Elisa. *Power Cards: Using Special Interests to Motivate Children and Youth with Asperger Syndrome and Autism.* Shawnee Mission, KS: Autism Asperger Publishing Company, 2001

Gerlack, Elizabeth K. *Autism Treatment Guide,* 3rd ed. Arlington, TX: Future Horizons, 2003.

———. *Just This Side of Normal: Glimpses into Life with Autism.* Arlington, TX: Future Horizons, 1999.

Gillberg, C., and Mary Coleman. *The Biology of the Autistic Syndromes,* 3rd ed. London, UK: Mac Keith Press, 2000.

Gilpin, R. Wayne. *Laughing & Loving with Autism: A Collection of "Real Life" Warm & Humorous Stories.* Arlington, TX: Future Horizons, 1993.

——. *More Laughing & Loving with Autism.* Arlington, TX: Future Horizons, 1994.

——. *Much More Laughing & Loving with Autism.* Arlington, TX: Future Horizons, 2002.

Goldstein, H. *Promoting Social Communication: Children with Developmental Disabilities from Birth to Adolescence.* Baltimore, MD: Paul Brookes Publishing, 2002.

Grandin, Temple. *Thinking in Pictures: And Other Reports from My Life with Autism.* New York, NY: Vintage, 1996.

Grandin, Temple, and Catherine Johnson. *Animals in Translation: Using the Mysteries of Autism to Decode Animal Behavior.* New York, NY: Scribner, 2005

Grandin, Temple, and Sean Barron. *Unwritten Rules of Social Relationships.* Arlington, TX: Future Horizons, 2004.

Grandin, Temple, Kate Duffy, and Tony Attwood (foreword). *Developing Talents: Careers for Individuals with Asperger Syndrome and High-Functioning Autism.* Shawnee Mission, KS: Autism Asperger Publishing Company, 2004.

Gray, Carol, ed. *My Social Stories Book.* London, U.K.: Jessica Kingsley Publishing, 2002.

——. *Taming the Recess Jungle.* Arlington, TX: Future Horizons, 1993.

——. *The New Social Story Book.* Arlington, TX: Future Horizons, 2000.

——. *What's Next?: Preparing the Student with Autism or Other Developmental Disabilities for Success in the Community.* Arlington, TX: Future Horizons, 1992.

——. *Comic Strip Conversations.* Arlington, TX: Future Horizons, 1994.

Greenspan, Stanley, Serena Weider, and Robin Simon (contributor). *The Child with Special Needs: Encouraging Intellectual and Emotional Growth.* New York, NY: Perseus Books, 1998.

Haddon, Mark. *The Curious Incident of the Dog in the Night-Time.* New York, NY: Doubleday, 2003.

Hamaguchi, Patricia McAleer. *Childhood Speech, Language, & Listening Problems,* 2nd ed. New York, NY: John Wiley & Sons, 2001.

Hamersky, Jean. *Cartoon Cut-Ups: Teaching Figurative Language and Humor.* Eau Claire, WI: Thinking Publications, 1995.

Hammeken, Peggy. *Inclusion: 450 Strategies for Success: A Practical Guide for All Educators Who Teach Students with Disabilities.* Minnetonka, MN: Peytral Publishers, 2000

Harland, Kelly. *A Will of His Own: Reflections on Parenting a Child with Autism.* Bethesda, MD: Woodbine House, 2002.

Harris, Sandra L., and Beth A. Glasberg. *Sibling of Children with Autism: A Guide for Families,* 2nd ed. Bethesda, MD: Woodbine House, 2003.

Harris, Sandra L., and Mary Jane Weiss. *Right from the Start: Behavioral Intervention for Young Children with Autism.* Bethesda, MD: Woodbine House, 1998.

Hart, Charles *Without Reason: A Family Copes with Two Generations of Autism.* Arlington, TX: Future Horizons, 1989.

——. *A Parent's Guide to Autism: Answers to the Most Common Questions.* New York, NY: Pocket Books, 1993.

Hermelin, Beate. *Bright Splinters of the Mind: A Personal Story of Research with Autistic Savants.* London, U.K.: Jessica Kingsley, 2001.

Hodgdon, Linda. *Solving Behavior Problems in Autism: Improving Communication with Visual Strategies.* Troy, MI: QuirkRoberts, 2003.

——. *Visual Strategies for Improving Communication: Volume 1: Practical Supports for School and Home.* Troy, MI: QuirkRoberts, 2004.

Holmes, David L. *Autism through the Life Span: The Eden Model.* Bethesda, MD: Woodbine House, 1998.

Hoskins, Barbara. *Conversations: A Framework for Language Intervention.* Eau Claire, WI: Thinking Publications, 1996.

Howlin, Patricia. *Teaching Children with Autism to Mind-Read: A Practical Guide for Teachers and Parents.* Hoboken, NJ: John Wiley & Sons, 1999.

——. *Children with Autism and Asperger Syndrome: A Guide for Practitioners and Carers.* Hoboken, NJ: John Wiley & Sons, 1999.

Howlin, Patricia, Simon Baron-Cohen, and Julie Hadwin. *All About Emotions.* Hoboken, NJ: John Wiley & Sons, 2000.

Holwlin, Patricia, and Michael Rutter. *Treatment of Autistic Children.* Hoboken, NJ: John Wiley & Sons, 1999.

Hyatt-Foley, Dean, and Matthew G. Foley. *Getting Services for Your Child on the Autism Spectrum.* London, U.K.: Jessica Kingsley, 2002.

Jackson, Luke. *Freaks, Geeks, and Asperger Syndrome: A User Guide to Adolescence.* London, U.K.: Jessica Kingsley Publishers, 2002.

Kaplan, Lawrence P, and Jay D. Burstein. *Diagnosis Autism: Now What?* Salt Lake City, UT: Etham Press, 2005

Kephart, Beth. *A Slant of Sun: One Child's Courage.* New York, NY: Quill, 1999.

Kirby, David. *Evidence of Harm: Mercury in Vaccines and the Autism Epidemic: A Medical Controversy.* New York, NY: St. Martin's. 2005.

Kluth, Paula. *You're Going to Love this Kid! Teaching Students with Autism in the Inclusive Classroom.* Baltimore, MD: Paul H. Brookes, 2003.

Koegel, Robert L., and Lynn Kern Koegel. *Pivotal Response Treatments for Autism: Communication, Social, and Academic Development.* Baltimore, MD: Paul H. Brookes Publishing Company, 2005.

——. *Teaching Children with Autism: Strategies for Initiating Positive Interactions and Improving Learning Opportunities.* Baltimore, MD: Paul H. Brookes Publishing Inc., 1995.

Kramer, Laura Shapiro. *Uncommon Voyage: Parenting a Special Needs Child.* Berkley CA. North Atlantic Books, 2001.

Kranowitz, Carol Stock. *The Out-of-Sync Child: Recognizing and Coping with Sensory Integration Dysfunction.* New York, NY: Skylight Press, 1998.

——. *The Out-of-Sync Child Has Fun: Activities for Kids with Sensory Integration Dysfunction.* New York, NY: The Berkley Publishing Group, 2003.

Kushner, H.S. *When Bad Things Happen to Good People.* New York, NY: Avon, 1981.

Leaf, Ron, and John McEachin, and Jaisom D. Harsh. *A Work in Progress: Behavior Management Strategies and a Curriculum for Intensive Behavioral Treatment of Autism.* New York, NY: DRL Books, 1999.

Lears, Laurie. *Ian's Walk: A Story About Autism.* Morton Grove, IL: Albert Whitman & Company, 1998.

Legge, Brenda. *Can't Eat, Won't Eat: Dietary Difficulties and the Autism Spectrum.* London, U.K.: Jessica Kingsley, 2002.

Lewis, Jackie, and Debbie Wilson. *Pathways to Learning in Rett Syndrome.* London, U.K.: David Fulton Publishers, 1998.

Lewis, Lisa. *Special Diets for Special Kids.* Arlington, TX: Future Horizons, 1998.

Lindberg, Barbro, and Rett, Andreas (foreword). *Understanding Rett Syndrome: A Practical Guide for Parents, Teachers, and Therapists.* Toronto; Lewiston, NY: Hogrefe & Huber Publishers, 1990.

Lovett, Herbert, ed. *Learning to Listen: Positive Approaches and People with Difficult Behavior.* Baltimore, MD: Paul H. Brookes, 1996.

Luckevich, Diana. *Language Targets to Teach a Child to Communicate: A Resource to Manage Language Instruction.* TalkingWords, 2004.

Marsh, Jayne D.B. *From the Heart: On Being the Mother of a Child with Special Needs.* Bethesda, MD: Woodbine House, 1994.

Martin Jr., Earle P., Earle P. Martin, and Gary B. Mesibov (foreword). *Dear Charlie: A Grandfather's Love Letter to His Grandson with Autism.* Arlington, TX: Future Horizons, 2000.

Maurice, Catherine, Gina Green, and Stephen Luce, eds. *Behavioral Intervention for Young Children with Autism: A Manual for Parents and Professionals.* Austin, TX: Pro-Ed, Inc., 1996.

Mayerson, Gary. *How To Compromise with Your School District Without Compromising Your Child: A Field Guide for Getting Effective Services for Children with Special Needs.* New York, NY: DRL Books, 2004.

McAfee, Jeanette. *Navigating the Social World: A Curriculum for Individuals with Asperger's Syndrome, High-Functioning Autism, and Related Disorders.* Arlington, TX: Future Horizons, 2002.

McClannahan, Lynn E., and Patricia J. Krantz. *Activity Schedules for Children with Autism: Teaching and Independent Behavior*. Bethesda, MD: Woodbine House, 1999.

McCoy, Elin. *What to Do . . . When Kids Are Mean to Your Child*. Pleasantville, NY: Reader's Digest, 1997

McEwan, Elaine K. *Nobody Likes Me: Helping Your Child Make Friends*. Wheaton, IL: Harold Shaw Publishers, 1996.

McGann, W., and G. Berven. *Social Communication Skills for Children*. Vero Beach, FL: The Speech Bin, 2001.

McGinnis, E., and A.P. Goldstein. *Skillstreaming the Elementary School Child: Strategies and Perspectives for Teaching Prosocial Skills*. Champaign, IL: Research Press, 1997.

——. *Skillstreaming in Early Childhood: Teaching Prosocial Skills to the Preschool and Kindergarten Child*. Champaign, IL: Research Press, 1990.

McKean, Thomas A. *Soon Will Come the Light: A View from Inside the Autism Puzzle*. Arlington, TX: Future Horizons, 1994.

Meyer, Donald, ed. *Uncommon Fathers: Reflections on Raising a Child with a Disability*. Bethesda, MD: Woodbine House, 1995.

——. *Views From Our Shoes: Growing Up with a Brother or Sister with Special Needs*. Bethesda, MD: Woodbine House, 1997.

Meyer, Donald, and Patricia Vadasy (contributor). *Living with a Brother or Sister with Special Needs: A Book for Sibs,* 2nd ed. Seattle, WA: University of Washington Press, 1996.

Moor, Julia. *Playing, Laughing, and Learning with Children on the Autism Spectrum: A Practical Resource of Play Ideas for Parents and Carers*. New York, NY: Jessica Kingsley Publishers, 2002.

Moore, Lorraine O. *Inclusion: A Practical Guide for Parents: Tools to Enhance Your Child's Success in Learning*. Minnetonka, MN: Peytral Publications, 2000.

Moyes, Rebecca A. *Incorporating Social Goals in the Classroom: A Guide for Teachers and Parents of Children with High-Functioning Autism and Asperger Syndrome*. London, U.K.: Jessica Kingsley Publishers, 2001.

——. *Addressing the Challenging Behavior of Children with High-Functioning Autism/Asperger Syndrome in the Classroom: A Guide for Teachers and Parents*. London, U.K.: Jessica Kingsley Publishers, 2002.

Mukhopadhyay, Tito Rajarshi. *The Mind Tree: A Miraculous Child Breaks the Silence of Autism*. New York: Arcade Publishing, 2003.

Myles, Brenda Smith, and Jack Southwick. *Asperger Syndrome and Difficult Moments: Practical Solutions for Tantrums, Rage, and Meltdowns*. Shawnee Mission, KS: Autism Asperger Publishing Company, 1999.

Naseef, Robert A. *Special Children, Challenged Parents: The Struggles and Rewards of Raising a Child with a Disability.* Baltimore, MD: Paul H. Brookes, 2001.

National Research Council. *Educating Children with Autism.* National Academies Press, 2001.

Newman, Bobby. *When Everybody Cares: Case Studies of ABA with People with Autism.* Dove & Orca, 1999.

Newport, Jerry, and Ron Bass (foreword). *Your Life Is Not a Label: A Guide to Living Fully with Autism and Asperger's Syndrome.* Arlington, TX: Future Horizons, 2001.

Nowicki, Stephen, and Marshall P. Duke. *Helping the Child Who Doesn't Fit In.* Atlanta, GA: Peachtree Publishers, 1992.

Notbohm, Ellen, and Veronica Zysk. *1001 Great Ideas for Teaching and Raising Children with Autism Spectrum Disorders.* Arlington, TX: Future Horizons, 2004.

O'Neill, Jasmine Lee. *Through the Eyes of Aliens: A Book About Autistic People.* London, UK: Jessica Kingsley Publishers, 1998.

Osman, Betty B. *No One to Play With: The Social Side of Learning Disabilities.* New York, NY: Random House, 1996.

Overton, Jennifer. *Snapshots of Autism: A Family Album.* London, U.K.: Jessica Kingsley, 2003.

Ozonoff, Sally, Geraldine Dawson, and James McPartland. *A Parent's Guide to Asperger Syndrome & High-Functioning Autism: How to Meet the Challenges and Help Your Child Thrive.* New York, NY: The Guilford Press, 2002.

Paradiz, Valerie. *Elijah's Cup: A Family's Journey into the Community and Culture of High-Functioning Autism and Asperger's Syndrome.* New York, NY: Free Press, 2002.

Park, Clara Claiborne. *Exiting Nirvana: A Daughter's Life with Autism.* Boston, MA: Little Brown & Company, 2001.

——. *The Siege: The First Eight Years of an Autistic Child with and Epilogue.* Boston, MA: Little Brown &Company, 1990.

Potter, Carol, and Chris Whittaker. *Enabling Communication in Children with Autism.* London, U.K.: Jessica Kingsley, 2001.

Powell, Stuart, and Rita Jordan, eds. *Autism and Learning: A Guide to Good Practice.* London, U.K.: David Fulton, 1997.

Quill, Kathleen Ann. *Teaching Children with Autism: Strategies to Enhance Communication and Socialization.* San Diego, CA: Singular Publishing, 1995.

Reisner, Helen. *Children with Epilepsy: A Parent's Guide.* Kensington, MD: Woodbine House, 1988.

Rief, Sandra F., and Julie A. Heimburge. *How to Reach and Teach All Students in the Inclusive Classroom: Ready-to-Use Strategies Lessons & Activities Teaching*

Students with Diverse Learning Needs. West Nyack, NY: The Center for Applied Research in Education, 1996.

Rimland, B. *Infantile Autism: The Syndrome and Its Implications for Neural Theory of Behavior.* Upper Saddle River, NJ: Prentice Hall Publishers, 1964.

Rutter, Michael. *Bright Splinters of the Mind.* London, U.K.: Jessica Kingsley, 2001.

Sacks, Oliver. *An Anthropologist on Mars: Seven Paradoxical Tales.* New York, NY: Vintage Books, 1995

Sands, Deanna J., Elizabeth Kozleski, and Nancy French. *Inclusive Education for the 21st Century.* Belmont, CA: Wadswort/ Thomson Learning, 2000.

Savner, Jennifer L., and Brenda Smith Myles. *Making Visual Supports Work in the Home and Community: Strategies for Individuals with Autism and Asperger Syndrome.* Shawnee Mission, KS: Autism Asperger Publishing Company, 2000.

Scholpler, Eric, ed. *Parent Survival Manual: A Guide to Crisis Resolution in Autism and Related Developmental Disorders.* New York, NY: Plenum Press, 1995.

Schopler, Eric, and Gary B. Mesibov, eds. *High Functioning Individuals with Autism.* New York, NY: Plenum Press, 1992.

——. *Current Issues in Autism Series.* 6 vols. New York, NY: Plenum Press, 1983–1988.

Schnurr, Rosina, Rosina G. Schnurr, and John Strachan. *Asperger's Huh? A Child's Perspective.* Anisor Publishing, 1999.

Scott, Jack, Claudia Clark, and Michael Brady. *Students with Autism: Characteristics and Instructional Programming for Special Educators.* San Diego, CA: Singular Publishing Group, 2000.

Seroussi, Karyn. *Unraveling the Mystery of Autism and Pervasive Developmental Disorder: A Mother's Story of Research and Recovery.* New York, NY: Simon & Schuster, 2000.

Shore, Stephen M. *Beyond the Wall: Personal Experiences with Autism and Asperger Syndrome.* Shawnee Mission, KS: Autism Asperger Publishing Company, 2001.

Shure, Myrna B. *I Can Problem Solve: An Interpersonal Cognitive Problem-Solving Program.* Champaign, IL: Research Pr Pub, 2001.

——. *Thinking Parent, Thinking Child.* New York, NY: McGraw-Hill, 2004.

Shure, Myrna B., Theresa Foy Digeronimo (contributor), and Amelia Sheldon (ed). *Raising a Thinking Child: Help Your Young Child to Resolve Everyday Conflicts and Get Along with Others: The "I Can Problem Solve" Program.* New York, NY: Pocket Books, 1996.

Shure, Myrna B., Theresa Foy Digeronimo (contributor), and Jackie Aher (illustrator). *Raising a Thinking Child Workbook: Teaching Young Children How to Resolve Everyday Conflicts and Get Along with Others.* Champaign, IL: Research Pr Press, 2000.

Sicile-Kira, Chantal. *Autism Spectrum Disorders: The Complete Guide.* London, U.K.: Vermilion, 2003.

Siegel, Bryna. *Helping Children with Autism Learn: Treatment Approaches for Parents and Professionals*. Oxford, U.K.: Oxford University Press, 2003.

——. *The World of the Autistic Child: Understanding and Treating Autistic Spectrum Disorders*. Oxford, U.K.: Oxford University Press, 1996.

Simmons, Karen. *Little Rainman*. Arlington, TX: Future Horizons, 1996.

Siperstein, G., and E. Richards. *Promoting Social Success*. Baltimore, MD: Paul H. Brookes, 2004.

Small, Mindy, and Lisa Kontente. *Everyday Solutions: A Practical Guide for Families of Children with Autism Spectrum Disorder*. Shawnee Mission, KS: Autism Asperger Publishing Company, 2003.

Spector, Cecile Cyrul. *Saying One Thing, Meaning Another: Activities for Clarifying Ambiguous Language*. Eau Claire, WI: Thinking Publications, 1997.

Stehli, Annabel. *The Sound of a Miracle: A Child's Triumph over Autism*. West Port, CT: Georgiana Organization, 1997.

Strohm, Kate. *Being the Other One: Growing Up with a Brother or Sister Who Has Special Needs*. Boston, MA: Shambhala, 2005.

Thompson, Mary. *Andy and His Yellow Frisbee*. Bethesda, MD: Woodbine House, 1996.

Thousand, J. *Creativity and Cooperative Learning*. Baltimore, MD: Paul H. Brookes, 2002.

Tilton, Adelle Jameson. *The Everything Parent's Guide to Children with Autism: Know What to Expect, Find the Help You Need, and Get through the Day*. Avon, MA: Adams Media, 2004.

Treffert, Darold A. *Extraordinary People: Understanding Savant Syndrome*. New York, NY: Harper & Row, 1989.

Volkmar, Fred, Paul Rhea, Ami Klin, and Donald J. Cohen, eds. *Handbook of Autism and Pervasive Developmental Disorders, Assessment, Interventions, and Policy*. Hoboken, NJ: John Wiley & Sons, 2005.

Volkmar, Fred, and Ian M. Goodyer, eds. *Autism and Pervasive Developmental Disorders*. Cambridge, U.K.: Cambridge University Press, 1998.

Wagner, Sheila. *Inclusive Programming for Middle School Students with Autism/Asperger's Syndrome*. Arlington, TX: Future Horizons, 2001

——. *Inclusive Programming for Elementary Students with Autism*. Arlington, TX: Future Horizons, 1999.

Waltz, Mitzi. *Autism Spectrum Disorders: Understanding the Diagnosis and Getting Help*, 2nd ed. Sebastopol, CA: O'Reilly & Associates, Inc., 2002.

——. *Pervasive Developmental Disorders: Diagnosis, Options, and Answers*. Arlington, TX: Future Horizons, 2003.

Weiss, Mary Jane, and Sandra L. Harris. *Reaching Out, Joining In: Teaching Social Skills to Young Children with Autism (Topics in Autism)*. Bethesda, MD: Woodbine House, 2001.

Welton, Jude, Elizabeth Newson (foreword), and Jane Telford (illustrator). *Can I tell you About Asperger Syndrome? A Guide for Friends and Family*. London, U.K.: Jessica Kingsley, 2004.

Wheeler, Maria. *Toilet Training for Individuals with Autism and Related Disorders: A Comprehensive Guide for Parents and Teachers*. Arlington, TX: Future Horizons, 1998.

Willey, Liane Holliday, and Tony Attwood (foreword). *Pretending to be Normal: Living with Asperger's Syndrome*. London, U.K.: Jessica Kingsley, 1999.

Williams, A. Lynn. *Speech Disorders Resource Guide for Preschool Children*. Clifton Park, NY: Singular Publishers Group, 2003.

Williams, Donna. *Nobody Nowhere: The Extraordinary Autobiography of an Autistic*. New York, NY: Avon Books, 1994.

——. *Somebody Somewhere: Breaking Free from the World of Autism*. New York, NY: Crown Publishing Group, 1995.

Winebrenner, Susan, and Pamela Espeland. *Teaching Kids with Learning Difficulties in the Regular Classroom: Strategies and Techniques Every Teacher Can Use to Challenge and Motivate Struggling Students*. Minneapolis, MN: Free Spirit Publishing, 1996

Wing, Lorna. *The Autistic Spectrum: A Parents' Guide to Understanding and Helping Your Child*. Berkeley, CA: Ulysses Press, 2001.

Wolfberg, Pamela J. *Play and Imagination in Children with Autism*. Teachers College Press, 1999.

Wright, Pam, and Peter Wright. *From Emotions to Advocacy: The Special Education Survival Guide*. Hartfield, VA: Harbor House Law Press, 2004.

Wrobel, Mary. *Taking Care of Myself: A Hygiene, Puberty, and Personal Curriculum for Young People with Autism*. Arlington, TX: Future Horizons, 2003.

Yapko, Diane. *Understanding Autism Spectrum Disorders: Frequently Asked Questions*. London, U.K.: Jessica Kingsley Publishers, 2003.

BOOK/PUBLISHER RESOURCES THAT SPECIALIZE IN BOOKS ON ASDs

You can access these websites for more information about books, products, and teaching tools specifically geared for ASDs.

Jessica Kingsley Publishers (www.jkp.com) publishes a range of books for parents and professionals. Based in England with a U.S. outlet.

Future Horizons (www.futurehorizons-autism.com) provides a range of publications, including those that are difficult to find at the usual bookstore/internet sites.

Woodbine House (www.woodbinehouse.com) publishes books on a range of disabilities/special needs, including ASDs. Most are written specifically for parents, although some books are focused on teachers and siblings.

Paul H. Brooks Publishing (www.pbrookes.com) publishes books for parents, teachers, and health care professionals.

Therapro Products (www.theraproducts.com) provides access to a range of materials. The OT/PT materials are particularly good.

DRL Books, Inc. (www.DRLbooks.com) provides publications that relate to the educational needs of the autism and developmental disability community.

GLOSSARY

ADAPTIVE BEHAVIOR (AB) The capability to familiarize oneself with new environments, people, and things while learning routines which allow coping with those new situations.

ADAPTIVE DEVELOPMENT How a child grows in behavioral skills as compared to other children of the same age. Among the benchmarks are dressing and feeding oneself, toilet training, social interaction with other children, responding to potentially dangerous situations, and behaving when unattended by adults.

ADAPTIVE PHYSICAL EDUCATION (APE) A personally tailored program of activities, games, and sports suitable to the special capacities of students with disabilities; an alternative to a general physical education program.

ADVOCATE Individual who promotes or reforms a cause that benefits an individual or groups, as in *educational advocate*.

AMERICANS WITH DISABILITIES ACT (ADA) Signed in 1990, this law legally forbids discrimination against people with disabilities in the areas of jobs, housing, and public service.

AMERICAN SIGN LANGUAGE (ASL) A system of communication for deaf adults through gestures, hand signals, and finger spelling. Prevalent in North America.

ANNUAL GOALS A set of reasonable expectations for pupils in a period of one year, as documented in the Individualized Education Plan (IEP).

ANNUAL REVIEW A re-examination of every twelve-month period of a pupil's IEP to determine if changes should made in next year's IEP.

APPLIED BEHAVIOR ANALYSIS (ABA) A treatment methodology pioneered by Dr. Ivar Lovaas and based on theories of operant conditioning by B. F. Skinner (see Appendix C for more information).

APHASIA The loss of ability to implement or comprehend language. Condition may be complete or partial.

APRAXIA A disorder in which the individual suffers partial or total loss of voluntary movement, while retaining muscular power and coordination. Disorder most frequently affects speech.

ASSESSMENT Includes tests and observations to determine a child's areas of strengths and weaknesses. Usually performed by an interdisciplinary team of professionals and parent to determine special education needs. Also called an evaluation.

ASSISTIVE AUGMENTATIVE COMMUNICATION (AAC) A method of communication utilizing a picture board or recorded messages, employed by speech and language therapists.

ATTENTION DEFICIT DISORDER (ADD) A neurological disorder marked by a severe shortness of attention span, cognitive disorganization, and sometimes hyperactivity (ADHD).

AUDITORY Relating to hearing skills and abilities.

AUDITORY INTEGRATION TRAINING (AIT) A treatment method of rehabilitation for the auditory system. Developed by Dr. Guy Berard, an eminent ear, nose, and throat physician (see Appendix C for more information).

AUTISM A condition marked by developmental delay in social skills, language, and behavior. Can present itself in varying degrees of severity.

AUTISM BEHAVIOR CHECKLIST (ABC) A method of measuring the level of autistic behaviors in individuals by giving each autistic behavior a weighted score.

AUDITORY INTEGRATION TRAINING (AIT) A technique in which the ear is retrained, thereby improving auditory processing (see Appendix C for more information).

AUDITORY PROCESSING The capability to understand aural stimuli, both words and nonverbal sounds.

AUGMENTATIVE COMMUNICATION Alternative methods of communication for those who are unable to communicate verbally. Tactics range from low-tech systems (e.g., sign language or pictures) to high-tech systems (e.g., voice output devices).

AUTISTIC SAVANT A person who expresses extraordinary mental abilities, often in the fields of numerical calculation, art, or music, but usually set within the context of autism or mental retardation.

AUTISM SPECTRUM DISORDERS Encompasses the following five disorders as defined in the DSM-IV-TR: Autistic Disorder, Asperger's Disorder, Childhood Disintegrative Disorder, Rett's Disorder, and Pervasive Developmental Disorder-Not Otherwise Specified (see Appendix B).

BASELINE The congenital level of function by a child before instruction is introduced.

BEHAVIOR An individual's personal set of actions and responses to the environment. These external movements are influenced by internal factors such as understanding, feelings, and emotions.

BEHAVIOR MODIFICATION A term that is sometimes used to describe ABA.

BEHAVIORIST OR BEHAVIORAL THERAPIST Certified individual who analyzes behaviors and designs and implements behavioral treatment programs to teach new skills.

BEST PRACTICE Strategies that reliably lead to a desired result or outcome, as confirmed through experience, research, and evaluation. The set of strategies that utilizes the best practices, knowledge, and technology to ensure success.

CENTRAL AUDITORY PROCESSING DISORDER (CAPD) While retaining hearing, an individual experiences difficulty in understanding and/or processing spoken language.

CHILDHOOD AUTISM RATING SCALE (CARS) A test developed at TEACCH to diagnose autism. The child is rated in fifteen areas of ability, resulting in an assessment of nonautistic, autistic, or severely autistic.

CHILDHOOD DISINTEGRATIVE DISORDER (CDD) A rare form of pervasive developmental disorder in which normally developing children suddenly lose language and social skills after age three.

CHRONOLOGICALLY AGE-APPROPRIATE Altering the activities and behaviors for disabled children to bring them into line with those of nondisabled children of the same age.

COEXISTING DISORDERS Condition in which individuals with ASDs possess additional disorders. Among them: impulse-control disorders, psychoses, obsessive-compulsive disorder, seizures, mood and anxiety disorders, and developmental delays. Also called Co-Morbid Disorders or Differential Diagnosis.

COGNITION Ability to acknowledge and understand the environment.

COGNITIVE Describes the process used for the tasks of remembering, reasoning, understanding, and using judgment; in special education, a cognitive disability refers to difficulty in learning.

COGNITIVE ABILITY An individual's intellectual ability or the aggregate skills of knowing and understanding.

COMMUNICATION The conveyance of gestures or information between people. As a social skill, communication offers autonomy as well as control over one's environment.

COMMUNICATIONS NOTEBOOK A notebook used by parents and teachers of a special education student, designed to facilitate daily communication between the two parties on student progress.

COMMUNITY ADVISORY COMMITTEE FOR SPECIAL EDUCATION (CACSE) A legally-empowered group of parents and professionals that advises the Board of Education, Superintendent of Schools, and school district administration about special education programs and policies.

COMPREHENSIVE EVALUATION A complete assessment of a child, based on his psychological, educational, social, and health status. Usually conducted by a team of professionals and complemented by information from parents and teachers.

CONCRETE THINKING Thinking that is grounded in facts and details, rather than ideas and concepts.

CONSENT Written permission provided by the parent to the local district to allow actions on behalf of the pupil.

CONSEQUENCE The direct result of action or effort. Consequences can be either pleasant and reinforcing or unpleasant and punishing.

CRITERION REFERENCED TEST Child is evaluated by his own performance, not in comparison to others.

CUE Stimulus that prompts a behavior or activity in an individual.

DAILY LIVING ACTIVITIES Routine maintenance or self-improvement tasks which include eating, dressing, grooming, cooking, and cleaning.

DEVELOPMENT The process of growth and learning during which a child acquires intellectual and social skills; includes interaction between psychosocial factors and stage by stage growth of the body.

DEVELOPMENTAL DISABILITY (DD) A handicap or impairment which occurs before the age of eighteen months and is expected to persist indefinitely. This includes pervasive developmental disorders, cerebral palsy, and mental retardation.

DEVELOPMENTAL MILESTONE A standard of growth against which one measures the progress of an individual or group over time.

DEVELOPMENTALLY DELAYED A condition in which the physical development of a person is slower than normal.

DIAGNOSIS The name of the disorder identified after an evaluation.

DIAGNOSTIC AND STATISTICAL MANUAL OF MENTAL DISORDERS, FOURTH EDITION, TEXT REVISION (DSM-IV-TR) The official system that classifies psychological and psychiatric disorders. Prepared by and published by the American Psychiatric Association (see Appendix B).

DIRECT THERAPY Process of work between therapist and child.

DISCRETE TRIAL Part of ABA therapy, a trial is a sequence composed of three parts: a direction, a behavior, and a consequence.

DISCRETE TRIAL TRAINING (DTT) Used in ABA therapy, DTT breaks down complex skills into small, easily manageable steps so that skills can be more easily mastered by the child with an ASD. Also referred to as Discrete Trial Therapy and Discrete Trial Teaching. (see Appendix C for more information).

DUE PROCESS HEARING A hearing at which parents present evidence that the school district is not properly educating their child.

DYSFLUENCY An interruption in the flow of speech, for example, stuttering.

DYSLEXIA A learning disability which affects one's ability to read. The results range from reversing written letters, numbers, and words to reading backwards and poor handwriting, to difficulty remembering and recognizing written text.

EARLY INTERVENTION SERVICES (EI) A collection of services provided by public and private agencies and designed by law to support eligible children and families in enhancing a child's potential for growth and development from birth to age three. (Services for three- to five-year-olds are called "preschool services.")

ECHOLALIA A condition in which an individual repeats words or phrases previously heard. Delayed echolalia can occur days or weeks after initially hearing the word or phrase.

ENGAGEMENT The ability to remain involved with a person or object.

EVALUATION See *Assessment*.

EVALUATION CRITERIA A component of the IEP. Provides a description of how the results of a pupil's IEP will determine the achievement of standard goals. Methods of obtaining information include teacher observation, interviews with parents, and standardized tests.

EXPRESSIVE LANGUAGE The language used to communicate to others. Oral expressive language is the child's expression of thoughts and feelings through oral speech. Expressive language also refers to gestures and signing, as well as communication through objects, pictures, and writing.

EXTENDED SCHOOL YEAR (ESY) Educational services specially crafted for students who need them beyond the regular school year. Not to be confused with summer school or year-round school.

FINE MOTOR SKILLS Activities that require the coordination of smaller body muscles, especially those of the hand, such as writing and drawing.

FRAGILE X SYNDROME A genetic cause of mental retardation, in which one part of the X-chromosome is defective.

FREE APPROPRIATE PUBLIC EDUCATION (FAPE) A program which mandates the provision of public school services to all school-aged children (up to age twenty-one), even if disabled.

FUNCTIONAL ANALYSIS The evaluation of individual behaviors through observation of what happens before and after the behavior occurs. Behaviors are further assessed for their appropriateness to the situation and to the individual.

GENERAL EDUCATION A curriculum of the arts and sciences courses that provides students with a broad educational experience. A general education school can include inclusion programs for children with ASDs, where children with ASDs are integrated into classes with typically developing children.

GENERALIZATION The ability to learn a skill in one situation and be able to apply it to other situations.

GENETIC Inherited.

GILLIAM AUTISM RATING SCALE (GARS) A rating scale to help identify and diagnose ASD in children and young adults. Standards are based on definitions of autism adopted by the Autism Society of America and the *Diagnostic and Statistical Manual of Mental Disorders, Fourth Edition* (DSM-IV).

GROSS MOTOR SKILLS Body movements which utilize larger muscle group of the body, such as sitting, walking, and jumping.

HIGH-FUNCTIONING AUTISM (HFA) Although not officially recognized as a diagnostic category, HFA refers to individuals with ASDs who have near-average to above-average cognitive abilities and can communicate through receptive and expressive language.

HYPERACTIVE A condition marked by chronic restlessness and the inability to concentrate for any length of time. Could be evidence of an attention deficit disorder.

HYPERLEXIA An ability to read at an early age, but without total comprehension.

HYPERSENSITIVITY Excessive, often painful, reaction to everyday auditory, visual, or tactile stimuli such as bright lights or loud noises.

HYPOSENSITIVITY A marked absence of reaction to everyday stimuli.

INCLUSION See *mainstreaming*.

IDENTIFICATION Evaluation of child as a candidate for special education services. Process requires proper screening and assessment to confirm whether child has an ASD or another disorder.

INDEPENDENT EDUCATION EVALUATION (IEE) Assessment of child requested by parent who believes that the school did not conduct a proper evaluation. In some instances, this evaluation may be conducted at the school's expense.

INDIVIDUAL TRANSITION PLAN (ITP) A plan which facilitates the transfer of a student from one setting to another, such as to a classroom, school, or work environment.

INDIVIDUALIZED EDUCATION PLAN (IEP) The written yearly plan for school-age children ages three to twenty-one that specifies the services that the local education agency has agreed to provide children with disabilities who are eligible under IDEA.

INDIVIDUAL FAMILY SERVICE PLAN (IFSP) Documents and guides the early intervention process for children with disabilities and their families, in accordance with Part C of the IDEA. Through the IFSP process, families and service providers work together as a team to plan, implement, and evaluate services to meet the specific needs of the child and family.

INDIVIDUALS WITH DISABILITIES EDUCATION ACT (IDEA) A federal law originally passed in 1975 that requires states to establish performance goals and indicators for children with disabilities consistent with the maximum extent appropriate with other goals and standards for all children established by the state and to report on progress toward meeting those goals. IDEA states that children with disabilities must be included in state and district-wide assessments of student progress with individual modifications and accommodations as needed. IDEA promotes improved educational results for children with disabilities through early intervention, preschool, and educational experiences that prepare them for later educational challenges and employment.

INDIVIDUALS WITH DISABILITIES EDUCATION IMPROVEMENT ACT 2004 (IDEIA) The IDEA of 1997 has been reauthorized and is now known as the IDEIA 2004, effective July 1, 2005. The goal of the IDEIA 2004 is to help children learn better by promoting accountability for results, enhancing parent involvement, using proven practices and materials, providing more flexibility, and reducing paperwork burdens for teachers, states, and local school districts.

INSTRUCTIONAL OBJECTIVES A game plan for desired achievements in the child's development, based on current level of performance and a broader annual goal.

INSTRUCTIONAL STRATEGIES Specific methods and materials employed in teaching the pupil.

INTEGRATION See *Inclusion* or *Mainstreaming*.

INTELLIGENCE QUOTIENT (IQ) A numerical measurement of intellectual capacity that compares an individual's chronological age to his or her mental age according to standardized tests.

INTERDISCIPLINARY TEAM A group of professionals from different disciplines (psychologist, speech therapist, occupational therapist, etc.) who assess a child and develop a comprehensive plan to address his needs.

INTERVENTION Action taken to attain an individual's developmental potential. The term is often used synonymously with Treatment.

INTRINSIC REINFORCEMENT The positive reinforcement that radiates from within, stemming from satisfaction or pride in accomplishing a task.

JOINT ATTENTION OR SHARED ATTENTION A social skill which develops early in typically developing children, in which two people—usually a young child and an adult—jointly observe an object or event and share the experience. This skill is crucial to later language and social development. Often referred to as Shared Attention.

LANGUAGE IMPAIRMENT A condition marked by difficulty in understanding and/or using language.

LEARNING DISABLED (LD) Having a compromised learning ability, manifested by a severe discrepancy between the student's intellectual ability and his level of academic achievement in one or more of the following areas: oral expression, listening, reading and writing comprehension, and mathematics calculation or reasoning.

LEAST RESTRICTIVE ENVIRONMENT (LRE) The requirement under the IDEA that all children receiving special education must be educated to the fullest extent possible with children who do not have disabilities.

LOCAL EDUCATION AGENCY (LEA) Agency responsible for providing educational services for children with ASDs on the local (city, county, and school district) level.

MAINSTREAMING The concept that students with disabilities should be integrated with their nondisabled peers to the maximum extent possible, when appropriate to the needs of the child with a disability. Mainstreaming is one point on a continuum of educational options. The term is sometimes used synonymously with *inclusion* and *integration*.

MEDIATION A resolution process. If parents disagree with the school district on providing services for a child with disabilities, a third party mediator will be assigned to help both parties resolve the issue.

MEDICAID A U.S.government–funded program that pays the medical expenses of people with limited financial means.

MENTAL AGE (MA) An assessment of intellectual functioning, based on the average standard for children of the same chronological age.

MENTAL RETARDATION (MR) A classification based upon three criteria: intellectual functioning level below 70, based on IQ test; significant limitations in two or more adaptive skill areas (e.g., communication, self-care, home living, social skills, self-health and safety, academics); and the presence of intellectual limitations from childhood (since the age of 18 or earlier).

MOTOR Muscle activity—especially voluntary muscle activity—and consequent body movements.

MOTOR PLANNING The brain's ability to conceive, organize, and execute a sequence of complex physical actions.

MULTIDISCIPLINARY A team approach involving specialists in more than one discipline, including but not limited to an occupational therapist, a speech and language pathologist, and a psychologist.

MULTIDISCIPLINARY EVALUATION TEAM (MDT) A group of people who evaluate the abilities and needs of a child to determine whether the child meets eligibility criteria for special needs.

MODELING Observing and imitating another's behaviors and actions to copy them in one's own actions.

NEUROLOGIST A physician who treats medical problems associated with the brain and spinal cord.

NEUROTRANSMITTER The chemical substance which allows the transmission of an impulse from one nerve cell to another in the brain.

NO CHILD LEFT BEHIND (NCLB) An act signed in 2002 to reform schools by encouraging stronger accountability for results, more freedom for states and communities, proven education methods, and more choices for parents. Under No Child Left Behind, states are working to close the achievement gap and make sure all students, including those who are disadvantaged, achieve academic proficiency. Annual state and school district report cards inform parents and communities about state and school progress. Schools that do not make progress must provide supplemental services, such as free tutoring or after-school assistance; take corrective actions; and, if still not making adequate yearly progress after five years, make dramatic changes to the way the school is run.

NORM REFERENCED TESTS Measurement of a child's performance as compared to others the same age.

NEUROTYPICAL (NT) Description applicable to person who does not suffer from a neurodevelopmental disorder such as an ASD. Often referred to as typical.

OBJECTIVES The intermediate steps that must be taken to reach the annual goals; a component of the IEP.

OBJECT PERMANENCE A child's awareness that an object still exists even when it is taken out of visual range.

OBSESSIVE COMPULSIVE DISORDER (OCD) A psychiatric disorder characterized by obsessive thoughts and compulsive behavior.

OCCUPATIONAL THERAPY (OT) A therapy that focuses on improving the development of fine and gross motor skills, sensory integration skills, and daily living skills.

ORAL MOTOR Movement of the muscles located in and around the mouth.

PEDANTIC SPEECH A longwinded, tiresome style of speaking, emphasizing self-absorption more than salient fact.

PERSERVERATIVE BEHAVIOR Repetitive movements, speech or play patterns, such as repeatedly opening and closing doors or eye tracking.

PERVASIVE DEVELOPMENTAL DISORDER (PDD) The official classification for Autism Spectrum Disorders that is documented in the DSM-IV-TR. Among the conditions belonging to this group are Autistic Disorder, Asperger's Disorder, Rett's Disorder, Childhood Disintegrative Disorder (CDD), and Pervasive Developmental Disorder-Not Otherwise Specified (PDD-NOS).

PERVASIVE DEVELOPMENTAL DISORDER-NOT OTHERWISE SPECIFIED (PDD-NOS) An autism spectrum disorder that includes most characteristics of Autistic Disorder but not enough to meet the specific criteria for Autistic Disorder or other Pervasive Developmental Disorders.

PHYSICAL THERAPY (PT) A therapy that specializes in the improvement of developing motor skills, with an emphasis on gross motor skills.

PICTURE EXCHANGE COMMUNICATION SYSTEM (PECS) A communication system for nonverbal or functionally nonverbal individuals, especially for young children with ASDs. For example, PECS allows a child to exchange a picture card for something he or she wants. (See Appendix C for more information).

PICA Ingestion of nonfood items.

PINCER GRASP The use of the thumb and forefinger to grasp small objects.

PIVOTAL RESPONSE TRAINING (PRT) A treatment intervention for children with ASDs that teaches behaviors central to wide areas of functioning, such as motivation and responsiveness. (See Appendix C for more).

PLACEMENT The selection of an appropriate educational program for a child with special needs.

PRAGMATICS The method of using language to communicate effectively in a natural context, focusing on considerations like eye contact between speaker and listener, how close to stand, taking turns, and selecting topics of conversation.

PRESCHOOL Full- or half-day school or day care program provided prior to kindergarten for children ages three to five.

PROMPT A stimulus or cue given to help a child compete a task. Prompts may be physical, verbal, visual, or location-appropriate.

PRONOUN REVERSAL Phenomenon where in child switches first- and second-person pronouns, replacing "I" or "me" with "you" or "them."

PROPRIOCEPTION A sense that informs us of the position of our body parts.

PROSODY The style of speech identified by pitch or intonation, loudness, and tempo of spoken words.

RECEPTIVE LANGUAGE The comprehension of spoken and written communication and gestures.

REINFORCEMENT A positive event which follows an action, thereby creating in the doer a pleasant feeling and increasing the likelihood that the action will be repeated. For example, reinforcement can occur by rewarding the individual with a toy, token, food treat, or social praise for a good behavior.

REINFORCEMENT MENU A list of extrinsic reinforcers from which the student may choose after successfully completing an assigned task.

REINFORCER Anything positive that follows a behavior and increases that behavior, including social praise, desired food, or toys. Conversely, a negative reinforcer will decrease behavior, as it prompts a reaction that the person will try to avoid.

REFERRAL The request to identify and assess a child's special education needs, usually made by a parent, teacher, or medical personnel.

RELATED SERVICES Auxiliary services for a disabled child, such as transportation, occupational, physical and speech pathology services, interpreters, and medical services.

RELATIONSHIP DEVELOPMENT INTERVENTION (RDI) A program that employs specific exercises and activities to teach interpersonal social skills. (See Appendix C for more.)

REMEDIATION In special education, programming which improves the student's performance.

RESOURCE ROOM A nonrestrictive environment for the child with special needs, where he or she may play for a portion of the day.

RESPITE CARE This service allows the primary caregiver (most often parents) of a severely disabled person an opportunity for a temporary break.

RETT'S DISORDER Features reduced head growth and usually profound cognitive delays. An extremely rare genetic disorder affecting only girls.

REVERSE MAINSTREAMING The placement of nondisabled children in a special education classroom to play and learn with disabled children.

SCREENING Brief assessments which identify children who may require comprehensive evaluation.

SEIT (SPECIAL EDUCATION ITINERANT TEACHER) (pronounced *see-it*) An aide who accompanies a child in the classroom to support the child's individual needs in areas such as social skills and academic skills. Also referred to as a *shadow*.

SELF-CONTAINED CLASS Classroom specifically designed for special education students.

SELF-STIMULATORY BEHAVIOR Actions used solely to stimulate one's own senses, such as body rocking and finger flicking. Theories suggest that "self-stims" serve to reduce sensory overload and increase concentration. Sometimes self-stimulatory behavior can create an arousal state. Other examples include hand flapping, toe walking, spinning, and echolalia. Often referred to as stimming.

SENSORIMOTOR Voluntary movement and senses like sight touch and hearing. Pertaining to brain activity other than automatic functions (respiration, circulation, sleep) or cognition.

SENSORY DEFENSIVENESS Involves a group of symptoms that signal an overreaction to stimuli. These include patterns of avoidance, sensory seeking, fear, anxiety, and even aggression.

SENSORY INTEGRATION (SI) The harmonic organization of parts of the nervous system so that an individual can effectively interact with the environment.

SENSORY INTEGRATION THERAPY Treatment focused on improving the way the brain processes and organizes the senses. Therapy is implemented by an occupational therapist and involves full-body movements that provide vestibular, proprioceptive, and tactile stimulation (see Appendix C for more information).

SERVICE COORDINATOR A coordinator of an infant's or toddler's services, working in partnership with the family and providers of special programs.

SHADOW See SEIT.

SHAPING Reinforcing behavior in successive approximations until desired behavior is attained.

SOCIAL ADAPTATION A child's ability to respond to and interact with others at a level appropriate for his or her age, including self-help skills like dressing, toileting, and eating, which lead to greater independence.

SOCIAL INTERACTION The process by which individuals act in relation to one another.

SOCIAL SECURITY DISABILITY INSURANCE (SSDI) Money entitled to disabled workers, obtained through the social security system. People who become disabled before the age of twenty-two may collect SSDI under a parent's account, if the parent is retired, disabled, or deceased.

SOCIAL SKILLS Positive, situation-appropriate behaviors that are necessary to communicate, interact, and form relationships with others.

SPECIAL EDUCATION (SPED) Specialized and personalized instruction of a disabled child, designed in response to educational disabilities determined by team evaluation.

SPEECH LANGUAGE IMPAIRMENT (SLI) Diminished communication or complete absence of speech or language.

SPEECH-LANGUAGE PATHOLOGIST (SLP OR S-LP) A qualified professional who improves communication skills as well as oral motor abilities.

STEREOTYPY/STEREOTYPIC BEHAVIOR Purposeless movement or speech in children with ASDs, such as hand flapping or echolalia, which are repetitive and odd. Also referred to as *perseveration*.

STIM/STIMMING See "Self-Stimulatory Behavior"

STUDENT ASSISTANCE TEAM (SAT) A group engaged in problem solving and intervention strategies to assist the teacher(s) in the provision of general education.

SUPPLEMENTAL SECURITY INCOME (SSI) Benefits available to low-income people who are disabled, blind, or aged. SSI is based on need and income, not past earnings paid into the system.

SYMPTOMS Tangible manifestations of an existing disorder.

SYNDROME A condition characterized by a group of co-occurring symptoms that have a recognizable and uniform effect on a group of individuals.

TACTILE Pertaining to the sense of touch on the skin.

TACTILE DEFENSIVENESS A marked overreaction to touch by a child.

TARGET SKILL An isolated task selected by a teacher or student for accomplishment.

THEORY OF MIND (TOM) The ability to empathize: to understand what another person thinks, feels, desires, intends, or believes.

TRANSITION PLAN A plan that details services and accommodations provided to children with disabilities when moving from early intervention services to preschool, and from school to the work setting at age twenty-one. Required under IDEA.

TRANSITIONS The changes from one environment to another, such as from an early childhood program to school. Transitions may also refer to changes from one activity to another.

TREATMENT AND EDUCATION OF AUTISTIC AND RELATED COMMUNICATION HANDICAPPED CHILDREN (TEACCH) A structured teaching intervention developed by Division TEACCH of the University of North Carolina (see Appendix C for more information).

TRIGGER An event that precipitates a certain behavior.

VESTIBULAR Pertaining to the sensory system located on the inner ear that governs posture and balance.

VISUAL ADAPTATIONS/VISUAL SUPPORTS Written schedules, lists, charts, and picture sequences that convey meaningful information that allow the person with autism to function more independently, without constant verbal direction.

VISUAL SCHEDULE A group of pictures or objects that guides a child through the order of events or activities.

VISUAL DISCRIMINATION The ability to distinguish and detect differences in objects, forms, letters, or words.

VISUAL MOTOR The skill and dexterity required to complete a task, such as fitting a piece into a puzzle or a key into a keyhole.

NOTES

CHAPTER 1

1 National Institutes of Mental Health www.nimh.nih.gov/publicat/ autism.cfm taken from: Newschaffer CJ (Johns Hopkins Bloomberg School of Public Health). "Autism Among Us: Rising Concerns and the Public Health Response" [Video on the Internet]. Public Health Training Network, 2003 June 20. Available from: www.publichealthgrandrounds.unc.edu/autism/webcast.htm.

2 Committee on Educational Interventions for Children with Autism, Division of Behavioral and Social Sciences and Education National Research Council, Catherine Lord and James P. McGee, eds., *Educating Children with Autism.* (Washington, DC: National Academy Press, 2001). (Note: read it free at: www.nap.edu/catalog/10017.html)

3 Molly Masland, "Children in the Grip of Autism: More Families Faced with a Difficult Diagnosis," part of the MSNBC News series, "Autism: The Hidden Epidemic?" February 23, 2005, www.msnbc.msn.com/id/6901860/.

4 Lorna Wing, M.D., *The Autism Spectrum: A Parent's Guide to Understanding and Helping Your Child.* (Berkeley, CA: Ulysses Press, 2001), 16.

5 Uta Frith. *Autism: Explaining the Enigma*, 2nd ed., Malden, MA: Blackwell Publishing, 2003, 173.

6 Peter Farley, "Mapping the Social Mind," *Yale Medicine*, Summer 2004: 22.

7 Committee on Educational Interventions for Children with Autism, Division of Behavioral and Social Sciences and Education National Research Council, Catherine Lord and James P. McGee, eds. *Educating Children with Autism*. Washington, DC: National Academy Press, 2001.

CHAPTER 2

1 Ivar O. Lovaas, "Behavioral Treatment and Normal Educational and Intellectual Functioning in Young Autistic Children," *Journal of Consulting and Clinical Psychology* 1987 Feb; 55 (1): 3–9.

2 The National Society for Epilepsy, "Epilepsy: Information on Seizures," October 2004. www.epilepsynse.org.uk/pages/info/leaflets/seizures.cfm

3 Carolyn Thorwarth Bruey, Psy.D. *Demystifying Autism Spectrum Disorders: A Guide to Diagnosis for Parents and Professionals* Bethesda, MD: Woodbine House, 2004, 109–119.

CHAPTER 3

1 Joseph Serwach, "Autism: Why Do Some Develop Then Regress?" *University Record Online.* Ann Arbor: University of Michigan News Service, November 18, 2004. www.umich.edu/~urecord/0405/Nov22_04/22.shtml

2 Ami Klin, Ph.D.; Warren Jones, BA; Robert Schultz, Ph.D.; Fred Volkmar, M.D.; Donald Cohen, M.D., "Visual Fixation Patterns During Viewing of Naturalistic Social Situations as Predictors of Social Competence in Individuals with Autism," *Archives of General Psychiatry*, Volume 59, No. 9, 331–340. American Medical Association: September, 2002.

3 K.A. Loveland, and S.H. Landry, "Joint Attention and Language in Autism and Developmental Language Delay," *Journal of Child Psychology and Psychiatry* 16 (1986): 335–49; M. Sigman, and L. Capps. *Children with Autism: A Developmental Perspective.* Cambridge, MA: Harvard University Press, 1997.

4 Simon Baron-Cohen, *Mindblindness: An Essay on Autism and Theory of Mind.* Cambridge, MA: MIT Press, 1997.

5 Heinz Wimmer and Josef Perner, "Beliefs about Beliefs: Representations and Constraining Function of Wrong Beliefs in Young Children's Understanding of Deception," *Cognition*, 13 (1983): 103–128.

6 C.D. Frith, and J. Done, "Stereotyped Behavior in Madness and in Health," *The Neurobiology of Behavioral Stereotypy* by S.J. Cooper and C.T. Dourish, eds. (Oxford: (Oxford, U.K. University Press, 1990), 232–59.

7 E. Ornitz, "Neurophysiology in Infantile Autism," *Journal of the American Academy of Child Psychiatry,* 24 (1985):251–262.

8 Jane Taylor McDonnell and Paul McDonnell. *News from the Border.* New York, NY: Ticknor & Fields, 1993.

9 Temple Grandin, *Thinking In Pictures: And Other Reports from My Life with Autism.* (New York: Vintage, 1996), 62.

10 Neil Walker and Margaret Whelan, Geneva Symposium on Autism, Toronto, Canada, October 27, 1994.

11 Lorna Wing. *The Autism Spectrum: A Parent's Guide to Understanding and Helping Your Child.* Berkeley, CA: Ulysses Press, 2001, 114–15.

12 Stephen M. Edelson, Ph.D., "Self-Injurious Behavior," Center for Autism, Salem, Oregon, 1995, www.autism.org/sib.html

13 Claudia Kalb, "When Does Autism Start?" *Newsweek.* Feb. 28, 2005. 53.

14 Lorna Wing, *The Autistic Spectrum: A Parent's Guide to Understanding and Helping Your Child.* (Berkeley: Ulysses Press, 2001), 105.

15 Lorna Wing, *The Autism Spectrum: A Parent's Guide to Understanding and Helping Your Child* (Berkeley, CA: Ulysses Press, 2001), 14–19.

16 Claudia Kalb, "When Does Autism Start?" *Newsweek* (February 28, 2005), 51.

17 Leo Kanner (1943) "Autistic Disturbances of Affective Contact," *Nervous Child* 2, 217–50, p.227. Reprinted in L. Kanner, *Childhood Psychosis: Initial Studies and New Insights* 1–43. Washington, DC: V.H. Winston, 1973, pp.1–43, 15.

18 Julie Osterling, and Geraldine Dawson, "Early Recognition of Children with Autism: A Study of First Birthday Home Videotapes," *Journal of Autism and Developmental Disorders*, 24 (1994): 247–57.

19 Julie Osterling, Geraldine Dawson, and J. Munson, "Early Recognition of One-Year-Old Infants with Autism Spectrum Disorder Versus Mental Retardation: A Study of First Birthday Party Home Videotapes," *Development and Psychopathology* 14 (2002): 239–52.

20 Anthony Attwood, Uta Frith, and B. Hermelin, "The Understanding and Use of Interpersonal Gestures by Autistic and Down's Syndrome Children," *Journal of Autism and Developmental Disorders*, 18 (1988): 241–57.

21 Uta Frith, *Autism: Explaining the Enigma* (Malden, MA: Blackwell Publishing, 2003), 106–8.

22 Philip Teitelbaum, Osnat Teitelbaum, Jennifer Nye, Joshua Fryman, and Ralph G. Maurer, "Movement Analysis in Infancy May Be Useful for Early Diagnosis of Autism," *Proceedings of the National Academy of Sciences of the United States of America*, 95 (1998): 13982–7.

23 Dr. Ralph Maurer, "Movement and Relationship in Autism" (presentation to the National Institutes of Health: The State of the Science Conference, April 1995) as seen in the 1995 year-end review by the Autism National Committee website: www.autcom.org/relationship.html.

24 Darold A. Treffert, M.D. *Extraordinary People: Understanding Savant Syndrome.* New York, NY: Ballantine, 2000.

25 L. Selfe, *Nadia, A Case of Extraordinary Drawing Ability in an Autistic Child* (London, U.K.: Academic Press, 1977).

26 Beate Hermelin, *Bright Splinters of the Mind: A Personal Story of Research with Autistic Savants.* London, U.K.: Jessica Kingsley Publishers, 2001, 78.

CHAPTER 4

1 M.A. Just, V.L. Cherkassky, T.A. Keller, and N. J. Minshew, "Cortical Activation and Synchronization during Sentence Comprehension in High-Functioning Autism: Evidence of Underconnectivity," *Brain* 127 (2004): 1811–21.

2 University of Washington, "Study Seeks to Pinpoint Genes Related to Autism," http://depts.washington.edu/autism/Outlook/STY6genes.html

3 UC Davis M.I.N.D. Institute, "Autism Conference Reports Advances in Early Diagnosis, Role of Immune System, Genes and Environmental Influences," Boston, MA, May 5, 2005.

4 The National Fragile X Foundation website: www.fragilex.org

5 The Associated Press, "Uncovering Autism's Mysteries," *CNN.com*, 2003. www.cnn.com/2003/HEALTH/conditions/03/02/autism.ap/

6 Yale Child Study Center Developmental Disabilities Clinic, "Frequently Asked Questions about Pervasive Developmental Disorders." http://info.med.yale.edu/chldstdy/autism/pddinfo.html#child

7 Diana Parsell, "Assault on Autism: Scientists Target Drugs and Other Environmental Agents that May Play a Role," *Science News Online*, Vol. 166, No. 20 (November 13, 2004): 311. www.sciencenews.org

8 UC Davis M.I.N.D. Institute conference, May 5, 2005.

9 Parsell, 311.

10 S. Limin Shi, Hossein Fatemi, Robert W. Sidwell, and Paul H. Patterson, "Maternal Influenza Infection Causes Marked Behavioural and Pharmacological Abnormalities in the Offspring," *The Journal of Neuroscience* 23 (2003): 297–302.

11 Bernard Rimland, *Infantile Autism: The Syndrome and Its Implications for a Neural Theory of Behavior* (New York: Prentice Hall, 1964).

12 D. H. Skuse, "Imprinting the X-Chromosome and the Male Brain: Explaining Sex Differences in the Liability to Autism," *Pediatric Research* 47 (2000): 9–16.

13 Dr. Dan Geschwind, associate professor of neurology; Rita Cantor, adjunct professor of human genetics; Stan Nelson, professor of human genetics; Jennifer Stone, graduate student researcher at The David Geffen School of Medicine at UCLA, "Gene Affects Boys Only: May Explain Autism's Low Incidence in Girls," *The American Journal of Human Genetics*. www.journals.uchicago.edu/AJHG/journal/issues/v76n6/42136/42136.html (June 2005).

14 Simon Baron-Cohen, *The Essential Difference: The Truth about the Male and Female Brain* (New York: Perseus, 2003).

15 David Whitney, "Rapid Spread of Autism Baffling: Increase Creates a Big Financial Burden for State, Summit Is Told," November 21, 2003, www.sacbee.com/content/politics/story/7823498p-8764252c.html

16 Autism Society of America website: www.ASA.org and Autism Speaks website: www.autismspeaks.org/autism/index.asp

17 Interview with Gary Goldstein, M.D., 2005, www.autismspeaks.org/autism/children.html

CHAPTER 5

1 American Academy of Pediatrics (2001). Policy Statement: The Pediatrician's Role in the Diagnosis and Management of Autistic Spectrum Disorder in Children (RE060018) Pediatrics, 107, 1221–1226. Committee on Children with Disabilities (2001). Technical Report: The Pediatrician's Role in the Diagnosis and Management of Autistic Spectrum Disorder in Children. Pediatrics, 107, e85. http://rsaffran.tripod.com/ieibt.html

2 Molly Masland, "Children in the Grip of Autism: More Families Faced with a Difficult Diagnosis," *MSNBC.com*, Feb. 23, 2005.

3 Suz Redfearn, "Seeking the First Signs of Autism Researchers Hope Early Diagnosis, Intervention Can Improve Outcomes," *The Washington Post*, April 15, 2003.

4 "Catching Them Young," *BrainWaves*, Johns Hopkins Neurology and Neurosurgery. Winter 2004, Vol. 16. Number 2. www.neuro.jhmi.edu/BrainWaves/Winter2004/autism_landa.htm

5 Claudia Kalb, "When Does Autism Start?" *Newsweek*, Feb. 28, 2005: 46.

6 C.A. Garland and Brenda Harris, "Aid for Autism," *Baltimore Sun*, January 25, 2005.

7 Committee on Educational Interventions for Children with Autism, Division of Behavioral and Social Sciences and Education National Research Council, Catherine Lord and James P. McGee, eds., *Educating Children with Autism* (Washington, DC: National Academy Press, 2001), 6.

8 Ibid. page 4.

CHAPTER 6

1 O.I. Lovaas, "Behavioral Treatment and Normal Educational and Intellectual Functioning in Young Autistic Children," *Journal of Consulting and Clinical Psychology*, 55 (1987): 3–9.

2 Gina Green, "Autism and ABA: Applied Behavior Analysis for Autism, 1997–2004" Concord, MA: Cambridge Center for Behavioral Studies. From website: www.behavior.org

3 "Mental Health: A Report of the Surgeon General," Rockville, MD: Department of Health and Human Services, Substance Abuse and Mental Health Services Administration, Center for Mental Health Services, National Institute of Mental Health, 1999. www.surgeongeneral.gov/library/mentalhealth/chapter3/sec6.html#autism

CHAPTER 7

1 Kathy Ward, "Health Insurance Reimbursement Tips & Tricks," Talk About Curing Autism (TACA) website: www.tacanow.com/health_ins_reimbursement_ tips.htm

CHAPTER 8

1 Sheila Wagner, *Inclusive Programming for Elementary Students with Autism* (Arlington, TX: Future Horizons, 1999).

2 E. Kelley, J. Paul, D. Fein, and L. Naigles (in press), "Residual Language Deficits in Optimal Outcome Children with a History of Autism;" and D. Fein, P. Dixon, J. Paul, and H. Levin (in press), "Brief Report: Pervasive Developmental Disorder Can Evolve into ADHD: Case Illustrations," *Journal of Autism and Developmental Disorders.*

CHAPTER 9

1 Elizabeth Kubler-Ross, *On Death and Dying.* New York, NY: Touchstone, 1969.

2 David Gray, "Gender and Coping: The Parents of Children with High Functioning Autism," *Social Science and Medicine*, Vol. 56, No. 3, 2003.

3 Carl Rogers, "Experiences in Communication," lecture at California Institute of Technology in Pasadena, CA. Fall, 1964.

CHAPTER 10

1 Bridget Taylor, (2001). Teaching peer social skills to children with autism. In C. Maurice, G. Green, & R.M. Foxx (Eds.), *Making a difference: Behavioral intervention for autism* (pp. 83–96). Austin Texas: PRO-ED.

2 D. Kamps, J. Royer, E. Dugan, T. Kravits, A Gonzalez-Lopez, J. Garcia, K. Carnazzo, L. Morrison& L. G. Kane (2002). "Peer training to facilitate social interaction for elementary students with autism and their peers." *Exceptional Children*, 68, 173–187.

3 Terese Dana in interviews with author 2005.

4 Lynn Kern Koegel, Robert Koegel, W.D. Frea & R.M. Fredeen, (2001). "Identifying early intervention targets for children with autism in inclusive school settings.: *Behavior Modification,* 25, 745–761.

CHAPTER 11

1 Elisa Gagnon, *Power Cards: Using Special Interests to Motivate Children and Youth with Asperger Syndrome and Autism.* Kansas: Autism Asperger Publishing Company, 2001.

2 Susan Boswell, and Debbie Gray, "Applied Structured Teaching Principles to Toilet Training," Division TEACCH, 2005, www.teaacch.com/toilet.htm

3 Brenda Smith Myles, and Jack Southwick. *Asperger Syndrome and Difficult Moments: Practical Solutions for Tantrums, Rage, and Meltdowns.* Shawnee Mission, KS: Autism Asperger Publishing Company, 1999, 2005, 25–40.

4 Ela Schwartz, "The Friendly Skies?" *NYC/United Spectrum*, NY: Spectrum Publications, January 2005. 21–3. (For more information the reader can call the U.S. Department of Transportation Consumer Protection Division at 1-800-778-4838).

CHAPTER 12

1 Sandra L. Harris, Ph.D., and Beth A. Glasberg, Ph.D., *Siblings of Children with Autism: A Guide for Families* (Bethesda, MD: Woodbine House, 2003), 60–61.

CHAPTER 13

1 Stephen R. Covey, *The Seven Habits of Highly Effective People* (New York: Free Press, 1989, 2004), 79–80.

2 Cindy N. Ariel, Ph.D., and Robert Naseef, Ph.D., "The Relationship Factor: When Special Needs Challenge a Household." Philadelphia: Alternative Choices, 2003, www.specialfamilies.com

3 Tracy Brown Wright, "Autistic Kids Benefit from Dads' Involvement," *The Post*, University of Florida Heath Science Center Newsletter, May 5, 2005, http://webapps.health.ufl.edu/HSCNews/Post/May%202005%20POST.pdf

ACKNOWLEDGMENTS

Thank You . . .

To all of the courageous and caring parents and siblings of children with ASDs who helped make this book special. Your candid stories about your families, marriages, and the realities of living with a child with an ASD were inspirational.

To Jake's extraordinary team of treatment therapists who will always be a part of our lives: Bridget Taylor, PhD.; Julie Fisher; Terese Dana; Diane Scott; Sandra Mackey; Anna Corbett; Laura Pinto; Lisa DiBari; Laura Wilkes; Stephanie Wendt; and Judy Palazzo.

To Dr. Fred Volkmar, for all of his support and encouragement, for answering my daily e-mails and phone calls about this book, and for the stellar work he and his colleagues are conducting on ASDs at the Yale Child Study Center.

To Bridget Taylor, ABA therapist extraordinaire, cofounder of the Alpine Learning Group, and friend, who offered valuable insights.

To Terese Dana and Diane Scott, gifted behavioral therapists, who also developed into gifted researchers and readers while helping me out on (too) many late nights with this book.

To Marlene Derasmo, the best ever preschool/elementary school chairperson of the Committee on Special Education, for all of the information she provided and for being the model of what a CSE chairperson should be: compassionate, caring, and a true team player.

To Gary Mayerson and Michelle Kule-Korgood, brilliant and concerned lawyers who are out there fighting every day to help parents get services for their children with ASDs and who offered valuable feedback on the legal information in the book.

To Dr. Cecelia McCarton, who upon giving me the news of Jake's diagnosis, also gave me a hug and great advice on how to get our treatment program started.

To Caren Zucker and Jon Donvan, who helped give us the courage to come out and share our family's story and who produced two poignant segments for ABC's *Nightline*.

To Liz Egloff and Sandi Gelles-Cole, who helped me organize my thoughts and reminded me to write this book from my heart.

To Judith Regan, my publisher at ReganBooks, who believed in this book right from the start. To Anna Bliss, my editor, for all of her encouragement, patience and diligence, and for asking all the right questions. Special thanks to Paul Crichton and Heidi Krupp, my publicists; Richard Ljeones, art director; Kelly Jones, online marketing manager; and Vivian Gomez, production editor.

To my agent, Bill Contardi of Brandt & Hochman, for all of his wonderful advice and support, and to Gail Hochman.

To those who contributed their expertise, advice, and support for the book, including Jonathan Shestack, Portia Iversen, Laura Slatkin, Dr. Deborah Fine, Ami Klin, Kathy Mannion, Deborah Hilibrand, Mark Gladstone, Rita Bigelow, Michelle Smigel, Karen Simmons, Stephen Shore, Lori Bechner, Mike Maloney, Amy Mahoney, Martin Schwartzman, Mike Brogioli, Susan Covert, James Twaite, Jane Gross, Jay Blotcher, Tristam Smith, Alisa Jones, Lauren Levine, David Kirby, Leslie Sharpe, Bette Ann Moscowitz, Emily Perl Kingsley, James Stovall, Toni Morrison, and to the wonderfully helpful people at the following: The Yale Child Study Center, Autism Society of America (ASA), Cure Autism Now (CAN), National Alliance for Autism Research (NAAR), Autism Coalition, Autism Speaks, Organization for Autism Research (OAR), The National Autistic Society, Unlocking Austism, The New York Center for Autism (NYCA), The Alpine Learning Group, and The Schafer Autism Report.

To those who helped Jake and our family along the way, including so many dear friends and loved ones: Robert and Shirley Siff, Larry and Joan Siff, Karen Humphries Sallick, Juan Acevedo-Lucio, Jodi Magee, Rich and Melissa Pacheco, David and Nancy Gross, Jonathan and Heather Schindler, Annette Azan, Ian Warburg, Sharyn Grobman, Beth Blatt, Mary Kaplan, Manny Group, Stacey Ringenary, Jeff Lee, Jon-Alec Raubeson, Leila and Jeffrey Masson, Patti Seminelli, Linda Russell, Margery Rappaport, Winsome Gregory, Donna Hesselgrave, Debra Arouesty, Dr. Mary Bayno, Debra Murphy Fisher, Jeffrey Friedberg, James Handlin, Chaffee Monell, Karen Tull, Elspeth Crowley, Rockland Country Day School, Preschool Playhouse, The Community Playgroup.

And last but certainly not least . . . I offer special thanks to my husband and best friend, Franklin, who held my hand during all the hard times and never let go and who is forever in my heart. And to Jake, who made me believe in miracles.

INDEX